Essentials of Cataract Surgery

Essentials of Cataract Surgery

Editor: Joanne Galbraith

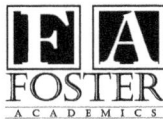

FA
FOSTER
ACADEMICS

www.fosteracademics.com

www.fosteracademics.com

FA
FOSTER
A C A D E M I C S

Cataloging-in-Publication Data

Essentials of cataract surgery / edited by Joanne Galbraith.
p. cm.
Includes bibliographical references and index.
ISBN 978-1-63242-942-1
1. Cataract--Surgery. 2. Cataract--Treatment. 3. Crystalline lens--Diseases.
4. Eye--Diseases--Treatment. I. Galbraith, Joanne.
RE451 .E87 2020
617.742--dc23

Foster Academics,
118-35 Queens Blvd., Suite 400,
Forest Hills, NY 11375, USA

ISBN 978-1-63242-942-1 (Hardback)

Contents

Preface

The world is advancing at a fast pace like never before. Therefore, the need is to keep up with the latest developments. This book was an idea that came to fruition when the specialists in the area realized the need to coordinate together and document essential themes in the subject. That's when I was requested to be the editor. Editing this book has been an honour as it brings together diverse authors researching on different streams of the field. The book collates essential materials contributed by veterans in the area which can be utilized by students and researchers alike.

Cataract surgery is the process for removing the natural lens of the eye that has developed an opacification and replacing it with an intraocular lens. The opacification, which is referred to as a cataract, is developed due to metabolic changes of the crystalline lens fibers over time. Early symptoms of cataract disease include reduced acuity at low light levels, and strong glare from lights and small light sources at night. The cloudy natural lens of the patient is either removed by the process of phacoemulsification or by extracapsular cataract extraction. In phacoemulsification, either a machine with an ultrasonic handpiece with titanium or steel tip, or a cracker machine is used. Extracapsular cataract extraction involves the technique where the entire lens is taken out while the elastic lens capsule is left intact. This enables the implantation of an artificial lens. An intraocular lens is inserted in the surgery through a small or enlarged incision. The ever-growing need for advanced technology is the reason that has fueled the research in the field of cataract surgery in recent times. This book includes some of the vital pieces of work being conducted across the world in this area of study. With state-of-the-art inputs by acclaimed experts of this field, it targets students and professionals.

Each chapter is a sole-standing publication that reflects each author's interpretation. Thus, the book displays a multi-facetted picture of our current understanding of application, resources and aspects of the field. I would like to thank the contributors of this book and my family for their endless support.

Editor

Early Results with a New Posterior Chamber Phakic Intraocular Lens in Patients with High Myopia

Dilek Yaşa [ID],[1] Ufuk Ürdem,[1] Alper Ağca [ID],[1] Yusuf Yildirim [ID],[1] Burçin Kepez Yildiz,[1] Nilay Kandemir Beşek,[1] Ulviye Yiğit,[2] and Ahmet Demirok[1]

[1]Beyoğlu Eye Research and Training Hospital, Bereketzade Mah., No. 2 Beyoglu, Istanbul, Turkey
[2]Dr. Sadi Konuk Bakirkoy Research and Training Hospital, Zuhuratbaba Mah., Tevfik Saglam Cad., No. 21 Bakirkoy, Istanbul, Turkey

Correspondence should be addressed to Dilek Yaşa; dilekyasa2@gmail.com

Academic Editor: Suphi Taneri

Purpose. To report clinical results of a foldable, hydrophilic acrylic, single-piece, injectable, posterior chamber phakic intraocular lens (pIOL). *Material and Methods.* Medical records of patients who underwent posterior chamber phakic IOL (Eyecryl Phakic IOL, Biotech Vision Care, Ahmedabad, India) implantation for surgical correction of myopia were retrospectively reviewed. Only patients with at least a one-year follow-up were included. Manifest refraction, uncorrected distance visual acuity (UDVA), corrected distance visual acuity (CDVA), endothelial cell density (ECD), and pIOL vault were analyzed at 1, 3, 6, and 12 months after surgery. Complications observed during and after surgery were also recorded. *Results.* The study included 58 eyes of 29 patients. Mean patient age was 32 ± 7 years. Spherical equivalent of manifest refraction was -13.41 ± 3.23 D preoperatively and -0.44 ± 0.55 D postoperatively. Preoperative CDVA was 0.29 ± 0.71 logMAR. Postoperative UDVA and CDVA were 0.21 ± 0.66 and 0.15 ± 0.69 logMAR, respectively, at the 12-month visit. At the 12-month visit, the efficacy index was 1.20 and the safety index was 1.39. Mean ECD was 2713 ± 339 cells/mm^2 at the preoperative visit and 2608 ± 362 cells/mm^2 at the 12-month visit (3.9% loss, $p < 0.001$). ECD loss from 3 months to 12 months was not statistically significant. No significant cataract formation, significant endothelial cell loss, glaucoma, uveitis, or any other vision-threatening complication was observed. *Conclusion.* Based on postoperative experience, we have found that Eyecryl Phakic IOL is safe and effective for treating high myopia.

1. Introduction

Phakic intraocular lens (IOL) implantation, corneal refractive surgery (small incision lenticule extraction and laser in situ keratomileusis), and refractive lens exchange are alternatives for the surgical treatment of high myopia [1]. Refractive lens exchange may correct a high amount of myopia; however, it results in loss of accommodation (in addition to its potential complications); thus, it is not usually considered in non-presbyopic individuals. Corneal refractive surgery is usually not considered for high myopia because the quality of vision decreases, and the complication rate increases after a certain degree. In addition, pIOL implantation may result a better quality of vision and offer significant vision-related quality-of-life advantages over corneal refractive surgery [2]. Phakic IOL implantation has the advantage of correcting greater myopia than corneal refractive surgery while preserving accommodation in contrast to refractive lens exchange.

A multitude of angle-supported and iris-fixated anterior chamber pIOLs have been taken off the market because of excessive endothelial cell loss and complications such as cataract, glaucoma, and pupil ovalization [3, 4]. However, some models of posterior chamber pIOL and iris-fixated pIOL are considered to have good safety and efficacy, yielding predictable and stable results [5–10]. Today, there are only a few commercially available options for posterior chamber and iris-supported pIOLs on the market. Eyecryl Phakic IOL (Biotech Vision Care, Ahmedabad, India) is a foldable, hydrophilic acrylic, single-piece, injectable, posterior chamber phakic IOL and, to the best of our knowledge, there are no published studies describing clinical outcomes following implantation of this lens.

In this study, we evaluated the efficacy and safety of Eyecryl posterior chamber phakic IOL implantation in patients with high myopia.

2. Patients and Methods

This study followed the tenets of the Declaration of Helsinki, and approval was obtained from the Ethics Committee of Bakirkoy Research and Training Hospital. At the time of the surgery, all patients were fully informed about the details and possible risks of the surgical procedure. Written informed consent was obtained from all patients before surgery. Medical records of patients who underwent Eyecryl Phakic IOL implantation were retrospectively evaluated. Only the patients with at least a 1-year follow-up were included in the study. The main outcome measures in this study were the spherical equivalent (SE) of manifest refractive error, UDVA, CDVA, and ECD at 1 month, 3 months, 6 months, and 1 year after surgery. Perioperative and postoperative complications were also recorded, giving special attention to cataract development. We defined cataract as a lens opacity of any type that results in the loss of ≥2 lines of CDVA or cataract surgery.

2.1. Preoperative and Postoperative Examinations. All patients underwent the standard detailed anterior and posterior segment examination procedure of our Refractive Surgery Clinic preoperatively and postoperatively. All patients were examined at postoperative day 1; week 1; and months 1, 6, and 12 because it is routine in our clinic. The patients were scheduled for yearly follow-up thereafter.

An autorefractometer (RM-8800 Autorefractor, Topcon, Tokyo, Japan) was used for keratometry measurements and objective refraction. An automated phoropter (CV-5000, Topcon, Tokyo, Japan) and a back-illuminated 19″ LED LCD monitor chart (CC-100 XP, Topcon, Tokyo, Japan) were used for uncorrected distance visual acuity (UDVA) and corrected distance visual acuity (CDVA) measurements. Visual acuities were converted to logMAR for statistical analysis. Corneal topography and corneal pachymetry mapping were performed with the Sirius topography platform (Schwind eye-tech-solutions GmbH, Germany). Endothelial cell density was measured with a specular microscope (CEM 530, NIDEK, Japan). Intraocular pressure was measured with a Goldmann applanation tonometer at every visit. All patients underwent a detailed anterior and posterior segment examination with a slit lamp. All these examinations were performed in preoperative and all postoperative visits except for the first postoperative day, when only UDVA, CDVA, slit lamp, and IOP measurements were performed. In addition, in all postoperative visits, the phakic IOL vault (distance between the phakic lens and the crystalline lens) was measured with an anterior segment optical coherence tomography (OCT) device (Visante OCT, Carl Zeiss AG, Germany). In our clinic, it is routine to implant pIOLs only in patients with an anterior chamber depth of at least 3 mm from the endothelium. Anterior chamber depth from the endothelium and white-to-white measurements was measured with an IOL Master (Carl Zeiss Meditec, Germany).

2.2. Phakic Intraocular Lens and Surgical Procedure. The Eyecryl Phakic IOL is a foldable, hydrophilic acrylic, single-piece, injectable, posterior chamber phakic IOL. It is designed to be placed in the posterior chamber behind the iris with the haptic zone resting on the ciliary sulcus. It is available in 3 overall lengths (12.0 mm, 12.5 mm, and 13.0 mm) and is designed to correct myopia in a dioptric power range of −3.00 to −23.00 diopters (D). It has an aspheric optic with zero aberration. The diameter of the optic is 4.65 to 5.50 mm. A 320 μm hole in the center of the optic prevents pupillary block and improves aqueous humor circulation. Power calculation for the phakic intraocular lens was performed using the modified vergence formula in the software provided by the manufacturer. Target was emmetropia in all cases. The lens size was determined based on the horizontal white-to-white (WTW) distance.

All surgeries were performed by the same surgeon (AA). The pupil was dilated with cyclopentolate and phenylephrine drops, instilled 30 minutes prior to surgery. After sub-Tenon anesthesia, a 2.8 mm clear corneal tunnel incision was performed in the horizontal temporal meridian. The anterior chamber was filled with sodium hyaluronate 1%. The Eyecryl Phakic IOL was implanted behind the iris through the incision, using the injector cartridge supplied by the manufacturer. A temporal clear corneal incision was used in all cases. As a result, the position of the pIOLs was horizontal immediately after implantation. To avoid any unnecessary trauma to intraocular structures (i.e., the crystalline lens, iris, ciliary sulcus, and zonula), pIOLs were left in this horizontal position. After the Eyecryl Phakic IOL was gently positioned in the sulcus, the remaining viscoelastic material was completely washed out of the anterior chamber with a balanced salt solution, and a miotic agent was instilled. No preoperative or intraoperative peripheral iridectomies were performed.

2.3. Statistical Methods. Statistical analysis and the associated tables and listings were performed using SAS®, version 9.4. Descriptive statistics were obtained. The assumption of normality was assessed by the Shapiro–Wilk test. If p value was >0.05, it was assumed that the data followed a normal distribution. Paired t-test was used to analyze data with normal distribution, and nonparametric Wilcoxon signed rank test was used to analyze the data with a non-normal distribution. One-way analysis of variance (ANOVA) was used to evaluate ECD and the vault changes over time.

3. Results

Fifty-eight eyes of 29 subjects were included in the study. Among 29 subjects, 6 (21%) subjects were male and 23 (79%) subjects were female. All patients had pIOL implantation bilaterally. Preoperative characteristics and distribution of preoperative SE of manifest refraction are shown in Table 1 and Figure 1, respectively.

Mean preoperative CDVA was 0.29 ± 0.69 logMAR. Mean UDVA was 0.20 ± 0.66 logMAR at 1 month, 0.21 ± 0.65 logMAR at 3 months, 0.18 ± 0.68 logMAR at 6 months, and 0.21 ± 0.66 logMAR at 12 months. Mean UDVA at 1 month was statistically significantly better than mean

TABLE 1: Preoperative patient characteristics.

	Mean ± SD	Minimum	Maximum
Age (years)	31 ± 6.92	23	49
SE (D)	−13.41 ± 3.22	−7.13	−22.00
Cylinder (D)	1.10 ± 0.70	0	2.25
DCVA (logMAR)	0.29 ± 0.72	1	0
WTW (mm)	11.72 ± 0.30	10.82	12.10
ECD (cells/mm^2)	2712 ± 338.50	2048	3227
ACD (mm)	3.63 ± 0.21	3.04	4.04
Mean Sim K (D)	44.48 ± 1.72	39.21	47.49
IOP (mmHg)	14 ± 2.35	10.00	21.00
AL (mm)	28.23 ± 1.23	24.15	31.12
Corneal thickness (μ)	530 ± 33.27	452	595

SE: spherical equivalent; DCVA: corrected distance visual acuity; WTW: white-to-white; ECD: endothelial cell density; Sim K: simulated keratometry; IOP: intraocular pressure; AL: axial length.

preoperative CDVA (paired samples t-test, two-tailed, $p < 0.001$). Efficacy index (ratio of postoperative CDVA to preoperative UDVA) was 1.20 at 1 year. Figure 2 shows preoperative and postoperative cumulative Snellen visual acuity (preoperative CDVA and postoperative UDVA). Preoperative CDVA was 0.29 ± 0.69 logMAR, and postoperative CDVA was 0.15 ± 0.69 at the last follow-up visit (1 year, paired sample t-test, two-tailed, p value <0.001). The safety index (ratio of postoperative CDVA to preoperative CDVA) was 1.39 at 1 year. No patient lost 2 or more lines of CDVA, and 62% of the eyes gained 2 or more lines of CDVA (Figure 3).

Figure 4 shows the attempted versus achieved refractive correction. At 12 months, 62% of the eyes were within ±0.50 D of the attempted correction, and 93% of the eyes were within ±1.00 D of the attempted correction (Figure 5). Figure 6 shows the stability of manifest refraction throughout follow-up.

Figure 7 shows the mean ECD at preoperative and different postoperative visits. ECD was 2713 ± 339 cells/mm^2 at the preoperative visit, and 2608 ± 362 cells/mm^2 at the 12-month visit (3.9% loss, paired sample t-test, $p < 0.001$). ECD loss from 3 months to 12 months was not statistically significant.

Figure 8 shows the mean vault of the pIOL during follow-up. The mean vault was 535 ± 137 (min: 270; max: 880) at 1 year. There was a statistically significant decrease in vault during follow-up (repeated measures ANOVA, $p < 0.001$). At the 12-month visit, the vault of the pIOL had decreased 57 ± 91 μ when compared to the 1-month visit (paired sample t-test, $p < 0.001$).

The mean preoperative central corneal thickness (thinnest) was 530 ± 33.26 μm. Postoperatively, the mean central corneal thickness (thinnest) was 532 ± 30.86 μm at 1 month, 529 ± 32.95 μm at 3 months, 528 ± 31.83 μm at 6 months, and 530 ± 32.18 μm at 12 months. No statistically significant difference was observed from preoperative visit to all postoperative visits (repeated measures ANOVA, $p = 0.9703$).

3.1. Complications. In both eyes of one patient, elevated intraocular pressure (IOP) (24 mmHg bilaterally) was detected at the one-month visit. The increase in IOP was considered steroid induced because there was no pupillary, block, inflammatory reaction, or pigment dispersion. The intraocular

pressures returned to their baseline levels after the cessation of topical steroid treatment. There were no cases of anterior subcapsular cataracts or opacities. There were no other intraoperative or postoperative complications.

4. Discussion

There are no published studies on the results of the IOL implanted in this study, and the amount of myopia in this study is higher when compared to other posterior chamber phakic IOL studies in the literature [2, 6–16]. In a multicenter, prospective study on refractive surgery in 15,011 eyes reported by Kamiya et al. [6], a pIOL with a very similar design (plate haptic posterior chamber IOL with a central hole) was implanted in 1319 eyes. They reported that the mean patient age was 32 years, and the mean SE was −8.42 ± 3.10 D. In our study, the mean patient age was similar (31 years), but the mean SE of manifest refraction was −13.41 ± 3.22 D, and 23% of our patients had myopia higher than −15.00 D. The refractive error in our study was relatively high because this retrospective case series reflects the practice in our clinic. We prefer implantation of phakic IOLs only in nonpresbyopic patients who are not suitable for corneal refractive surgery (mainly small incision lenticule extraction).

As expected, we found that SE decreased and UDVA increased after implantation of phakic IOL. We obtained predictable postoperative refractive results in line with previous studies on other types of phakic IOLs. At 12 months, 62% of the eyes were within ±0.50 D of the attempted correction, and 93% of the eyes were within ±1.00 D of the attempted correction. Lee et al. [8] reported that in a series of 281 eyes, 69% and 87.2% were within ±0.50 D and ±1.00 D of the desired refraction 5 years after surgery, respectively. Alfonso et al. [12] reported that 86.7% were within ±0.50 D one month after surgery. However, only 64.1% and 38% were within ±0.50 D 3 and 5 years after surgery, respectively. Our patient groups had a considerably higher level of mean SE and lower DCVA than in other studies in the literature. For example, Huseynova et al. [14] reported that 75% and 100% were within ±0.50 D and ±1.00 D of the desired refraction 3 months after surgery, respectively. However, the CDVA of their patients was 0.12 logMAR (decimal notation: 0.76), whereas the mean preoperative CDVA in our patients was 0.29 logMAR (decimal notation: 0.51). We believe that the percentage of eyes within ±0.50 D would be higher if SE were lower and DCVA were better in our patient group. In contrast to cataract surgery, refractive vergence formulas are used to determine the power of the IOL to be implanted in phakic eyes. As a result, precise determination of manifest refraction is critical in these patients to calculate the pIOL to correct that manifest refractive error [17]. However, precise determination of manifest refraction gets more difficult as the CDVA decreases. For example, a patient with a visual acuity of 20/40 may not respond to 0.50 D changes during subjective manifest refraction.

In this study, we found the efficacy index to be 1.20, indicating that the mean postoperative UCVA was better than preoperative CDVA after implantation of Eyecryl

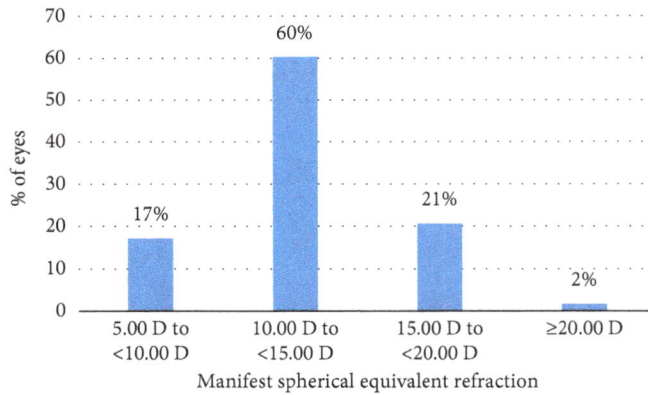

FIGURE 1: Distribution of manifest spherical equivalent for the patients preoperatively.

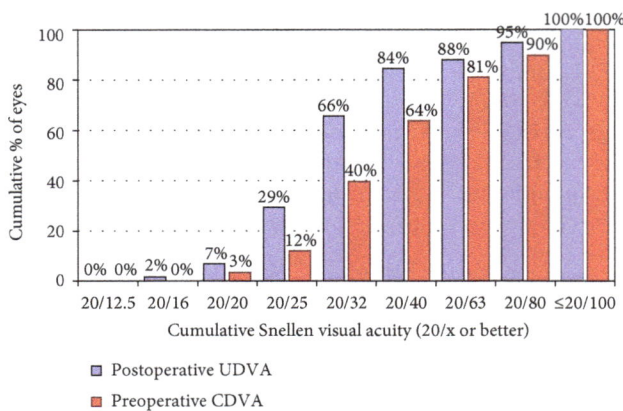

FIGURE 2: Postoperative uncorrected distance visual acuity (UDVA) versus preoperative corrected distance visual acuity (CDVA).

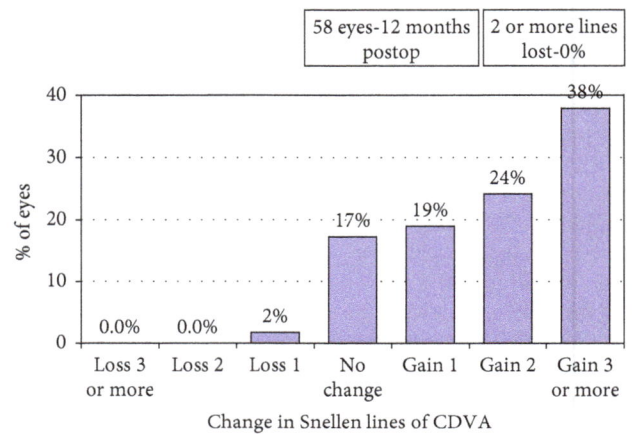

FIGURE 3: Change in corrected distance visual acuity (CDVA).

Phakic IOL. Lisa et al. [10] evaluated a posterior chamber pIOL with a similar design and a central hole implanted in 147 eyes and found an efficacy index of 1.04, whereas Shimizu et al. [13] and Cao et al. [7] found efficacy indices of 1.13 and 1.11, respectively, with the same lens model. In addition to the expected increase in UDVA, there was an improvement in CDVA of the patients. Eighty-one percent of the eyes gained 1 line, 62% percent of the eyes gained 2 or more lines of CDVA, and none of the eyes lost 2 or more lines; the safety index was 1.39. Previous studies have also found that 35% to 100% of the pIOL implanted in patients experienced 1 or more lines of CDVA increase after pIOL implantation [5–10, 12–14, 18, 19]. Although the exact mechanism is unclear, the relative magnification of the image and the reduction in visual aberrations after an anterior chamber pIOL implantation when compared to spectacle lenses may be the reason for the improvement [20]. In addition, the studies in the literature that evaluate CDVA improvement in adult amblyopic eyes after laser-assisted in situ keratomileusis (LASIK), photorefractive keratectomy (PRK), or pIOL implantation agree that improvement occurs; however, the rates vary over a wide range [19, 21, 22].

The amount of endothelial cell loss after pIOL implantation has always been a topic of discussion. In the present study, the cumulative mean percentage of endothelial cell loss was 3.9% at 3, 6, and 12 months after the surgery. The most detailed data with the highest level of evidence on the ECD loss after a posterior chamber pIOL (Visian implantable Collamer lens, STAAR Surgical, Nidau, Switzerland) were reported during the prospective, multi-center U.S. FDA trial and showed that it was $3.3 \pm 7.6\%$ at one year (90% confidence limits: 2.4% to 4.3%) and 9.7 ± 9.3 at 4 years [11, 23]. Moya et al. [16] published a cumulative 12-year retrospective study, including data from 144 eyes implanted with the same pIOL model of implantable contact lenses (ICLs) between 1998 and 2001 and estimated a 6.46% surgically induced ECD decrease during the first year and an average yearly decrease rate of 1.20% after that. Other studies in the literature report much lower levels of ECD loss during the first year; they all agree that endothelial damage occurs primarily during the surgical procedure, and the rate of ECD loss decreases after a certain time [10, 12, 15, 24]. In line with all these studies, absence of a statistically significant difference in ECD after three months postoperatively in this study reflects the fact that the power of the statistical test is insufficient to reveal the small amount of normal endothelial loss. On the contrary, detection of an acute loss early after the surgery and stabilization after the 3-month visit suggests that the main reason for the cell loss is surgical trauma and

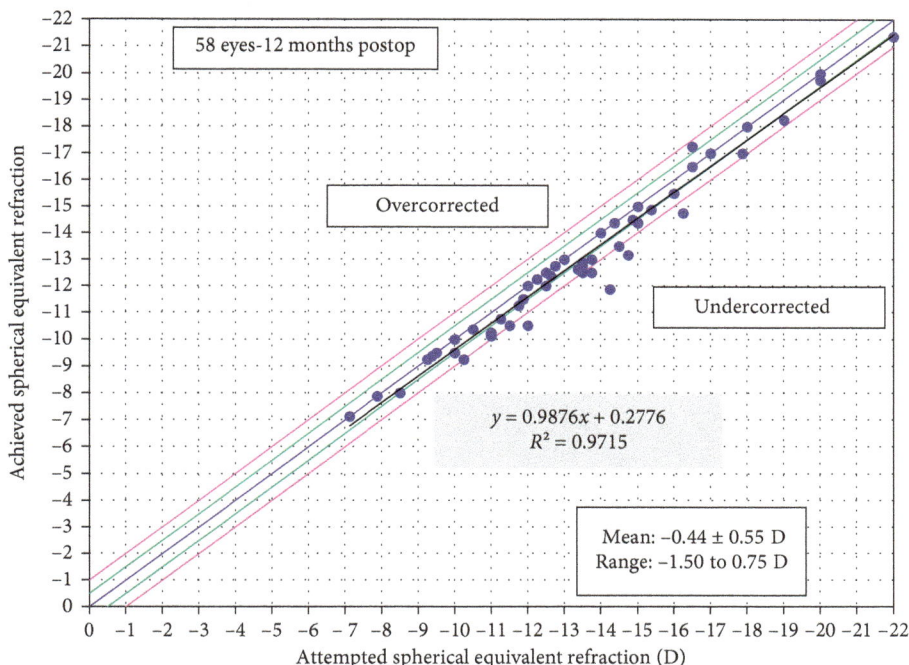

FIGURE 4: Attempted versus achieved spherical equivalent of manifest refraction.

that the pIOL does not induce a *clinically* significant amount of ECD loss by itself, *at least in the patients included in this study*. Previous studies show that a smaller ACD is a significant risk factor for increased ECD loss in both anterior and posterior chamber pIOLs [11, 25]. Accordingly, it is routine in our clinic to implant pIOLs of any type in only patients who have a ACD greater than 3.00 mm and the minimum anterior chamber depth (ACD) in this study was 3.04 mm from the endothelium.

Cataract formation is another major concern when implanting a pIOL in a young, highly myopic patient because cataract surgery results in loss of accommodation and increases the rate of retinal complications. Asymptomatic anterior subcapsular lens opacities (ASCLO) are recorded between 0% and 18% after surgery, and the difference is probably related to surgical technique, the retrospective nature of the studies, and to the definition of cataract. In this retrospective study, we defined cataract as a lens opacity of any type that results in loss of ≥2 lines of CDVA or cataract surgery. None of the patients in this study had a cataract at the 1-year visit. Also, there were no cases of anterior subcapsular opacities. However, because of the retrospective nature of the study, very mild anterior subcapsular opacities without clinical significance could have gone unnoticed and could only have been revealed in a prospective study. This result is in line with previous reports that the incidence of a visually significant cataract after pIOL implantation is low in the early postoperative years [26]. However, recent studies show that the rate of cataract formation is higher in longer follow-up. In a retrospective study, Lee et al. [8] reported that 2.1% of 281 eyes in their study developed a cataract at 5 years. Guber et al. [27] reported that phacoemulsification was performed in 4.9% and 18.3% of 133 eyes at 5 and 10

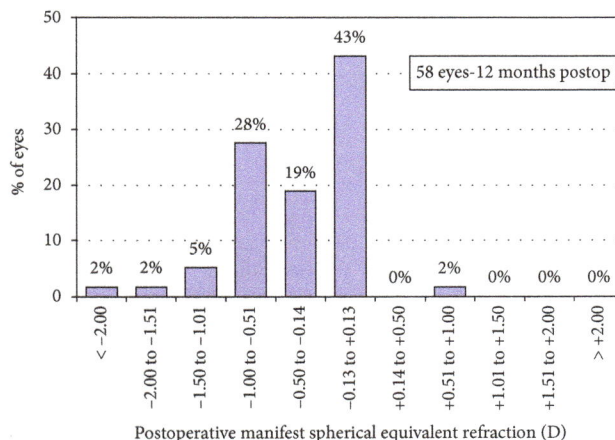

FIGURE 5: Distribution of manifest spherical equivalent for the patients postoperatively.

years after ICL implantation, respectively. Low vault, higher levels of myopia, and older patient age are risk factors for cataract formation after pIOL implantation [28].

Extremes of vault are risk factors for complications such as cataract, pigment dispersion, pupillary block, and glaucoma. However, precise definitions of excessive and insufficient vault are not clear. In the literature, the lower limit of safe vault is reported to be between 50 and $250\,\mu$ by different authors, and the upper limit is around $1000\,\mu$, as long as the anterior chamber structure and pupillary function are normal [10, 28–30]. However, given the yearly increase in crystalline lens rise and the young age of the patients, we believe that it is advisable to be as close to $250\,\mu$ as possible. The lens vault is closely related to appropriate

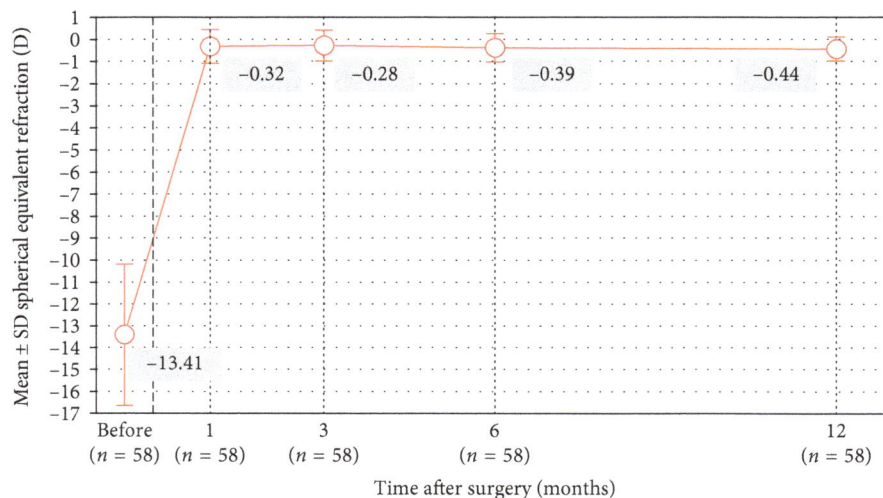

Figure 6: Mean manifest refraction throughout follow-up.

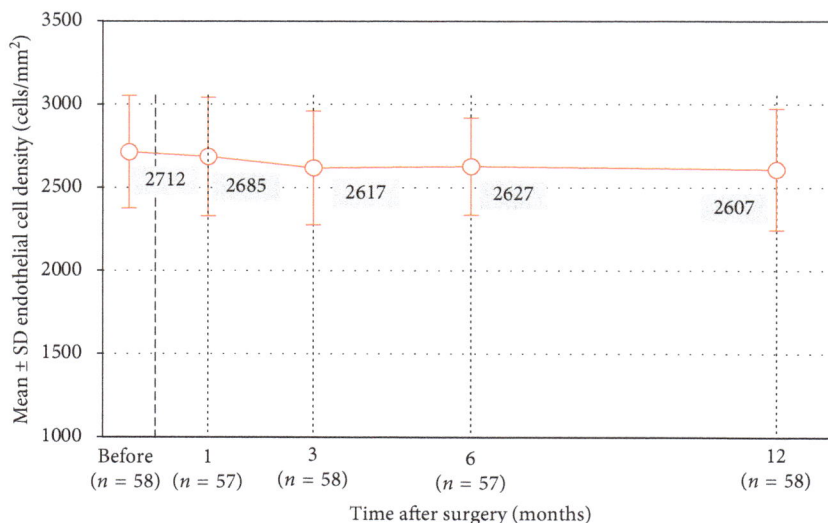

Figure 7: Mean endothelial cell count ($n = 58$, repeated measures ANOVA, all visits, $p < 0.001$). Statistically significant difference was observed from preoperative visit to postoperative month 3 ($p = 0.001$), postoperative month 6 ($p < 0.001$), and postoperative month 12 ($p = 0.003$). No statistically significant difference was observed from preoperative visit to postoperative month 1 ($p = 0.1267$). ECD loss from three months to 12 months was not statistically significant ($p = 0.674$).

sizing of the pIOL to the posterior chamber. Mean vault in our patient group was 535 ± 137 (min: 270; max: 880) at 1 year, indicating that the sizes of the pIOLs matched well with the posterior chambers of the patients in our study.

In line with the previous studies on posterior chamber phakic IOLs, there were no sight-threatening intraoperative or postoperative complications in our patients up to 1 year after surgery.

The only complication was a bilateral, steroid-induced, transient IOP rise in one patient. Glaucoma may occur after anterior or posterior pIOL implantation due to pupillary block or pigment dispersion. Although preoperative or intraoperative peripheral iridectomies were not performed in our patients, no pupillary block was seen during follow-up. This is probably due to the central hole in the optic, which prevents pupillary block despite the lack of

a peripheral iridectomy. In addition, no pigment dispersion or pigment dispersion glaucoma was observed. However, gonioscopy was not performed preoperatively and postoperatively because this study was retrospective, and gonioscopy was not a routine part of our preoperative and postoperative examinations. Thus, very mild clinical pigment dispersion in some patients could have gone unnoticed.

The weak points of this study are its retrospective nature and the relatively short follow-up to draw conclusions on two specific issues: long-term endothelial safety and rate of cataract formation at long term. However, it would take many years before the exact incidences of these two complications are revealed, and we would like to underline the fact that no conclusions can be drawn regarding long-term ASC formation based on the short 12-month follow-up used in the study.

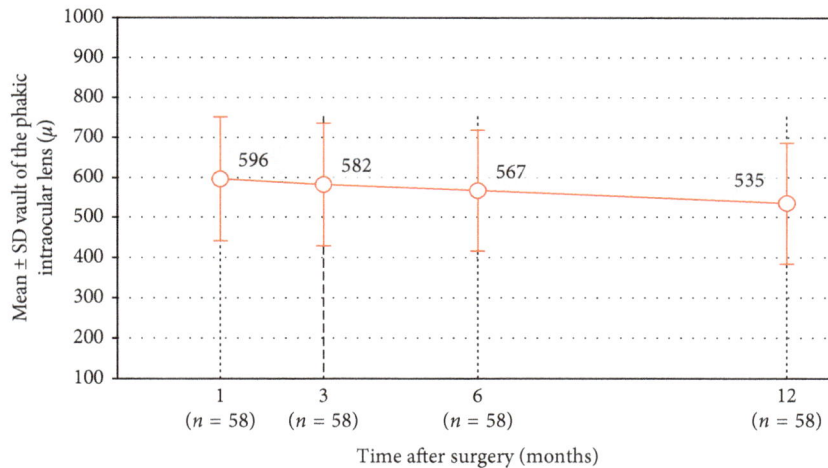

FIGURE 8: Mean vault of the phakic IOL ($n = 58$, repeated measures ANOVA, all visits, $p < 0.001$). Statistically significant difference was observed from the 1-month visit to the 6-month visit ($p = 0.04$) and from the 6-month visit to the 12-month visit ($p < 0.001$).

We have found that Eyecryl Phakic IOL is safe and effective for treating high myopia, similar to other models of posterior chamber IOLs. Prospective studies with larger patient groups and longer follow-up are needed to reveal long-term efficacy and safety.

Conflicts of Interest

The authors declare that there are no conflicts of interest regarding the publication of this article.

References

[1] M. Lundstrom, S. Manning, P. Barry, U. Stenevi, Y. Henry, and P. Rosen, "The European registry of quality outcomes for cataract and refractive surgery (EUREQUO): a database study of trends in volumes, surgical techniques and outcomes of refractive surgery," *Eye and Vision*, vol. 2, p. 8, 2015.

[2] H. Kobashi, K. Kamiya, A. Igarashi, K. Matsumura, M. Komatsu, and K. Shimizu, "Long-term quality of life after posterior chamber phakic intraocular lens implantation and after wavefront-guided laser in situ keratomileusis for myopia," *Journal of Cataract and Refractive Surgery*, vol. 40, no. 12, pp. 2019–2024, 2014.

[3] J. L. Guell, M. Morral, D. Kook, and T. Kohnen, "Phakic intraocular lenses part 1: historical overview, current models, selection criteria, and surgical techniques," *Journal of Cataract and Refractive Surgery*, vol. 36, no. 11, pp. 1976–1993, 2010.

[4] T. Kohnen, D. Kook, M. Morral, and J. L. Guell, "Phakic intraocular lenses: part 2: results and complications," *Journal of Cataract and Refractive Surgery*, vol. 36, no. 12, pp. 2168–2194, 2010.

[5] K. Kamiya, A. Igarashi, K. Hayashi, K. Negishi, M. Sato, and H. Bissen-Miyajima, "Survey Working Group of the Japanese Society of C, Refractive S: a multicenter retrospective survey of refractive surgery in 78,248 eyes," *Journal of Refractive Surgery*, vol. 33, no. 9, pp. 598–602, 2017.

[6] K. Kamiya, A. Igarashi, K. Hayashi, K. Negishi, M. Sato, and H. Bissen-Miyajima, "Survey Working Group of the Japanese Society of C, Refractive S: a multicenter prospective cohort study on refractive surgery in 15,011 eyes," *American Journal of Ophthalmology*, vol. 175, pp. 159–168, 2017.

[7] X. Cao, W. Wu, Y. Wang, C. Xie, J. Tong, and Y. Shen, "Posterior chamber collagen copolymer phakic intraocular lens with a central hole for moderate-to-high myopia: first experience in China," *Medicine*, vol. 95, no. 36, article e4641, 2016.

[8] J. Lee, Y. Kim, S. Park et al., "Long-term clinical results of posterior chamber phakic intraocular lens implantation to correct myopia," *Clinical and Experimental Ophthalmology*, vol. 44, no. 6, pp. 481–487, 2016.

[9] K. Shimizu, K. Kamiya, A. Igarashi, and H. Kobashi, "Long-term comparison of posterior chamber phakic intraocular lens with and without a central hole (hole ICL and conventional ICL) implantation for moderate to high myopia and myopic astigmatism: consort-compliant article," *Medicine*, vol. 95, no. 14, article e3270, 2016.

[10] C. Lisa, M. Naveiras, B. Alfonso-Bartolozzi, L. Belda-Salmeron, R. Montes-Mico, and J. F. Alfonso, "Posterior chamber collagen copolymer phakic intraocular lens with a central hole to correct myopia: one-year follow-up," *Journal of Cataract and Refractive Surgery*, vol. 41, no. 6, pp. 1153–1159, 2015.

[11] D. R. Sanders, K. Doney, and M. Poco, "Group ICLiToMS: United States Food and Drug Administration clinical trial of the Implantable Collamer Lens (ICL) for moderate to high myopia: three-year follow-up," *Ophthalmology*, vol. 111, no. 9, pp. 1683–1692, 2004.

[12] J. F. Alfonso, B. Baamonde, L. Fernandez-Vega, P. Fernandes, J. M. Gonzalez-Meijome, and R. Montes-Mico, "Posterior chamber collagen copolymer phakic intraocular lenses to correct myopia: five-year follow-up," *Journal of Cataract and Refractive Surgery*, vol. 37, no. 5, pp. 873–880, 2011.

[13] K. Shimizu, K. Kamiya, A. Igarashi, and T. Shiratani, "Early clinical outcomes of implantation of posterior chamber phakic intraocular lens with a central hole (hole ICL) for moderate to high myopia," *British Journal of Ophthalmology*, vol. 96, no. 3, pp. 409–412, 2012.

[14] T. Huseynova, S. Ozaki, T. Ishizuka, M. Mita, and M. Tomita, "Comparative study of 2 types of implantable collamer lenses, 1 with and 1 without a central artificial hole," *American Journal of Ophthalmology*, vol. 157, no. 6, pp. 1136–1143, 2014.

[15] A. Igarashi, K. Shimizu, and K. Kamiya, "Eight-year follow-up of posterior chamber phakic intraocular lens implantation for moderate to high myopia," *American Journal of Ophthalmology*, vol. 157, no. 3, pp. 532–539, 2014.

[16] T. Moya, J. Javaloy, R. Montes-Mico, J. Beltran, G. Munoz, and R. Montalban, "Implantable collamer lens for myopia: assessment 12 years after implantation," *Journal of Refractive Surgery*, vol. 31, no. 8, pp. 548–556, 2015.

[17] J. T. Holladay, "Refractive power calculations for intraocular lenses in the phakic eye," *American Journal of Ophthalmology*, vol. 116, no. 1, pp. 63–66, 1993.

[18] D. Yasa, A. Agca, Z. Alkin et al., "Two-year follow-up of Artisan iris-supported phakic anterior chamber intraocular lens for correction of high myopia," *Seminars in Ophthalmology*, vol. 31, no. 3, pp. 280–284, 2016.

[19] S. W. Kwon, H. S. Moon, and K. H. Shyn, "Visual improvement in high myopic amblyopic adult eyes following phakic anterior chamber intraocular lens implantation," *Korean Journal of Ophthalmology*, vol. 20, no. 2, pp. 87–92, 2006.

[20] I. S. Barequet, T. Wygnanski-Jaffe, and A. Hirsh, "Laser in situ keratomileusis improves visual acuity in some adult eyes with amblyopia," *Journal of Refractive Surgery*, vol. 20, no. 1, pp. 25–28, 2004.

[21] A. Agca, E. B. Ozgurhan, O. Baz et al., "Laser in situ keratomileusis in adult patients with anisometropic amblyopia," *International Journal of Ophthalmology*, vol. 6, no. 3, pp. 362–369, 2013.

[22] N. Cagil, N. Ugurlu, H. B. Cakmak, S. Ilker Kocamis, D. Turak, and S. Simsek, "Photorefractive keratectomy in treatment of refractive amblyopia in the adult population," *Journal of Cataract and Refractive Surgery*, vol. 37, no. 12, pp. 2167–2174, 2011.

[23] H. F. Edelhauser, D. R. Sanders, R. Azar, and H. Lamielle, "Group ICLiToMS: corneal endothelial assessment after ICL implantation," *Journal of Cataract and Refractive Surgery*, vol. 30, no. 3, pp. 576–583, 2004.

[24] H. Goukon, K. Kamiya, K. Shimizu, and A. Igarashi, "Comparison of corneal endothelial cell density and morphology after posterior chamber phakic intraocular lens implantation with and without a central hole," *British Journal of Ophthalmology*, vol. 101, no. 11, pp. 1461–1465, 2017.

[25] S. M. R. Jonker, T. Berendschot, A. E. Ronden, I. E. Y. Saelens, N. J. C. Bauer, and R. Nuijts, "Long-term endothelial cell loss in patients with artisan myopia and artisan toric phakic intraocular lenses: 5- and 10-year results," *Ophthalmology*, vol. 125, no. 4, pp. 486–494, 2017.

[26] K. Kamiya, K. Shimizu, W. Ando, A. Igarashi, K. Iijima, and A. Koh, "Comparison of vault after implantation of posterior chamber phakic intraocular lens with and without a central hole," *Journal of Cataract and Refractive Surgery*, vol. 41, no. 1, pp. 67–72, 2015.

[27] I. Guber, V. Mouvet, C. Bergin, S. Perritaz, P. Othenin-Girard, and F. Majo, "Clinical outcomes and cataract formation rates in eyes 10 years after posterior phakic lens implantation for myopia," *JAMA Ophthalmology*, vol. 134, no. 5, p. 487, 2016.

[28] H. S. Maeng, T. Y. Chung, D. H. Lee, and E. S. Chung, "Risk factor evaluation for cataract development in patients with low vaulting after phakic intraocular lens implantation," *Journal of Cataract and Refractive Surgery*, vol. 37, no. 5, pp. 881–885, 2011.

[29] G. Schmidinger, B. Lackner, S. Pieh, and C. Skorpik, "Long-term changes in posterior chamber phakic intraocular collamer lens vaulting in myopic patients," *Ophthalmology*, vol. 117, no. 8, pp. 1506–1511, 2010.

[30] Q. Y. Zeng, X. L. Xie, and Q. Chen, "Prevention and management of collagen copolymer phakic intraocular lens exchange: causes and surgical techniques," *Journal of Cataract and Refractive Surgery*, vol. 41, no. 3, pp. 576–584, 2015.

2

Effect of Reformation of the Anterior Chamber by Air or by a Balanced Salt Solution (BSS) on Corneal Endothelium after Phacoemulsification

Alahmady Hamad Alsmman [ID],[1] **Mohammed Ezzeldawla,**[1] **Amr Mounir** [ID],[1] **Ashraf Mostafa Elhawary,**[1] **Osama Ali Mohammed,**[1] **Mahmoud Farouk** [ID],[1] **and Ahmed Mohamed Sherif** [ID][2]

[1]*Department of Ophthalmology, Sohag Faculty of Medicine, Sohag University, Sohag, Egypt*
[2]*Department of Ophthalmology, Cairo Faculty of Medicine, Cairo University, Cairo, Egypt*

Correspondence should be addressed to Alahmady Hamad Alsmman; alahmady20@yahoo.com

Academic Editor: Van C. Lansingh

Aim. To study the effect of reformation of the anterior chamber by air or by a balanced salt solution, after smooth phacoemulsification on the corneal endothelial count and morphology. *Methods.* A prospective interventional nonrandomized comparative study included 500 eyes of 500 patients with age range between 50 and 60 years, prepared for cataract surgery and presented to the Ophthalmology department of Sohag University Hospital in the period from October 2016 to May 2017. Corneal endothelial morphology and count were examined, and the results were recorded for all cases before the surgery. Patients were divided into two groups, and both groups were diagnosed with grade 2 cataract and underwent uncomplicated phacoemulsification performed by well-trained surgeons. At the end of the surgery, group 1 was subjected to a reformation of the anterior chamber via a balanced salt solution (BSS) injection while group 2 was subjected to a reformation of the anterior chamber via air injection. Corneal endothelial morphology and count were evaluated in the first and 3rd month postoperatively. *Results.* The study included 500 patients (250 in each group), 220 males (44%) and 280 females (56%) with no significant statistical age differences. Both preoperative and postoperative (3 months after the operation) recorded parameters of the corneal endothelium did not show any significant statistical differences. The cumulative dissipated energy was recorded, for all cases of both groups, during phacoemulsification with no significant statistical differences ($P = 0.7$). *Conclusion.* There is no difference between the effect of reformation of the anterior chamber after phacoemulsification, using air or using a BSS injection, on the corneal endothelial count and morphology.

1. Introduction

Cataract surgery is one of the most frequently performed surgeries worldwide. It is well established that this surgery has a negative effect on corneal endothelium, as it decreases the endothelial cell count. The severity of the affection depends on many variables, as phacoemulsification time and energy, surgical technique, anterior chamber depth, and the use of ophthalmic viscoelastic devices (OVDs) [1].

The corneal endothelium functions as an active pump and also as a barrier against the aqueous humor of the anterior chamber; thus, it holds an important role in the process of corneal tissue hydration. It has no ability of regeneration, so any decrease in its density is irreversible and can lead to permanent blurring of vision and pain [2].

The corneal injury caused by phacoemulsification usually leads to corneal edema, and if it is severe enough, it might result in irreversible bullous keratopathy, making corneal tissue transplantation the only effective treatment [2].

Corneal endothelial injury associated with phacoemulsification is assessed by specular microscopy through measuring changes of the cell density (CD) and the cell morphology [3].

Air injection has become widely used in many anterior segment surgeries [4], for example, restoration of normal intraocular pressure and reformation of the anterior chamber and many other surgical procedures [5].

Direct contact between gases and the corneal endothelial layer is not natural, and many experimental and clinical studies have proved the occurrence of corneal injury as a result of air injection into the anterior chamber [6].

Nowadays, most surgeons prefer to use a balanced salt solution to avoid the harms of air injection, even though there were no reported complications of air injection over the long term [7].

This study aims at comparing the effect of reformation of the anterior chamber after phacoemulsification, using air and BSS injection, on corneal endothelial count and morphology.

2. Patient and Methods

This is a prospective interventional nonrandomized comparative study, which included 500 eyes of 500 patients with age range between 50 and 60 years, prepared for cataract surgery and presented to the Ophthalmology department of Sohag University Hospital in the period from October 2016 to May 2017. The study only included cases diagnosed with grade 2 cataract according to the Lens Opacities Classification System III (LOCS III) [8].

Exclusion criteria included the following: patients aged less than 50 years or more than 60 years; patients with a history of previous corneal pathology, pseudoexfoliation, ocular trauma or intraocular surgery, or intraocular inflammation; and patients having preoperative endothelial cell count < 1500 cells per square millimeter, preoperative anterior chamber depth < 2.5 mm, or short axial length eyes < 21 mm and long axial length > 25 mm.

The ethical committee of Sohag University approved this study protocol, which was carried out according to the Declaration of Helsinki. A written informed consent was obtained from each included case.

All patients were divided into two groups; group 1 was subjected to phacoemulsification with a reformation of the anterior chamber using a balanced salt solution (BSS) injection at the end of the surgery, while group 2 was subjected to phacoemulsification with a reformation of the anterior chamber by air injection at the end of the surgery.

Patients who fit the criteria were allocated to each group in turn.

All patients were subjected to a full ophthalmological evaluation before the operation The evaluation included a slit-lamp examination, measurement of the best corrected visual acuity, measurement of the intraocular pressure (IOP), and specular microscopic examination (using Specular Microscope, SP-3000P, Topcon, Tokyo, Japan, with the IMAGEnet system (version 2.1, Topcon)). Also, central corneal endothelium morphology assessment was conducted, which includes central corneal thickness (CCT), endothelial cell density (ECD), corneal endothelial cell size variations as the percentage of the abnormal sizes (corneal polymegathism), and corneal cell shape variations as the percentage of the hexagonal cells (corneal pleomorphism). Postoperative follow-up occurred on the first day (after 6 hours), second day, one week, and one month and after three months.

Specular microscopic examination postoperatively occurred twice after one month and three months.

All patients received the same regimen of 1 drop of cyclopentolate 1%, 1 drop of phenylephrine 10%, and 1 drop of diclofenac 0.1% 20 minutes before surgery. Also, a dose of 5-6 ml lidocaine hydrochloride 2% with adrenaline 1 : 200,000 was used for the peribulbar anesthesia.

All operations were performed by three well-experienced surgeons (first three authors) using the standard divide and conquer technique and the same phacoemulsification equipment (INFINITI Vision System; Alcon Laboratories Inc., Fort Worth, TX, USA) at similar settings. Any cases that developed intraoperative complications were excluded from the study.

The patients were allocated to different surgeons in turn, the first surgeon 167 eyes, second surgeon 167 eyes, and third surgeon 166 eyes.

All cases were operated on using the same standardized surgical technique, which includes the use of a sterile drape with speculum, application of the corneal topical anesthesia (lidocaine 2% in gel suspension), performance of a 2.75 mm self-sealing corneal incision, injection of a viscoelastic agent (Healon; Advanced Medical Optics Inc., Santa Ana, CA), application of capsulorrhexis, application of hydrodissection, application of the conventional phacoemulsification (longitudinal ultrasound) (divide and conquer), irrigation and aspiration of the cortical material, introduction of viscoelastic in a bag to implant a foldable acrylic lens (AcrySof SA60AT; Alcon Laboratories), implantation of the lens through a 2.8 mm incision with the use of injector, and aspiration of the viscoelastic. Closure of the incision was done by hydration using a 30-gauge cannula with no sutures. The cumulative dissipated energy (CDE; phaco energy) was documented for all patients.

In the postoperative period, all patients received the same treatment including topical antibiotic (moxifloxacin) at a rate of 5 times per day for one week and prednisolone acetate at a rate of 5 times per day for one week with a gradual decrease in the second week, then replaced by nonsteroidal anti-inflammatory drops at a rate of three times per day for the following two weeks.

2.1. Statistical Analysis. The data were analyzed using SPSS for Windows version 18.0 software (SPSS Inc., Chicago, IL, USA). The data are shown as the mean and standard deviation. The results were analyzed using Student's *t*-test to compare the mean values of both groups. The qualitative data was

TABLE 1: Preoperative demographics and corneal endothelial parameters.

| | Group 1 (BSS) | | Group 2 (air) | | |
	Mean ± SD	Range	Mean ± SD	Range	P value
Sample size (male : female)	250 (120 : 130)		250 (100 : 150)		
Age (year)	56 ± 2.3	52 to 60	57.9 ± 3.9	53 to 60	0.1
CDE (joules)	7.19 ± 1.1	4.96 to 9.14	6.51 ± 1	4.97 to 8.52	0.7
Cell density (cells/mm^2)	2646 ± 284	1858 to 2890	2604 ± 367	1998 to 3209	0.16
Coefficient of variance % (polymegathism)	38.2 ± 6	27 to 49	40.3 ± 8.4	31 to 61	0.8
Hexagonality % (pleomorphism)	49 ± 8	39 to 64	51 ± 10	34 to 73	0.3
Central corneal thickness (micron)	508 ± 22	474 to 571	509 ± 34	450 to 571	0.28

TABLE 2: Pre- and postoperative corneal endothelial parameters.

| | Group 1 (BSS) Mean ± SD | | | Group 2 (Air) Mean ± SD | | | P value |
	Preoperative	Post 1 month	Post 3 month	Preoperative	Post 1 month	Post 3 month	
Cell density (cells/mm^2)	2646 ± 284.1	2523 ± 311	2479 ± 303	2605 ± 367	2465 ± 351	2424 ± 336	0.16
Endothelial cell loss	—	146 ± 84 5.5%	189 ± 132 7.1%	—	164 ± 125 6.3%	172 ± 95 6.6%	0.1
Coefficient of variance % (polymegathism)	38.2 ± 6	1644±	39.8 ± 10	40.3 ± 8.4	35.8 ± 11	34.4 ± 11	0.8
Hexagonality % (pleomorphism)	49 ± 8	39 ± 15	45 ± 10	51 ± 10	42 ± 8	43 ± 9	0.3
Central corneal thickness, micron	508 ± 22	518 ± 23	508 ± 20	509 ± 34	530 ± 40	510 ± 41	0.28

expressed in the form of numbers and percentages and compared using the chi-square test. The multivariable regression analysis was done to identify the different corneal endothelial parameters. *P* value was considered significant if it was less than 0.05.

3. Results

The study included 500 patients (250 on each group), 220 males (44%) and 280 females (56%); group 1 included 120 males and 130 females with age range between 52 and 60 years, while group 2 included 100 males and 150 females with age range between 53 and 60 years. No significant statistical differences were recorded in the preoperative data about the age and the corneal parameters which include endothelial cell density, the coefficient of variance, hexagonality, and central corneal thickness (Table 1).

The cumulative dissipated energy was recorded for all cases during the phacoemulsification; the mean CDE in group 1 was 7.19 with SD 1.1, while the mean CDE in group 2 was 6.51 with SD 1. There was no significant statistical difference between both groups with *P* value = 0.7 (Table 1).

In group 1, the mean endothelial cell loss was 146 with SD 84 in the first month and 189 with SD 132 in the third month, while in group 2, the mean endothelial cell loss was 164 with SD 125 in the first month and 172 with SD 95 in the third month, with *P* value = 0.1 for both groups at the 3rd month.

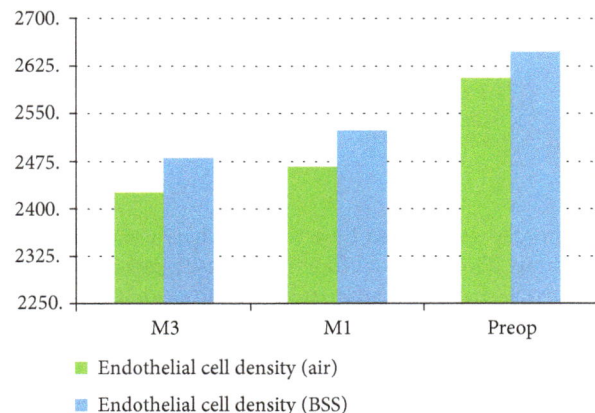

FIGURE 1: Pre- and post mean endothelial cell density.

There were no operative complications reported for all cases. There was no significant statistical difference between both groups regarding the corneal endothelial data in the 3rd month postoperatively. The postoperative corneal parameters are summarized in Table 2 and Figures 1–3.

4. Discussion

Normally the cornea is transparent. This state is maintained by the corneal endothelium, which keeps the corneal stroma

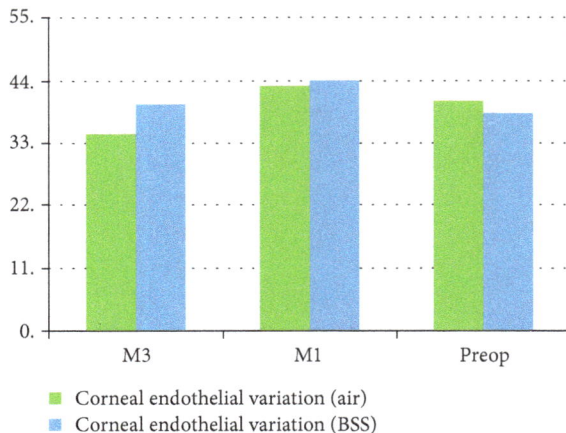

FIGURE 2: Pre- and post mean corneal endothelial variation.

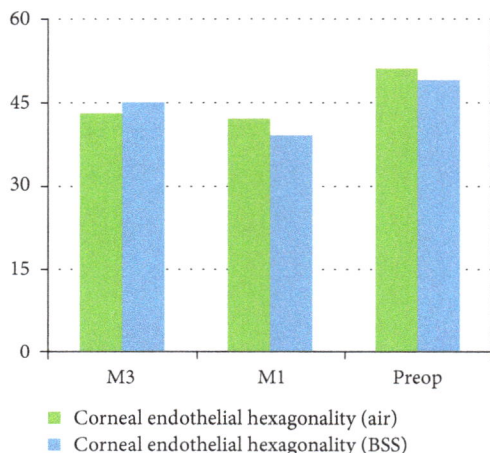

FIGURE 3: Pre- and post mean corneal endothelial hexagonality.

continuously dehydrated by acting as a barrier and an active fluid pump. This essential function is easily compromised by any damage that could happen during any eye surgery, especially phacoemulsification surgeries. This has prompted many studies to compare the severity of the damage that results from different cataract operation techniques [9].

Although the safety of the phacoemulsification has been markedly improved, the prevention of the corneal endothelial damage during phacoemulsification is still an important interest for all cataract surgeons [10].

In this study, we investigated the effect of reformation of the anterior chamber by air injection and by BSS injection on different corneal endothelial cell parameters, which were evaluated using the specular microscope to detect any damage resulting from the injection.

All preoperative data as regards age, the degree of cataract, and corneal endothelial cell parameters showed no statistical significance between both groups. Patients with other factors which might affect the corneal endothelial count were excluded, for example, patients older than 60 years and patients with advanced grades of cataract [11].

Sutureless corneal wounds have become the standard technique in cataract surgery, based on the fact that a watertight wound is an airtight wound and not vice versa. Hence, air injection is used for the reformation of the anterior chamber after phacoemulsification [12]. However, some studies reported air leakiness in 1/3 of the included cases [13].

In this study, we proved that there is no statistically significant difference between air and BSS injection in the anterior chamber reformation.

Our results agree with the study of Galin et al. [14] which were performed on rabbits' eyes. The authors examined the effect of air injection in the anterior chamber on the corneal endothelium. They used a light microscope and an electronic microscope for their study. They reported that the presence of air in the anterior chamber in contact with the corneal endothelium has no toxic effect on the corneal endothelium but even stimulates the proliferation of the corneal endothelial cells.

Also, our results are similar to the results of the Ventura et al. study [15], who confirmed that the air has no damaging effect on the corneal endothelium of the cat. Our results coincide with the results of the Norn study [5]. Norn studied the effect of reformation of the anterior chamber, after cataract extraction, using air injection on the corneal endothelium of humans. His study included an examination of the patients before and after the surgery. He proved that the corneal thickness was thinner in patients injected with air with no other adverse effects over a six-month period following the operation.

This study disagreed with the study of Olson et al. [16], who compared the effect of air and balanced saline solution injection into the anterior chamber on the corneal endothelium of cats. They reported a significant decrease in the endothelial cell density after air injection into the anterior chamber. He also noted significant endothelial damage during corneal perfusion studies.

Corneal pachymetry is assessed as the occurrence of edema is an indirect tool to evaluate corneal endothelial changes. It is important in cases of surgically induced endothelial cell loss [17].

Although, in this study, an initial increase in the corneal thickness caused by postoperative edema was reported. But the difference between both groups was not of statistically significance.

A significant positive correlation was found in many studies between the endothelial cell loss and the nuclear sclerosis grade, also between the endothelial cell loss and phacoemulsification power and time [18]. So only cases with grade 2 cataract were included in this study. Also, the power used in the surgery did not show a significant difference between both groups. So the endothelial cell loss reported in our study was not affected by the previous factors, and as a result, the effect of air on the corneal endothelium had not been masked by any factor.

Corneal endothelial parameters as regards cell density, endothelial cell loss, hexagonality, and coefficient of variance did not show any significant difference between both groups, which means that the reformation of the anterior chamber by air injection has no toxic effect on the corneal endothelium.

This was expected as thousands of phacoemulsification surgeries with air use in the anterior chamber reformation have been performed in our society "South Egypt" with satisfactory results.

5. Conclusions

There is no difference between the effect of reformation of the anterior chamber, after phacoemulsification, using air or using BSS injection on the corneal endothelial count and morphology. Also, there is no reported toxic effect of air on corneal endothelial parameters evaluated by specular microscope.

Conflicts of Interest

The authors declare that they have no conflicts of interest.

References

[1] I. Conrad-Hengerer, F. H. Hengerer, T. Schultz, and H. B. Dick, "Effect of femtosecond laser fragmentation on effective phacoemulsification time in cataract surgery," *Journal of Refractive Surgery*, vol. 28, no. 12, pp. 879–884, 2012.

[2] T. Igarashi, I. Ohsawa, M. Kobayashi et al., "Hydrogen prevents corneal endothelial damage in phacoemulsification cataract surgery," *Scientific Reports*, vol. 6, no. 1, article 31190, 2016.

[3] G. O. Waring III, W. M. Bourne, H. F. Edelhauser, and K. R. Kenyon, "The corneal endothelium. Normal and pathologic structure and function," *Ophthalmology*, vol. 89, no. 6, pp. 531–590, 1982.

[4] H. Landry, A. Aminian, L. Hoffart et al., "Corneal endothelial toxicity of air and SF6," *Investigative Ophthalmology & Visual Science*, vol. 52, no. 5, pp. 2279–2286, 2011.

[5] M. S. Norn, "Corneal thickness after cataract extraction with air in the anterior chamber," *Acta Ophthalmologica*, vol. 53, no. 5, pp. 747–750, 1975.

[6] D. A. Sim, R. Wong, and M. F. P. Griffiths, "Injecting an air bubble at the end of sutureless cataract surgery to prevent inflow of ocular surface fluid," *Eye*, vol. 21, no. 11, pp. 1444-1445, 2007.

[7] D. A. Lee, M. R. Wilson, M. O. Yoshizumi, and M. Hall, "The ocular effects of gases when injected into the anterior chamber of rabbit eyes," *Archives of Ophthalmology*, vol. 109, no. 4, pp. 571–575, 1991.

[8] G. Bencić, M. Zorić-Geber, D. Sarić, M. Čorak, and Z. Mandić, "Clinical importance of the lens opacities classification system III (LOCS III) in phacoemulsification," *Collegium Antropologicum*, vol. 29, Supplement 1, pp. 91–94, 2005.

[9] P. K. Sahu, G. K. Das, S. Agrawal, and S. Kumar, "Comparative evaluation of corneal endothelium in patients with diabetes undergoing phacoemulsification," *Middle East African Journal of Ophthalmology*, vol. 24, no. 2, pp. 74–80, 2017.

[10] H. Takahashi, "Corneal endothelium and phacoemulsification," *Cornea*, vol. 35, pp. S3–S7, 2016.

[11] M. Orski, A. Synder, D. Pałenga-Pydyn, W. Omulecki, and M. Wilczyński, "The effect of the selected factors on corneal endothelial cell loss following phacoemulsification," *Klinika Oczna*, vol. 116, no. 2, pp. 94–99, 2014.

[12] D. Calladine and R. Packard, "Clear corneal incision architecture in the immediate postoperative period evaluated using optical coherence tomography," *Journal of Cataract & Refractive Surgery*, vol. 33, no. 8, pp. 1429–1435, 2007.

[13] C. Matossian, S. Makari, and R. Potvin, "Cataract surgery and methods of wound closure: a review," *Clinical Ophthalmology*, vol. 9, pp. 921–928, 2015.

[14] M. A. Galin, E. Fetherolf, L. Lin, and D. L. Van Horn, "Experimental cataract surgeryelectron microscopy," *Ophthalmology*, vol. 86, no. 4, pp. 608–620, 1979.

[15] A. S. Ventura, R. Walti, and M. Bohnke, "Corneal thickness and endothelial density before and after cataract surgery," *British Journal of Ophthalmology*, vol. 85, no. 1, pp. 18–20, 2001.

[16] L. E. Olson, J. Marshall, N. S. Rice, and R. Andrews, "Effects of ultrasound on the corneal endothelium: I. The acute lesion," *British Journal of Ophthalmology*, vol. 62, no. 3, pp. 134–144, 1978.

[17] A. Assaf and M. Roshdy, "Comparative analysis of corneal morphological changes after transversal and torsional phacoemulsification through 2.2 mm corneal incision," *Clinical Ophthalmology*, vol. 7, pp. 55–61, 2013.

[18] M. Mahdy, Eid, Bhatia, Mohammed, and Hafez, "Relationship between endothelial cell loss and microcoaxial phacoemulsification parameters in noncomplicated cataract surgery," *Clinical Ophthalmology*, vol. 6, pp. 503–510, 2012.

3

A Meta-Analysis Comparing Postoperative Complications and Outcomes of Femtosecond Laser-Assisted Cataract Surgery versus Conventional Phacoemulsification for Cataract

Zi Ye, Zhaohui Li, and Shouzhi He

Department of Ophthalmology, The PLA General Hospital, 28 Fuxing Road, Beijing 100853, China

Correspondence should be addressed to Zhaohui Li; puxiongqiang259438@163.com

Academic Editor: Van C. Lansingh

Objective. This meta-analysis aimed to compare the outcomes and postoperative complications between femtosecond laser-assisted cataract surgery (FLACS) and conventional phacoemulsification cataract surgery (CPCS). *Methods.* Bibliographic databases, including PubMed, Embase, and Cochrane library, were systematically searched for references on or before September 2015 regarding the outcomes and complications by FLACS or CPCS. Data on corneal endothelial cell loss, uncorrected distance visual acuity (UDVA), corrected distance visual acuity (CDVA), refractive outcomes, and postoperative complications were retrieved. *Results.* A total of 9 trials were included in this analysis. Refractive outcomes (MD = −0.21, 95% CI: −0.39~0.03, $P = 0.02$) were significantly improved after FLACS. Although corneal endothelial cell loss was not significantly reduced after FLACS, there was a trend towards lower corneal endothelial cell loss (mean difference (MD) = 197.82, 95% confidence interval (CI): 2.66~392.97, $P = 0.05$) after FLACS. There was no significant difference in UDVA (MD = −0.01, 95% CI: −0.13~0.10, $P = 0.80$) or CDVA (MD = −0.03, 95% CI: 0.07~0.00, $P = 0.09$) between the two surgeries. Elevated intraocular pressure and macular edema were most commonly developed complications after cataract surgery, and the incidence of these complications associated with the two surgeries was similar. *Conclusion.* Compared with CPCS, FLACS might achieve higher refractive stability and corneal endothelial cell count. Nevertheless, further study is needed to validate our findings.

1. Introduction

Cataract is responsible for 48% of worldwide blindness, especially in developed countries [1, 2]. Conventional phacoemulsification cataract surgery (CPCS) is the most common surgical treatment for cataract. CPCS is generally effective for cataract but may cause a few complications such as elevated intraocular pressure and macular edema probably due to the heat generated by ultrasound during the procedure [3]. Femtosecond laser-assisted cataract surgery (FLACS), a new technology that was firstly introduced in 2008 [4], has shown promising treatment outcomes. To date, many studies have attempted to compare the outcome and complications of FLACS and CPCS. Some studies have shown better visual acuity recovery and lower endothelial cell loss after FLACS when compared with CPCS [5, 6], whereas others have detected no significant difference between the

two technologies [7, 8]. We herein performed this systematic study in order to evaluate the treatment efficacy and complications of FLACS and CPCS, including visual recovery, corneal cell integrity, and functionality in an aim to provide guidance for clinical practice.

2. Material and Methods

2.1. Literature Search. Bibliographic databases, including PubMed, Embase, and Cochrane library, were systematically searched to identify eligible studies until September 2015. The search key words were used including "femtosecond" AND "phaco OR phacoemulsification OR phakoemulsification" AND "cataract."

2.2. Selection Criteria. Studies meeting the following criteria were included in the meta-analysis: (1) studies designed as

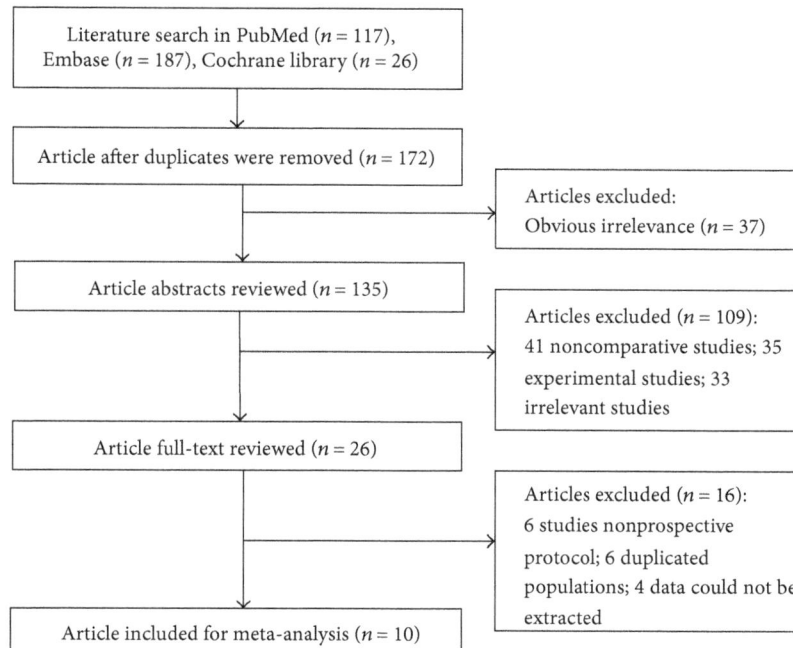

FIGURE 1: Flow chart of literature search and study selection.

prospective studies; (2) cataract patients were divided into FLACS and CPCS groups; (3) at least one of the following outcomes was reported: corneal endothelial cell counts, central corneal thickness, uncorrected distance visual acuity, corrected distance visual acuity, and refractive outcomes. Only the study with the longest follow-up time was included if the data was used in several studies. In addition, nonoriginal studies, including reviews, letters, and comments, were excluded.

2.3. Data Extraction and Quality Assessment. Two authors independently extracted data according to a predefined information sheet. The information, including the first author's name, publication year, study location, sample size, patients' characteristics, the number of cases, and controls, as well as outcome data, were extracted from each individual study. The Cochrane risk assessments tool was used to evaluate the quality of studies [9], including random sequence generation, allocation concealment, blinding of participants and personnel, blinding of outcome assessment, incomplete outcome data, selective reporting, and other biases.

2.4. Statistic Analysis. The outcomes and complications of FLACS versus CPCS were performed using RevMan 5.2. The pooled weighted mean differences (WMD) with 95% confidence intervals (CIs) were calculated to evaluate the differences between the two techniques. The potential heterogeneity across studies was evaluated by Cochran's Q and I^2 statistics [10]. $P < 0.05$ and/or $I^2 > 50\%$ was considered statistically significant. The random effect model was used in case of significant heterogeneity. Otherwise, the fixed-effect model was used. Sensitivity analysis was performed through omitting one study each time to evaluate the stability of the meta-analysis.

3. Results

3.1. Study Selection and Characteristic. The study selection process was illustrated in Figure 1. The search strategy originally yielded a total of 330 articles (117 articles from Embase database, 187 from PubMed database, and 26 from Cochrane library). After eliminating duplicated articles, 172 articles were included. Thirty-seven articles were removed after reviewing article titles. After reviewing the article abstracts, 109 articles were excluded, including 41 noncomparative studies, 35 experimental studies, and 33 noncataract patients. After reviewing the full-text of the 26 remaining articles, 10 prospective studies were finally selected for this meta-analysis ([5–7, 11–17], Table 1), including 8 from European countries, 1 from China [16], and 1 from Tasmania [7].

3.2. Evaluation of Risk of Bias. The risk of bias was shown in Figure 2. Generation of the randomization sequence was adequate in four trials. Blinding design was described in none of the enrolled studies. One study had a high risk of selective reporting because the author did not report all the outcome data that were described in the protocol.

3.3. Meta-Analysis of Operation Outcomes. Five studies evaluated corneal endothelial cell count as an outcome measure [5–7, 11, 17]. Evidence of heterogeneity was observed across these trials ($I^2 = 92\%$, $P < 0.00001$), and a random effect model was applied to pool the results (Figure 3). Corneal endothelial cell counts after CPCS was significantly less than FLACS (MD = 190.58, 95% CI: −1.70–342.86, $P = 0.05$). Heterogeneity was reduced to 0% after the study by Mastropasqua et al. was removed [6], and the results showed that FLACS significantly reduced corneal endothelial

TABLE 1: Characteristics of studies included in the meta-analysis.

Study	Area	Follow-up	Design	n, age (experimental)	n, age (control)	Main outcomes	Complications
Takacs et al. [11]	Hungary	4 weeks	Prospective case-control	38, 65.8 (12.4) ys	38, 66.9 (11.0) ys	Central corneal thickness, endothelial cell count	NA
Kranitz et al. [13]	Hungary	48 weeks	Prospective, randomized study	20, 68.2 (10.8) ys	25, 63.6 (13.7) ys	Refractive outcomes	NA
Filkorn et al. [12]	Germany	1 month	Prospective case-control	77, 65.2 (12.6) ys	57, 64.4 (12.4) ys	CDVA and refractive	NA
Abell et al. [7]	Tasmania	3 weeks	Prospective, consecutive, single-surgeon case-control	150, 72.8 (10.5) ys	51, 71.8 (10.8) ys	Corneal endothelial cell loss, CDVA, intraocular pressure, and refractive outcomes	NA
Conrad-Hengerer et al. [5]	Germany	3 months	Randomized intraindividual cohort study	73, 70.9 ys	73, 70.9 ys	Endothelial cell counts and corneal thickness	FLACS: EIP in 3 eyes; macular edema in 2 eyes CPCS: EIP in 2 eyes, macular edema in 5 eyes
Mastropasqua et al. [6]	Italy	24 weeks	Prospective randomized study	30, 70.2 (2.9) ys	30, 70.5 (3.2) ys	UDVA, CDVA, and corneal endothelial cell counts	NA
Mastropasqua et al. [14]	Italy	24 weeks	Prospective randomized clinical study	60, 69.3 (3.2) ys	30, 69.1 (3.9) ys	UDVA, CDVA, refractive outcomes	NA
Krarup et al. [17]	Denmark	3 months	Prospective case-control	47	47	UDVA, CDVA, central corneal endothelialcell count	NA
Conrad-Hengerer et al. [15]	Germany	6 months	Prospective randomized intraindividual cohort study	100, 71.6 ys	100, 71.6 ys	Manifest refraction, corrected distance visual acuity, and anterior chamber depth	FLACS: 1 eye developed macular edema; EIP in 3 eyes; CPCS: 2 eyes developed macular edema, 1 eye developed subclinical macular edema, EIP in 2 eyes
Yu et al. [16]	China	3 months	Prospective study	25, 62.3 (11.6) ys	29, 56.5 (16.6) ys	CDVA, refractive outcomes	FLACS: pupil miosis in 1 eye, mild subconjunctival hemorrhage in 5 eyes, EIP in 1 eye; CPCS: posterior capsular opacification in 2 eyes

ys: years; FLACS: femtosecond laser-assisted cataract surgery; UDVA: uncorrected distance visual acuity; CDVA: corrected distance visual acuity; EIP: elevated intraocular pressure; NA: not available.

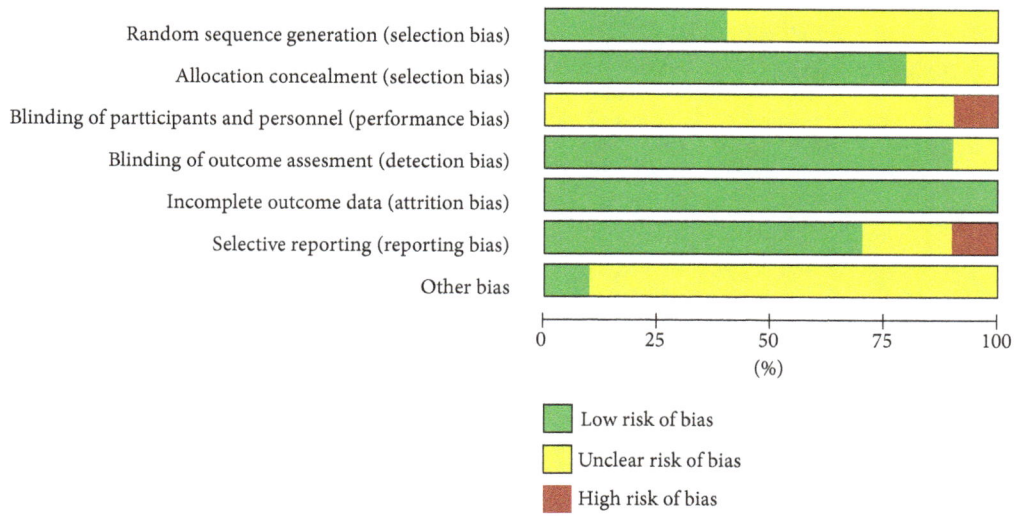

FIGURE 2: Risk of bias evaluation. (a) Risk of bias graph. (b) Risk of bias summary.

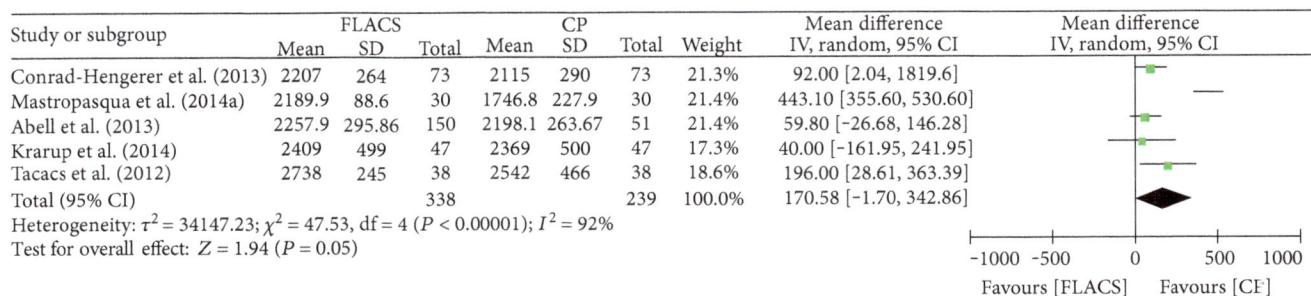

Study or subgroup	FLACS			CP			Weight	Mean difference IV, random, 95% CI	Mean difference IV, random, 95% CI
	Mean	SD	Total	Mean	SD	Total			
Conrad-Hengerer et al. (2013)	2207	264	73	2115	290	73	21.3%	92.00 [2.04, 1819.6]	
Mastropasqua et al. (2014a)	2189.9	88.6	30	1746.8	227.9	30	21.4%	443.10 [355.60, 530.60]	
Abell et al. (2013)	2257.9	295.86	150	2198.1	263.67	51	21.4%	59.80 [−26.68, 146.28]	
Krarup et al. (2014)	2409	499	47	2369	500	47	17.3%	40.00 [−161.95, 241.95]	
Tacacs et al. (2012)	2738	245	38	2542	466	38	18.6%	196.00 [28.61, 363.39]	
Total (95% CI)			338			239	100.0%	170.58 [−1.70, 342.86]	

Heterogeneity: $\tau^2 = 34147.23$; $\chi^2 = 47.53$, df = 4 ($P < 0.00001$); $I^2 = 92\%$
Test for overall effect: $Z = 1.94$ ($P = 0.05$)

FIGURE 3: Forest plots displaying the effect of femtosecond laser-assisted cataract surgery (FLACS) versus conventional phacoemulsification cataract surgery (CPCS) on corneal endothelial cell.

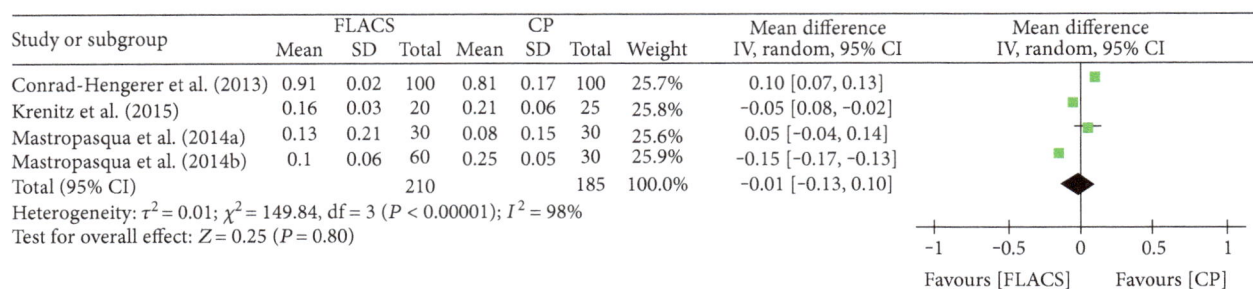

Study or subgroup	FLACS			CP			Weight	Mean difference IV, random, 95% CI	Mean difference IV, random, 95% CI
	Mean	SD	Total	Mean	SD	Total			
Conrad-Hengerer et al. (2013)	0.91	0.02	100	0.81	0.17	100	25.7%	0.10 [0.07, 0.13]	
Krenitz et al. (2015)	0.16	0.03	20	0.21	0.06	25	25.8%	−0.05 [0.08, −0.02]	
Mastropasqua et al. (2014a)	0.13	0.21	30	0.08	0.15	30	25.6%	0.05 [−0.04, 0.14]	
Mastropasqua et al. (2014b)	0.1	0.06	60	0.25	0.05	30	25.9%	−0.15 [−0.17, −0.13]	
Total (95% CI)			210			185	100.0%	−0.01 [−0.13, 0.10]	

Heterogeneity: $\tau^2 = 0.01$; $\chi^2 = 149.84$, df = 3 ($P < 0.00001$); $I^2 = 98\%$
Test for overall effect: $Z = 0.25$ ($P = 0.80$)

(a)

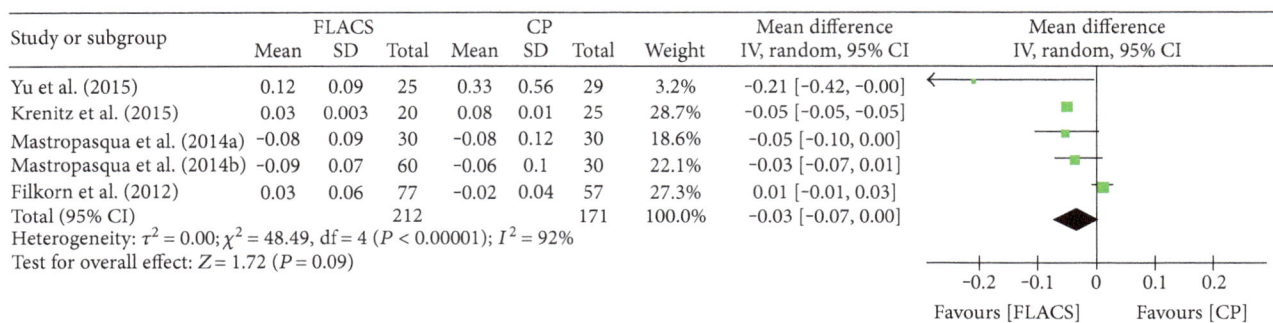

Study or subgroup	FLACS			CP			Weight	Mean difference IV, random, 95% CI	Mean difference IV, random, 95% CI
	Mean	SD	Total	Mean	SD	Total			
Yu et al. (2015)	0.12	0.09	25	0.33	0.56	29	3.2%	−0.21 [−0.42, −0.00]	
Krenitz et al. (2015)	0.03	0.003	20	0.08	0.01	25	28.7%	−0.05 [−0.05, −0.05]	
Mastropasqua et al. (2014a)	−0.08	0.09	30	−0.08	0.12	30	18.6%	−0.05 [−0.10, 0.00]	
Mastropasqua et al. (2014b)	−0.09	0.07	60	−0.06	0.1	30	22.1%	−0.03 [−0.07, 0.01]	
Filkorn et al. (2012)	0.03	0.06	77	−0.02	0.04	57	27.3%	0.01 [−0.01, 0.03]	
Total (95% CI)			212			171	100.0%	−0.03 [−0.07, 0.00]	

Heterogeneity: $\tau^2 = 0.00$; $\chi^2 = 48.49$, df = 4 ($P < 0.00001$); $I^2 = 92\%$
Test for overall effect: $Z = 1.72$ ($P = 0.09$)

(b)

FIGURE 4: Forest plots displaying the effect of femtosecond laser-assisted cataract surgery (FLACS) versus conventional phacoemulsification cataract surgery (CPCS) on visual acuity. (a) Uncorrected distance visual acuity. (b) Corrected distance visual acuity.

cell counts compared to CPCS (MD = 86.11, 95% CI: 29.99–142.23, $P = 0.003$).

Visual acuity was compared in 6 studies [6, 12–16], of which 4 evaluated uncorrected distance visual acuity (UDVA) and 5 compared corrected distance visual acuity (CDVA). As shown in Figure 4(a), significant heterogeneity was observed among the studies evaluating UDVA ($I^2 = 98\%$, $P < 0.00001$) and no significant difference in UDVA was observed between FLACS and CPCS (MD = −0.01, 95% CI: −0.13–0.10, $P = 0.80$). Figure 4(b) shows significant difference of postoperative CDVA using random effects model (MD = −0.03, 95% CI: 0.07–0.00, $P = 0.09$). Heterogeneity was reduced to 8% after the study by Filkorn et al. was omitted [12], and the result was not inversed when we removed other studies.

Mean absolute error (MAE) was adopted to assess refractive outcomes in 5 articles [7, 12, 14, 16, 17]. As shown in Figure 5, significant heterogeneity was calculated among studies evaluating refractive outcomes ($I^2 = 73\%$, $P = 0.05$) and FLACS that showed MAE in FLACS group was significantly lower than that in CP group (MD = −0.17, 95% CI: −0.32–0.02, $P = 0.02$). Heterogeneity was reduced to 8% after the study by Yu et al. was omitted [16], and the result was not inversed when we removed other studies.

3.4. Postoperative Complications. Among the enrolled studies, 3 described the occurrence of complications associated with the two surgeries [5, 15, 16]. Complications, including elevated intraocular pressure and macular edema, were most commonly reported. Moreover, the study by Yu et al.

Study or subgroup	FLACS			CP			Weight	Mean difference IV, random, 95% CI	Mean difference IV, random, 95% CI
	Mean	SD	Total	Mean	SD	Total			
Yu et al. (2015)	0.16	0.16	25	0.74	0.65	29	15.9%	-0.58 [-0.82, -0.34]	
Mastropasqua et al. (2014b)	0.39	0.33	60	0.54	0.43	30	20.3%	-0.15 [-0.033, 0.03]	
Abell et al. (2013)	-0.51	0.5	150	-0.45	0.71	51	18.0%	-0.06 [-0.27, 0.15]	
Filkorn et al. (2012)	-0.38	0.28	77	-0.5	0.38	57	24.1%	-0.12 [-0.24, -0.00]	
Krarup et al. (2014)	0.07	0.33	47	-0.41	0.42	47	21.8%	-0.04 [-0.19, 0.11]	
Total (95% CI)			359			214	100.0%	-0.17 [-0.32, -0.02]	

Heterogeneity: $\tau^2 = 0.02$; $\chi^2 = 14.74$, df = 4 ($P < 0.005$); $I^2 = 73\%$
Test for overall effect: $Z = 2.27$ ($P = 0.02$)

Favours [FLACS]   Favours [CP]

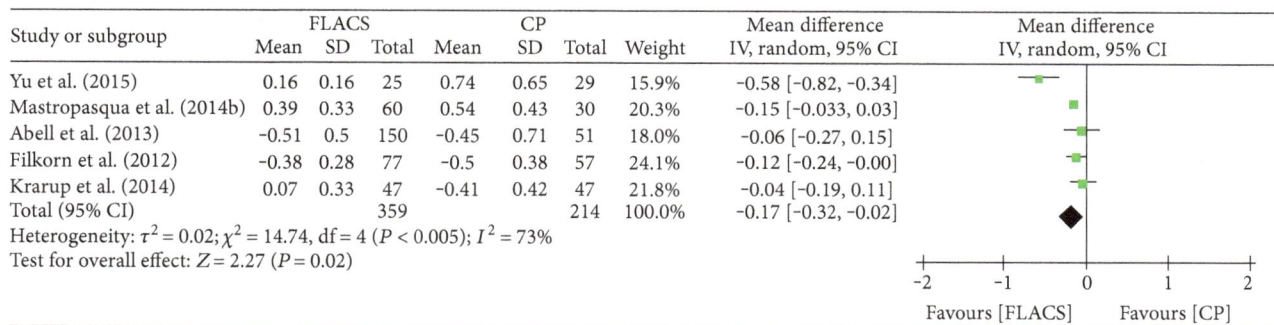

FIGURE 5: Forest plots displaying the effect of femtosecond laser-assisted cataract surgery (FLACS) versus conventional phacoemulsification cataract surgery (CPCS) on refractive outcome.

reported that pupil miosis occurred in 1 eye and mild subconjunctival hemorrhage occurred in 5 eyes after FLACS [16]. In total, 3 patients in FLACS group and 7 CPCS group developed macular edema. Additionally, elevated intraocular pressure was observed in 4 patients after FLACS and 7 patients after CPCS. Overall, the incidence of elevated intraocular pressure and macular edema during FLACS and CPCS was similar.

4. Discussion

A previous study by Chen et al. has suggested that FLACS is superior to CPCS for the reduction of mean phaco energy and effective phacoemulsification time [18]. Ultrasound energy introduced by conventional phacoemulsification may damage surrounding structures, resulting in endothelial cell loss [19, 20]. Therefore, a reduction in ultrasound phacoemulsification may markedly reduce postoperative corneal endothelial cell loss [21, 22]. In this study, FLACS was not superior to CPCS on postoperative corneal endothelial cell loss (MD = 197.82, 95% CI: 2.66~392.97, $P = 0.05$). However, when the study by Mastropasqua et al. was removed [6], corneal endothelial cell loss after FLACS was significantly lower than that in CPCS (MD = 86.11, 95% CI: 29.99~142.23, $P = 0.003$). Nevertheless, the conclusion needs to be validated by future studies. The positioning of intraocular lens is the most critical factor influencing the refractive outcomes [15]. Previous studies have suggested earlier stabilization of refraction after FLACS [23]. Consistently, our study found that refractive stability was significantly improved after FLACS (MD = -0.21, 95% CI: -0.39~0.03, $P = 0.02$).

It has been previously suggested that FLACS has a lower complication rate compared with CPCS [24]. In this study, we found that elevated intraocular pressure and macular edema were the most commonly reported complications. Although our study revealed a slightly lower number of cases with elevated intraocular pressure and macular edema, the incidence of elevated intraocular pressure and macular edema during FLACS and CPCS was similar. FLACS might slightly reduce the occurrence of macular edema when compared with CPCS, which might be associated with a slightly higher risk for elevated intraocular pressure probably due to the heat generated by ultrasound during the procedure [3].

Notably, significant heterogeneity was observed among the enrolled studies, which would weaken the strength of our conclusions. The heterogeneity might be attributed to various regional background, follow-up period, and surgical expertise. For instance, heterogeneity in refractive outcomes was significantly reduced (0%) after we removed the Chinese patients in Yu et al. [16]. Further, we performed sensitivity analysis, and the nonreversed results confirmed that the conclusion of our meta-analysis was reliable.

There are several limitations in the current study. First, the number of selected studies and patients are relatively small, which might affect the accuracy of our results. Furthermore, although sensitive analysis has shown the stability of our conclusions, significant heterogeneities were detected in initial analysis. Finally, given that surgical expertise could not be adjusted rigorously, our conclusions need to be verified by a study in a much larger population.

In summary, our meta-analysis found that FLACS could significantly improve refractive outcomes. Although FLACS was not superior to CPCS in reducing corneal endothelial cell loss, there was a trend towards reduced corneal endothelial cell loss after FLACS. Elevated intraocular pressure and macular edema were the most commonly developed complications. The incidence of these complications was similar after FLACS and CPCS. Our study provided evidence supporting higher treatment efficacy of FLACS based on refractive stability and corneal endothelial cell protection. However, further study is needed to validate our findings.

Conflicts of Interest

All authors declare that they have no conflict of interests.

References

[1] A. Churg, R. D. Wang, C. Xie, and J. L. Wright, "Alpha-1-antitrypsin ameliorates cigarette smoke-induced emphysema in the mouse," American Journal of Respiratory and Critical Care Medicine, vol. 168, no. 2, pp. 199–207, 2003.

[2] H. S. Dua, D. G. Said, and A. M. Otri, "Are we doing too many cataract operations? Cataract surgery: a global perspective," The British Journal of Ophthalmology, vol. 93, no. 1, pp. 1-2, 2009.

[3] Z. Nagy, A. Takacs, T. Filkorn, and M. Sarayba, "Initial clinical evaluation of an intraocular femtosecond laser in cataract surgery," *Journal of Refractive Surgery*, vol. 25, no. 12, pp. 1053–1060, 2009.

[4] E. Chan, O. A. Mahroo, and D. J. Spalton, "Complications of cataract surgery," *Clinical & Experimental Optometry*, vol. 93, no. 6, pp. 379–389, 2010.

[5] I. Conrad-Hengerer, M. Al Juburi, T. Schultz, F. H. Hengerer, and H. B. Dick, "Corneal endothelial cell loss and corneal thickness in conventional compared with femtosecond laser-assisted cataract surgery: three-month follow-up," *Journal of Cataract and Refractive Surgery*, vol. 39, no. 9, pp. 1307–1313, 2013.

[6] L. Mastropasqua, L. Toto, A. Mastropasqua et al., "Femtosecond laser versus manual clear corneal incision in cataract surgery," *Journal of Refractive Surgery*, vol. 30, no. 1, pp. 27–33, 2014.

[7] R. G. Abell, N. M. Kerr, and B. J. Vote, "Toward zero effective phacoemulsification time using femtosecond laser pretreatment," *Ophthalmology*, vol. 120, no. 5, pp. 942–948, 2013.

[8] R. Khandekar, A. Behrens, A. E. Al Towerki et al., "Determinants of visual outcomes in femtosecond laser assisted cataract surgery and phacoemulsification: a nested case control study," *Middle East African Journal of Ophthalmology*, vol. 22, no. 3, pp. 356–361, 2015.

[9] J. P. Higgins and S. Green, *Cochrane Handbook for Systematic Reviews of Interventions*, The Cochrane Collaboration John Wiley & Sons, Ltd., Chichester, UK, 2008.

[10] J. P. Higgins, S. G. Thompson, J. J. Deeks, and D. G. Altman, "Measuring inconsistency in meta-analyses," *Bmj*, vol. 327, no. 7414, pp. 557–560, 2003.

[11] A. I. Takacs, I. Kovacs, K. Mihaltz, T. Filkorn, M. C. Knorz, and Z. Z. Nagy, "Central corneal volume and endothelial cell count following femtosecond laser-assisted refractive cataract surgery compared to conventional phacoemulsification," *Journal of Refractive Surgery*, vol. 28, no. 6, pp. 387–391, 2012.

[12] T. Filkorn, I. Kovacs, A. Takacs, E. Horvath, M. C. Knorz, and Z. Z. Nagy, "Comparison of IOL power calculation and refractive outcome after laser refractive cataract surgery with a femtosecond laser versus conventional phacoemulsification," *Journal of Refractive Surgery*, vol. 28, no. 8, pp. 540–544, 2012.

[13] K. Kranitz, K. Mihaltz, G. L. Sandor, A. Takacs, M. C. Knorz, and Z. Z. Nagy, "Intraocular lens tilt and decentration measured by Scheimpflug camera following manual or femtosecond laser-created continuous circular capsulotomy," *Journal of Refractive Surgery*, vol. 28, no. 4, pp. 259–263, 2012.

[14] L. Mastropasqua, L. Toto, P. A. Mattei et al., "Optical coherence tomography and 3-dimensional confocal structured imaging system-guided femtosecond laser capsulotomy versus manual continuous curvilinear capsulorhexis," *Journal of Cataract and Refractive Surgery*, vol. 40, no. 12, pp. 2035–2043, 2014.

[15] I. Conrad-Hengerer, M. Al Sheikh, F. H. Hengerer, T. Schultz, and H. B. Dick, "Comparison of visual recovery and refractive stability between femtosecond laser-assisted cataract surgery and standard phacoemulsification: six-month follow-up," *Journal of Cataract and Refractive Surgery*, vol. 41, no. 7, pp. 1356–1364, 2015.

[16] A. Y. Yu, L. Y. Ni, Q. M. Wang et al., "Preliminary clinical investigation of cataract surgery with a noncontact femtosecond laser system," *Lasers in Surgery and Medicine*, vol. 47, no. 9, pp. 698–703, 2015.

[17] T. Krarup, L. M. Holm, M. la Cour, and H. Kjaerbo, "Endothelial cell loss and refractive predictability in femtosecond laser-assisted cataract surgery compared with conventional cataract surgery," *Acta Ophthalmologica*, vol. 92, no. 7, pp. 617–622, 2014.

[18] X. Chen, W. Xiao, S. Ye, W. Chen, and Y. Liu, "Efficacy and safety of femtosecond laser-assisted cataract surgery versus conventional phacoemulsification for cataract: a meta-analysis of randomized controlled trials," *Scientific Reports*, vol. 5, p. 13123, 2015.

[19] H. B. Dick, T. Kohnen, F. K. Jacobi, and K. W. Jacobi, "Long-term endothelial cell loss following phacoemulsification through a temporal clear corneal incision," *Journal of Cataract and Refractive Surgery*, vol. 22, no. 1, pp. 63–71, 1996.

[20] M. Ecsedy, K. Mihaltz, I. Kovacs, A. Takacs, T. Filkorn, and Z. Z. Nagy, "Effect of femtosecond laser cataract surgery on the macula," *Journal of Refractive Surgery*, vol. 27, no. 10, pp. 717–722, 2011.

[21] N. J. Friedman, D. V. Palanker, G. Schuele et al., "Femtosecond laser capsulotomy," *Journal of Cataract and Refractive Surgery*, vol. 37, no. 7, pp. 1189–1198, 2011.

[22] Y. J. Shin, Y. Nishi, C. Engler et al., "The effect of phacoemulsification energy on the redox state of cultured human corneal endothelial cells," *Archives of Ophthalmology*, vol. 127, no. 4, pp. 435–441, 2009.

[23] L. Toto, R. Mastropasqua, P. A. Mattei et al., "Postoperative IOL axial movements and refractive changes after femtosecond laser-assisted cataract surgery versus conventional phacoemulsification," *Journal of Refractive Surgery*, vol. 31, no. 8, pp. 524–530, 2015.

[24] M. Chen, C. Swinney, and M. Chen, "Comparing the intraoperative complication rate of femtosecond laser-assisted cataract surgery to traditional phacoemulsification," *International Journal of Ophthalmology*, vol. 8, no. 1, pp. 201–203, 2015.

4

Combined Phacoemulsification and Intravitreal Dexamethasone Implant (Ozurdex®) in Diabetic Patients with Coexisting Cataract and Diabetic Macular Edema

Claudio Furino,[1] **Francesco Boscia,**[2] **Alfredo Niro,**[1] **Ermete Giancipoli,**[2] **Maria Oliva Grassi,**[1] **Giuseppe D'amico Ricci,**[2] **Francesco Blasetti,**[2] **Michele Reibaldi,**[3] **and Giovanni Alessio**[1]

[1]Department of Medical Science, Neuroscience and Sense Organs, Eye Clinic, University of Bari, Bari, Italy
[2]Department of Surgical, Microsurgical and Medical Sciences, Eye Clinic, University of Sassari, Sassari, Italy
[3]Eye clinic, University of Catania, Catania, Italy

Correspondence should be addressed to Alfredo Niro; alfred.nir@tiscali.it

Academic Editor: Lisa Toto

Purpose. To investigate the effectiveness and safety of combined phacoemulsification and dexamethasone intravitreal implant in patients with cataract and diabetic macular edema. *Methods.* In this two-center, retrospective, single-group study, the charts of 16 consecutive patients who underwent combined phacoemulsification and intravitreal dexamethasone implant were retrospectively reviewed. These 16 patients, 7 men and 9 women, were observed at least 3 months of follow-up. Primary outcome was the change of the central retinal thickness (CRT); secondary outcome was the change of best-corrected visual acuity (BCVA). Any ocular complications were recorded. *Results.* Mean CRT decreased significantly from 486 ± 152.4 μm at baseline to 365.5 ± 91 μm at 30 days ($p = .005$), to 326 ± 80 μm at 60 days ($p = .0004$), and to 362 ± 134 μm at 90 days ($p = .001$). Mean BCVA was 20/105 (logMAR, 0.72 ± 0.34) at baseline and improved significantly ($p \le .007$) at all postsurgery time points. One case of ocular hypertension was observed and successfully managed with topical therapy. No endophthalmitis or other ocular complications were observed. *Conclusion.* Intravitreal slow-release dexamethasone implant combined with cataract surgery may be an effective approach on morphologic and functional outcomes for patients with cataract and diabetic macular edema for at least three months after surgery.

1. Introduction

Diabetes mellitus is associated with a 5-fold higher prevalence of cataract compared to the nondiabetic population [1]. Thus, cataract extraction is a frequently performed surgical procedure in patients with diabetes. Compared to nondiabetic cataract patients, this surgery is associated with a higher risk of complications in diabetic patients, including postsurgical development of cystoid macular edema (also called Irvine-Gass syndrome) or worsening of preexisting macular edema [2–4]. Diabetic macular edema (DME) is a complication of diabetic retinopathy and is the most common cause of visual loss in both proliferative and nonproliferative diabetic retinopathy. Approximately 20% of the patients with diabetic retinopathy are affected by macular edema [5].

Currently, there is no standard treatment approach for improving outcomes of cataract extraction in diabetic patients with different degrees of clinically significant macular edema. Previous papers proposed a combined approach with intravitreal injection of humanized anti-VEGF monoclonal antibodies (ranibizumab, bevacizumab) or triamcinolone acetonide and cataract surgery in patient with DME [6–12]. In a prospective, randomized clinical trial of intravitreous bevacizumab versus triamcinolone when administered at the time of cataract surgery, both groups gained vision but only triamcinolone acetonide was associated with a sustained reduction in central macular thickness after six months [13].

Dexamethasone intravitreal implant (Ozurdex®; Allergan Inc., Irvine, CA, USA) is a biodegradable implant that releases a small amount (700 μg) of the glucocorticoid dexamethasone over a period of up to six months. Ozurdex is indicated for the treatment of adult patients with visual impairment due to diabetic macular edema who are pseudophakic or who are considered insufficiently responsive to or unsuitable for non-corticosteroid therapy or macular edema following either branch retinal vein occlusion or central retinal vein occlusion, or inflammation of the posterior segment of the eye presenting as noninfectious uveitis.

In a prospective controlled, randomized interventional pilot trial, the intravitreal dexamethasone implant at the beginning of phacoemulsification significantly reduced central macular thickness and increased visual acuity after a 24-week follow-up [14]. But only two papers analyzed the safety and efficacy of Ozurdex implant at the end of cataract surgery in patients with diabetic macular edema [15, 16].

So, in this study, we contribute to analyze the effectiveness of intravitreal administration of dexamethasone implant at the end of cataract surgery in diabetic patients with coexisting cataract and clinical significant macular edema in order to avoid any increase of macular edema following uncomplicated phacoemulsification and to obtain the better functional outcome.

2. Methods

This was a two-center, non-randomized, retrospective, single-group study of combined cataract surgery with intravitreal dexamethasone implant (Ozurdex) in consecutive diabetic patients with a diagnosis of cataract and clinically significant diabetic macular edema as defined by the Early Treatment Diabetic Retinopathy Study (ETDRS) [17].

The primary objective was to assess if intravitreal dexamethasone implant (Ozurdex) injection immediately after cataract surgery was able to reduce or stabilize central retinal thickness (CRT). The secondary objective was to assess changes of best-corrected visual acuity (BCVA) throughout the follow-up.

Safety evaluation has also been performed as regard intraocular pressure (IOP) variations throughout the follow-up period and incidence of other ocular adverse events (ocular inflammation and other complications, such as retinal detachment or endophthalmitis).

Patients who met all of the following criteria were considered for inclusion into the study: glycated haemoglobin ≤ 9%, controlled blood pressure (≤130/80 mmHg), visually significant cataract diagnosed using a slit lamp; nonproliferative diabetic retinopathy and clinically significant macular edema; tomographic features of nontractional diabetic macular edema, cystoid pattern, and retinal detachment pattern as described by Koleva-Georgieva [18], regardless of central retinal thickness; and proliferative diabetic retinopathy whose proliferative component had been previously treated with laser photocoagulation. Patients who met any of the following criteria were excluded from study entry: treatment of diabetic macular edema with intravitreal anti-VEGF in 3 months before surgery or any type of intravitreal corticosteroid in the 6 months before surgery; presence of untreated proliferative diabetic retinopathy; history of ocular hypertension or glaucoma; and presence of associated conditions, such as uveitis,

retinal vein occlusion, and neovascular glaucoma, that could worsen macular edema. Patients who experienced intraoperative complications, such as posterior capsular tear or vitreous loss, were also excluded.

All patients underwent uneventful phacoemulsification in bag hydrophilic acrylic intraocular lens (IOL) implant using a 2.5 mm clear cornea tunnel and dispersive ophthalmic viscoelastic device. Ozurdex (700 μg dexamethasone) was administered via intravitreal injection under topical anesthesia directly at the end of cataract surgery, in the inferotemporal quadrant. Patient data (age, gender, and medical history with regard to diabetes and diabetic retinopathy) were recorded from the patient's medical file. CRT was measured using optical coherence tomography (TOPCON 3D OCT-2000 or CIRRUS, Zeiss). BCVA was measured by using a standardized ETDRS protocol [17]. Testing was done at a standardized distance (4 m) under standardized lighting conditions. ETDRS values were converted into Snellen fraction and then in logMAR values for the purpose of statistical analysis. IOP was measured using a Goldmann tonometer. Measurements of BCVA and CRT at different time points of interest (baseline, 30, 60, and 90 days after surgery) were retrospectively reviewed. IOP measurements at baseline, 10, 20, 30, 40, 50, 60, and 90 days after surgery were reviewed. Ocular and systemic complications were recorded. A total of 20 patients underwent combined phacoemulsification and dexamethasone implant and met inclusion criteria. All functional and morphologic data at baseline and at all post-baseline time points up to 90 days after surgery were available for only 16 patients. Four patients missed the follow-up at 90 days. 16 consecutive patients were included in this study. Statistical analysis was based on all patients included in the study. Baseline was defined as the day before surgery. Data processing, summaries, and analyses were performed using the statistical software package SAS version 9.1 or higher. A t-test was performed on the change from baseline in CRT to evaluate a reduction or stabilization of CRT and on the change from baseline in BCVA to evaluate an improvement of visual acuity. No formal sample size calculation was performed.

3. Results

Population's characteristics and relevant medical history data with regard to the underlying disease are summarized in Table 1. 16 consecutive patients out of 20 diabetic patients who underwent combined phacoemulsification and dexamethasone slow-release implant were included in this study. Mean age of the 7 men and 9 women included in this study was 62.5 ± 13.4 years (range: 31–76). Most patients ($n = 15$) had type 2 diabetes mellitus; only 1 patient had type 1 diabetes mellitus. The mean duration of diabetes was 20.1 ± 7.6 years and ranged between 2 and 30 years. The mean value of glycated haemoglobin (HbA1c) was $7.76 \pm 0.7\%$ (range: 6.3–9). All patients were treated for diabetes with insulin. Fourteen patients had nonproliferative diabetic retinopathy, and 2 patients with type 2 diabetes had proliferative diabetic retinopathy. The mean CRT decreased significantly from 486 ± 152.4 μm at baseline to 365.5 ± 91 μm at 30 days ($p = .005$),

TABLE 1: Demographic characteristics and relevant medical history with regard to diabetes.

		Total population ($N = 16$)
	N	16
Age [years]	Mean (SD)	62.5 (13.4)
	Median (min, max)	67.0 (31, 76)
Gender [n (%)]*	Male	7 (43.7%)
	Female	9 (56.3%)
Duration of diabetes [years]	Mean (SD)	20.1 (7.6)
	Median (min, max)	21.5 (2, 30)
Type of diabetes mellitus [n (%)]*	Type 1	1 (6.3%)
	Type 2	15 (93.7%)
Treatment of diabetes [n (%)]*	Insulin	16 (100.0%)
Hba1c [%]	Mean (SD)	7.76 (0.7)
	Median (min, max)	7.70 (6.3, 9)
Classification of diabetic retinopathy [n (%)]*	Nonproliferative	14 (87.5%)
	Proliferative	2 (12.5%)

*Percentages are based on the total number of patient.

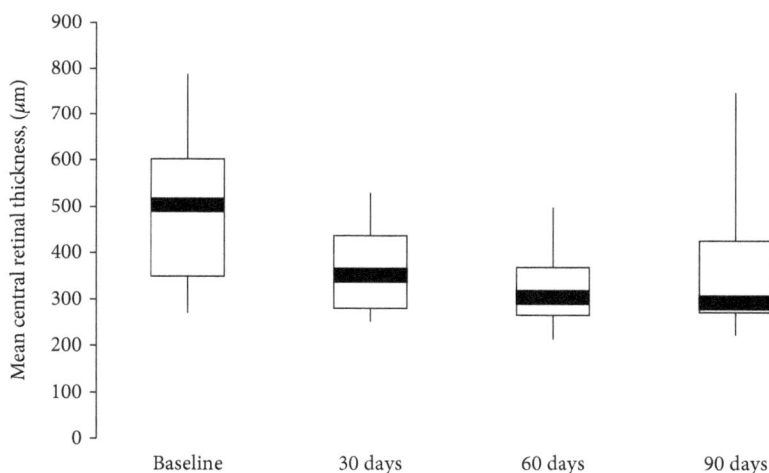

FIGURE 1: Boxplot of central retinal thickness (CRT) (μm) over 90 days. Mean CRT significantly decreased ($p \leq .005$), mainly at 60 days after combined approach.

to 326 ± 80 μm at 60 days ($p = .0004$), and to 362 ± 134 μm at 90 days ($p = .001$) after surgery (Figure 1). The largest mean (160 ± 142 μm) and median (116 μm) reduction were observed at 60 days. A large standard deviation for the changes from baseline in CRT was observed (Table 2).

The mean BCVA was 20/105 (logMAR, 0.72 ± 0.34) at baseline. At the postsurgery time points, the mean BCVA improved significantly to 20/60 (logMAR, 0.48 ± 0.28) at 30 days ($p = .007$), 20/53 (logMAR, 0.42 ± 0.30) at 60 days ($p = .0008$), and 20/57 (logMAR, 0.46 ± 0.39) at 90 days ($p = .004$) (Figure 2). The largest mean and median improvement of 0.30 logMAR were seen at 60 days (Table 3).

Measurements of IOP over time are summarized in Table 4. Mean and median IOP values were within normal ranges at baseline and at all postsurgery time points.

Ocular hypertension (28 mmHg) was observed in only one patient 10 days after surgery. The condition was well controlled with local therapy (dorzolamide/timolol fixed combination 2 times/day). No other ocular or systemic complications were observed.

4. Discussion

Phacoemulsification with in-the-bag IOL implantation, in general, do not cause progression of diabetic retinopathy [19–21]. However, previous studies suggested that diabetic patients with macular edema who were undergoing cataract surgery have poorer visual outcomes [20, 21]. So thanks to intravitreal dexamethasone implant after cataract surgery, patients with coexisting cataract and DME can benefit from downregulation of inflammatory mediators and reduction

TABLE 2: Central retinal thickness (CRT) over time.

Visit	Baseline	30 days	60 days	90 days
		Measured CRT [μm]		
Mean (SD)	486 (152.4)	365.5 (90.9)	325.8 (80.4)	361.7 (133.8)
Median (min, max)	503 (270, 789)	351 (251, 531)	305 (213, 499)	294 (222, 750)
		Change from baseline in CRT [μm]		
Visit	Baseline	30 days	60 days	90 days
Mean (SD)		−120.5 (147)	−160.0 (142)	−124 (125)
Median (min, max)	Not applicable	−81 (431, −41)	−116 (456, 0)	−103 (422, −18)
*p value**		*0.005*	*0.0004*	*0.001*

*Weighted *t*-test for change versus baseline.

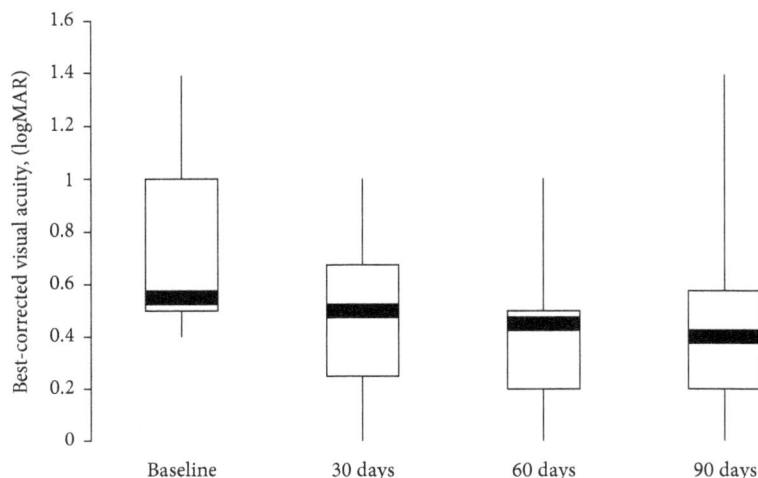

FIGURE 2: Boxplot of best-corrected visual acuity (BCVA) (logMAR) over 90 days. Mean BCVA increased significantly at all follow-up ($p \le .007$), mainly at 60 days after surgery.

of breakdown of the blood-retinal barrier due to diabetic status and surgical inflammatory stress.

With regard to the treatment of DME, dexamethasone slow-release implant (Ozurdex) has been shown to achieve a similar rate of visual acuity improvement compared with the anti-VEGF monoclonal antibody bevacizumab, with superior anatomic outcomes and fewer injections [22].

In previous studies, we successfully experienced the use of dexamethasone implant in refractory postsurgical macular edema [23, 24]. The study reported here investigated the effect of combining an intravitreal dexamethasone implant (Ozurdex) with cataract surgery in patients with coexisting cataract and clinically significant diabetic macular edema on visual acuity, retinal thickness, and safety parameters. Sixteen patients (7 men and 9 women) with cataract and DME were included.

In a small prospective clinical trial on 18 eyes with DME, dexamethasone implant was performed at the beginning of phacoemulsification [14]. We considered performing safer implant at the end of cataract surgery when potential intraoperative complications were overcome and a better visualization of implant in the vitreous was possible.

A prospective study published by Panozzo et al. [15] suggested that intravitreal dexamethasone implant performed at the end of phacoemulsification and IOL implantation was safe and effective in naïve and refractory DME. Same results were reported in a small case series which included 12 patients with macular edema secondary to diabetic retinopathy and 12 patients with macular edema secondary to retinal vein occlusion [16].

In our study, mean preoperative CRT (486 ± 152.4 μm) was higher than that reported in previous papers (335.9 ± 90.6 μm [14], $451 \pm$ NR μm [15], and 393 ± 166.5 μm [16]) with a wide range of value (270–789 μm) suggesting the heterogeneity of DME feature as a target for steroid therapy.

In our study, the mean reduction in CRT was statistically significant at 30, 60, and 90 days ($p \le .005$). Similar to previous reports [14–16], the greatest mean reductions in CRT occurred at 30 (120.5 μm) and 60 days (160 μm) after implant, with a recurrence of macular edema from the third month. After the mean reduction in CRT reaches the highest point, when dexamethasone reaches the highest concentration in the vitreous humor, the reduction in retinal thickness decreases in line with the known pharmacodynamics of the Ozurdex [25].

TABLE 3: Best-corrected visual acuity (BCVA) over time.

	Measured BCVA			
Visit	Baseline	30 days	60 days	90 days
Mean (logMAR ± SD)	20/105 (0.72 ± 0.34)	20/60 (0.48 ± 0.28)	20/53 (0.42 ± 0.30)	20/57 (0.46 ± 0.39)
Median, logMAR (min, max)	0.55 (0.4, 1.39)	0.50 (0.00, 1)	0.45 (0.00, 1)	0.40 (0.00, 1.39)
	Change from Baseline in BCVA			
Visit	Baseline	30 days	60 days	90 days
Mean, logMAR ± SD		−0.24 ± 0.30	−0.30 ± 0.28	−0.26 ± 0.30
Median, logMAR (min, max)	not applicable	0.15 (−0.20, 0.99)	0.30 (−0.10, 0.99)	0.25 (−0.30, 0.99)
*p value**		*0.007*	*0.0008*	*0.004*

*Weighted t-test for change versus baseline.

TABLE 4: Intraocular pressure (IOP) over time.

	Measured IOP [mmHg]			
Visit	Baseline	10 days	20 days	30 days
Mean (SD)	15.7 (2.0)	16.0 (5.0)	14.2 (2.8)	14.5 (2.3)
Median (min, max)	15.5 (13, 20)	15.5 (9, 28)	14 (9, 18)	15 (10, 18)
Visit	40 days	50 days	60 days	90 days
Mean (SD)	15.1 (3.0)	14.9 (1.7)	14.9 (2.5)	16.4 (3.1)
Median (min, max)	15 (10, 20)	15 (11, 17)	16 (10, 18)	16.5 (11, 25)

The mean change from baseline in BCVA was statistically significant at all follow-up visits ($p \leq .007$) as reported by different authors [14–16]. A clinically significant improvement in BCVA has been defined as ≥ 0.3 logMAR [26]. Agarwal et al. [14] reported a mean visual gain of 18 letters at 12 weeks. Panozzo et al. [15] reported a stable mean visual improvement of 18 letters at month 2 after treatment. In this study, according to this cut-off value, the mean or median visual change (0.30 ± 0.28 logMAR; 0.30 logMAR) indicated a clinically significant improvement at 60 days (2 months). An improvement ≥ 0.3 logMAR at at least 1 postsurgery time point was reported in 8 patients (50%) who maintained that improvement up to 90 days. Comparing the variations in BCVA at different follow-up visits, no significant difference was observed. These results could be attributed to the weak correlation between reduction in CRT and improvement in BCVA, as reported by previous studies [27, 28]. Also, clinical characteristics such as increasing age, female sex, duration of diabetes, high HbA1c level at the time of surgery, and moderate to severe retinopathy have been associated with poor prognosis after cataract surgery in diabetic patients [29–31]. So our functional outcomes should be analyzed considering that nine patients (56.3%) were female, the mean HbA1c level before surgery was 7.76, and the mean duration of diabetes mellitus was 20.1 years.

In previous reports [14–16], the injection of Ozurdex in combination with cataract surgery raised no safety concerns with regard to IOP or other ocular or systemic complications. So, in this study, there was only one case of elevated IOP (28 mmHg) occurring 10 days after cataract extraction, which returned to normal after topic treatment. No case of endophthalmitis was observed.

The power of this study is limited by the retrospective design, small sample size, and lack of a control group. In addition, the follow-up time is too short to decide on retreatment with dexamethasone implant if macular edema should recur even if these patients were sent to injection service for the next follow-up. Another limitation was the high interpatient variability regarding the study variables CRT and BCVA at baseline, which ranged between 270 μm and 789 μm and between 0.09 logMAR (normal vision) and 1.00 logMAR (severe vision loss), respectively. However, that interpatient variability could suggest the efficacy of combined approach regardless of the severity of cataract and macular edema.

In conclusion, the results of this study indicate that intravitreal dexamethasone implant administration in combination with phacoemulsification and IOL implantation may be safe and effective for morphologic and visual outcomes in cataract and DME during the first 3 months after surgery.

Disclosure

The authors alone are responsible for the content and writing of the paper.

Conflicts of Interest

The authors report no conflicts of interest.

References

[1] I. G. Obrosova, S. S. Chung, and P. F. Kador, "Diabetic cataracts: mechanisms and management," *Diabetes/Metabolism Research and Reviews*, vol. 26, no. 3, pp. 172–180, 2010.

[2] N. M. Haddad, J. K. Sun, S. Abujaber, D. K. Schlossman, and P. S. Silva, "Cataract surgery and in diabetic its complications patients," *Seminars in Ophthalmology*, vol. 29, no. 5-6, pp. 329–337, 2014.

[3] S. J. Kim, R. Equi, and N. M. Bressler, "Analysis of macular edema after cataract surgery in patients with diabetes using optical coherence tomography," *Ophthalmology*, vol. 114, no. 5, pp. 881–889, 2007.

[4] C. Suto, S. Hori, and S. Kato, "Management of type 2 diabetics requiring panretinal photocoagulation and cataract surgery," *Journal of Cataract and Refractive Surgery*, vol. 34, no. 6, pp. 1001–1006, 2008.

[5] J. W. Yau, S. L. Rogers, R. Kawasaki et al., "Global prevalence and major risk factors of diabetic retinopathy," *Diabetes Care*, vol. 35, no. 3, pp. 556–564, 2012.

[6] P. I. Rauen, J. A. S. Ribeiro, F. P. P. Almeida, I. U. Scott, A. Messias, and R. Jorge, "Intravitreal injection of ranibizumab during cataract surgery in patients with diabetic macular edema," *Retina*, vol. 32, no. 9, pp. 1799–1803, 2012.

[7] A. Lanzagorta-Aresti, E. Palacios-Pozo, J. L. Menezo Rozalen, and A. Navea-Tejerina, "Prevention of vision loss after cataract surgery in diabetic macular edema with intravitreal bevacizumab: a pilot study," *Retina*, vol. 29, no. 4, pp. 530–535, 2009.

[8] Y. Takamura, E. Kubo, and Y. Akagi, "Analysis of the effect of intravitreal bevacizumab injection on diabetic macular edema after cataract surgery," *Ophthalmology*, vol. 116, no. 6, pp. 1151–1157, 2009.

[9] A. Akinci, C. Batman, E. Ozkilic, and A. Altinsoy, "Phacoemulsification with intravitreal bevacizumab injection in diabetic patients with macular edema and cataract," *Retina*, vol. 29, no. 10, pp. 1432–1435, 2009.

[10] C. H. Chen, Y. C. Liu, and P. C. Wu, "The combination of intravitreal bevacizumab and phacoemulsification surgery in patients with cataract and coexisting diabetic macular edema," *Journal of Ocular Pharmacology and Therapeutics*, vol. 25, no. 1, pp. 83–89, 2009.

[11] M. S. Habib, P. S. Cannon, and D. H. Steel, "The combination of intravitreal triamcinolone and phacoemulsification surgery in patients with diabetic foveal oedema and cataract," *BMC Ophthalmology*, vol. 5, p. 15, 2005.

[12] A. Akinci, O. Muftuoglu, A. Altınsoy, and E. Ozkılıc, "Phacoemulsification with intravitreal bevacizumab and triamcinolone acetonide injection in diabetic patients with clinically significant macular edema and cataract," *Retina*, vol. 31, no. 4, pp. 755–758, 2011.

[13] L. L. Lim, J. L. Morrison, M. Constantinou et al., "Diabetic Macular Edema at the time of Cataract Surgery trial: a prospective, randomized clinical trial of intravitreous bevacizumab versus triamcinolone in patients with diabetic macular oedema at the time of cataract surgery - preliminary 6 month results," *Clinical and Experimental Ophthalmology*, vol. 44, no. 4, pp. 233–242, 2016.

[14] A. Agarwal, V. Gupta, J. Ram, and A. Gupta, "Dexamethasone intravitreal implant during phacoemulsification," *Ophthalmology*, vol. 120, no. 1, p. 211, 2013, 211.e1-5.

[15] G. A. Panozzo, E. Gusson, G. Panozzo, and M. G. Dalla, "Dexamethasone intravitreal implant at the time of cataract surgery in eyes with diabetic macular edema," *European Journal of Ophthalmology*, vol. 27, no. 4, pp. 433–437, 2017.

[16] A. M. Sze, F. O. Luk, T. P. Yip, G. K. Lee, and C. K. Chan, "Use of intravitreal dexamethasone implant in patients with cataract and macular edema undergoing phacoemulsification," *European Journal of Ophthalmology*, vol. 25, no. 2, pp. 168–172, 2015.

[17] "Photocoagulation for diabetic macular edema. Early Treatment Diabetic Retinopathy Study report number 1. Early Treatment Diabetic Retinopathy Study research group," *Archives of Ophthalmology*, vol. 103, no. 12, pp. 1796–1806, 1985.

[18] D. Koleva-Georgieva, "Optical coherence tomography findings in diabetic macular edema," in *Diabetic Retinopathy*, M. S. Ola, Ed., InTech, Vienna, Austria, 2012.

[19] A. S. Shah and S. H. Chen, "Cataract surgery and diabetes," *Current Opinion in Ophthalmology*, vol. 21, no. 1, pp. 4–9, 2010.

[20] D. Squirrell, R. Bhola, J. Bush, S. Winder, and J. F. Talbot, "A prospective, case controlled study of the natural history of diabetic retinopathy and maculopathy after uncomplicated phacoemulsification cataract surgery in patients with type 2 diabetes," *The British Journal of Ophthalmology*, vol. 86, no. 5, pp. 565–571, 2002.

[21] M. D. Somaiya, J. D. Burns, R. Mintz, R. E. Warren, T. Uchida, and B. F. Godley, "Factors affecting visual outcomes after small-incision phacoemulsification in diabetic patients," *Journal of Cataract and Refractive Surgery*, vol. 28, no. 8, pp. 1364–1371, 2002.

[22] M. C. Gillies, L. L. Lim, A. Campain et al., "A randomized clinical trial of intravitreal bevacizumab versus intravitreal dexamethasone for diabetic macular edema: the BEVORDEX study," *Ophthalmology*, vol. 121, no. 12, pp. 2473–2481, 2014.

[23] C. Furino, F. Boscia, N. Recchimurzo, C. Sborgia, and G. Alessio, "Intravitreal dexamethasone implant for macular edema following uncomplicated phacoemulsification," *European Journal of Ophthalmology*, vol. 24, no. 3, pp. 387–391, 2014.

[24] C. Furino, F. Boscia, N. Recchimurzo, C. Sborgia, and G. Alessio, "Intravitreal dexamethasone implant for refractory macular edema secondary to vitrectomy for macular pucker," *Retina*, vol. 34, no. 8, pp. 1612–1616, 2014.

[25] J. E. Chang-Lin, M. Attar, A. A. Acheampong et al., "Pharmacokinetics and pharmacodynamics of a sustained-release dexamethasone intravitreal implant," *Investigative Ophthalmology & Visual Science*, vol. 52, no. 1, pp. 80–86, 2011.

[26] N. Feltgen, A. Neubauer, B. Jurklies et al., "Multicenter study of the European Assessment Group for Lysin in Eye (EAGLE) for the treatment of central retinal artery occlusion: design issues and implications. EAGLE study report no.1," *Graefe's Archive for Clinical and Experimental Ophthalmology*, vol. 244, no. 8, pp. 950–956, 2006.

[27] M. S. Blumenkranz, J. A. Haller, B. D. Kuppermann et al., "Correlation of visual acuity and macular thickness measured by optical coherence tomography in patients with persistent macular edema," *Retina*, vol. 30, no. 7, pp. 1090–1094, 2010.

[28] Diabetic Retinopathy Clinical Research Network, D. J. Browning, A. R. Glassman et al., "Relationship between optical coherence tomography-measured central retinal thickness and visual acuity in diabetic macular edema," *Ophthalmology*, vol. 114, no. 3, pp. 525–536, 2007.

[29] G. H. Bresnick, "Diabetic maculopathy: a critical review highlighting diffuse macular edema," *Ophthalmology*, vol. 90, no. 11, pp. 1301–1317, 1983.

[30] M. L. Nelson and A. Martidis, "Managing cystoids macular edema after cataract surgery," *Current Opinion in Ophthalmology*, vol. 14, pp. 39–43, 2003.

[31] P. Massin, F. Audren, B. Haouchine et al., "Intravitreal triamcinolone acetonide for diabetic diffuse macular edema," *Ophthalmology*, vol. 111, no. 2, pp. 218–225, 2004.

5

Changes in Intraocular Straylight and Visual Acuity with Age in Cataracts of Different Morphologies

Sonia Gholami,[1] Nicolaas J. Reus,[2] and Thomas J. T. P. van den Berg[3]

[1]*Rotterdam Ophthalmic Institute, Rotterdam, Netherlands*
[2]*Amphia Hospital, Breda, Netherlands*
[3]*Netherlands Institute for Neuroscience and Royal Netherlands Academy of Arts and Sciences, Amsterdam, Netherlands*

Correspondence should be addressed to Sonia Gholami; sonia.gholami@googlemail.com

Academic Editor: Jose M. González-Meijome

Purpose. To investigate the significance of difference in straylight of cataract eyes with different morphologies, as a function of age and visual acuity. *Methods.* A literature review to collect relevant papers on straylight, age, and visual acuity of three common cataract morphologies leads to including five eligible papers for the analysis. The effect of morphology was incorporated to categorize straylight dependency on the two variables. We also determined the amount of progression in a cataract group using a control group. *Results.* The mean straylight was 1.22 log units $\pm$ 0.20 (SD) in nuclear (592 eyes), 1.26 log units $\pm$ 0.23 in cortical (776 eyes), and 1.48 log units $\pm$ 0.34 in posterior subcapsular (75 eyes) groups. The slope of straylight-age relationship was 0.009 ($R^2 = 0.20$) in nuclear, 0.012 ($R^2 = 0.22$) in cortical, and 0.014 ($R^2 = 0.11$) in posterior subcapsular groups. The slope of straylight-visual acuity relationship was 0.62 ($R^2 = 0.25$) in nuclear, 0.33 ($R^2 = 0.13$) in cortical, and 1.03 ($R^2 = 0.34$) in posterior subcapsular groups. *Conclusion.* Considering morphology of cataract provides a better insight in assessing visual functions of cataract eyes, in posterior subcapsular cataract, particularly, in spite of notable elevated straylight, visual acuity might not manifest severe loss.

1. Introduction

The eye is an optical system with imperfections. Entering this optical system, light is refracted by the ocular media (e.g., cornea and crystalline lens) to form an image on the retina. However, part of this light is scattered by optical imperfections. Depending on the direction of scattering (forward or backward), it can have different influences on vision. The forward light scattering causes (intraocular) straylight or disability glare [1]. It produces undesired veiling of the retinal image which leads to reduced vision, glare, and other visual impairments. In young healthy eyes, almost 10% of the inbound light is scattered [2]. However, in eyes older than 50 years of age, this number increases considerably [3]. A phakic norm curve has been established that can be used as a reference for clinical practice [3]. Some pathological conditions, in particular cataract, increase the amount of intraocular straylight above normal. In clinical practice, a patient's visual complaints, ophthalmic examination with a slit-lamp, and measurement of

visual acuity are the predominant scales for managing cataract. It should be noted that a slit-lamp examination provides only backscatter-based assessments. As the correlation between forward and backward light scattering has been shown to be small, methods that measure the amount of backscatter, such as slit-lamp examination, cannot reliably quantify straylight and glare [4–7]. Various studies have shown that straylight is a vision impairment that is not directly related to visual acuity and is only weakly correlated to it [3, 8]. A computerized purpose-built device, called C-Quant (Oculus Optikgeräte GmbH), measures the amount of ocular straylight and renders a parameter in the logarithmic unit (log(s)) with good reliability and repeatability [9–11].

As mentioned earlier, visual acuity is an important criterion in the cataract surgical decision-making process. However, various studies [12, 13] have shown that in a significant number of cataract cases, visual acuity is not an adequate measure to judge visual performance. Subsequent studies have supported this notion [14, 15]. Moreover, there have been reports of no change or even an increase in straylight after cataract surgery when the decision was made solely based on visual acuity [16]. The reason for this is that visual acuity only evaluates the impact of narrow-angle light spreading due to refractive errors and therefore can only measure a limited part of a patient's vision [13, 17]. Elliot et al. [7] expressed that additional visual tests were needed that could mirror visual loss but at the same time should be unrelated to visual acuity. They acknowledged the direct compensation method to quantify straylight as a standard technique to evaluate the validity of disability glare tests.

Recently, a literature review [18] established a norm curve for pseudophakic eyes and also a reference curve to estimate the amount of straylight to be expected after cataract surgery by introducing *straylight improvement* as a function of age and preoperative straylight. Although this reference is a good measure for cataract management in an average eye, it may overlook the influence of the type, location, and intensity of the cataract on the outcome because the type of cataract was not specified in the norm curve. To establish morphologically categorized references, we need a phakic norm stratified to the type of cataract. In the present study, we performed a literature review to identify relevant papers on straylight, age, and visual acuity in three common types of cataract. In addition, we recalculated the significance of the relation between straylight and visual acuity with taking cataract morphology into account. The published studies included in this literature review were evidenced individually that such correlation varies from one type of cataract to another. The population sizes and severities of the cataracts were different across these studies. We consider the relatively large final number of observations and their diverse degrees of cataract intensity as the strength of this study to improve the generalizability of the results.

2. Materials and Methods

This study includes two parts. The first part encompasses a comprehensive literature review to study the effect of different cataract morphologies on straylight and to determine models for straylight values as a function of age for different types of cataract. Second, we calculated the correlations between straylight and visual acuity, the amount of progression of straylight and visual acuity from those of a normal group, and the ratios of straylight to age and visual acuity in each cataract group.

A literature examination was carried out including all available studies that reported straylight values, measured with a C-Quant instrument (Oculus Optikgeräte GmbH), in cataract eyes with specification of its morphology. The language of the articles and age, gender, and race of the participants had no influence in this process. All papers provided information on intraocular straylight, age, and visual acuity of participants with the specification of the type of cataract. All papers had excluded patients with a history of ocular surgery or diseases, diabetic retinopathy, glaucoma, and age-related macular degeneration. We considered data with expected standard deviation (ESD) of 0.12 log units or less reliable for analysis.

TABLE 1: Red circles show deficient data, and green circles show available data in each individual study.

Cataract	Study (year)	Age	SL	VA
Nuclear	Filgueira et al. (2016)	🟢	🟢	🟢
	Congdon et al. (2012)	🟢	🟢	🟢
	Bal et al. (2011)	🟢	🟢	🟢
	Nischler et al. (2010)	🟢	🟢	🟢
	de Waard et al. (1992)	🔴	🟢	🟢
Cortical	Filgueira et al. (2016)	🔴	🔴	🔴
	Congdon et al. (2012)	🔴	🔴	🔴
	Bal et al. (2011)	🟢	🟢	🟢
	Nischler et al. (2010)	🟢	🟢	🟢
	de Waard et al. (1992)	🔴	🟢	🟢
Posterior subcapsular	Filgueira et al. (2016)	🟢	🟢	🟢
	Congdon et al. (2012)	🔴	🔴	🔴
	Bal et al. (2011)	🟢	🟢	🟢
	Nischler et al. (2010)	🟢	🟢	🟢
	de Waard et al. (1992)	🔴	🟢	🟢

PubMed, Medline, and Google Scholar were the scientific databases we screened using the following keywords: *straylight, C-Quant, age, visual acuity, cataract, cataract morphology, cataract classification, LOCS III, nuclear cataract, cortical cataract and posterior subcapsular cataract (PSC)*. In case of overlapping data in the studies, the one with the larger population was included for the review. Five papers met the eligibility criteria: de Waard et al., Nischler et al., Bal et al., Congdon et al., and Filgueira et al. [6, 19–22]. Because of lack of the desired data in four cases, we contacted the corresponding authors. In one case, there was no response; therefore GSYS2.4 (a graph digitizing system developed by Nuclear Reaction Data Center, University of Hokkaido, Japan) was used to extract data from the published graphs. Table 1 shows which data were reported by the five included studies. It has to be noted that the various studies classified the types of cataract differently based on LOCS (Table 2).

Data from all five articles were used to develop the log(s)-age normative curves for the three types of cataract. The correlations between the two variables were calculated and compared with each other. We calculated the normally expected mean straylight value for each cataract type, all types of cataract combined and the control group by using the log(s)-age normative equation obtained by van den Berg et al. [23], which reads

$$\log (\text{straylight parameter}) = \log(s) \qquad (1)$$
$$= 0.9 + \log \left(1 + (\text{age}/65)^4\right).$$

TABLE 2: Range of intensity defined for each type of cataract in the studies.

Study	Cataract definition
Filgueira et al. (2016)	Early age-related cataracts: nuclear (NO = 1 and 2), posterior subcapsular (P = 1 and 2)
Congdon et al. (2012)	Nuclear (NO ≥ 3)
Bal et al. (2011)	Nuclear (NO > 2, NC > 2, $C \leq 2$, $P \leq 1$), cortical (NO ≤ 2, NC ≤ 2, C > 2, $P \leq 1$), posterior subcapsular ($C \leq 2$, P > 1)
Nischler et al. (2010)	Nuclear (2 ≤ NO ≤ 4, 2 ≤ NC ≤ 4, C < 2, $P \leq 1.5$), cortical (NO < 2, NC < 2, 2 ≤ C ≤ 4, $P \leq 1.5$), posterior subcapsular (NO < 2, NC < 2, C < 2, $1.5 \leq P \leq 4$)
de Waard et al. (1992)	Advanced age-related cataracts (morphologically not categorized)

The results were compared with the measured straylight values. The residuals are displayed by using histograms. To study the possible differentiative impact of morphology on the progressive process of cataract, we used the largest control group—which belonged to Nischler et al.—with the best straylight and visual acuity values. We then compared the straylight and visual acuity of each cataract group in each study by connecting the mean values to those of the control group using arrows to show the magnitude and direction of progression. The slopes and lengths of the arrows were compared with each other. The correlations between log(s) and logMAR visual acuity values were calculated and compared with each other. We also calculated the ratio of straylight to age and visual acuity for each type of cataract; the results are illustrated using box-and-whisker plots. The log(s)-logMAR normative curves for each type of cataract are also derived using data from all five articles.

Linear regression analysis was performed with Excel software (2010, Microsoft Corporation) and SPSS Statistics 21 (IBM Corporation) on the straylight values—log(s)—to describe it as a function of age and logMAR visual acuity. Unpaired t-tests were used to calculate the significance of differences in means (±95% CI) between each study and the normative curve of each cataract type. The significance level was set at P value less than 0.05.

3. Results

3.1. Comprehensive Review. As explained in Materials and Methods, five reports fulfilled the eligibility criteria. Table 3 shows a summary of outcomes of each study. Table 4 shows the outcomes for each type of cataract, all types of cataract combined, and the control group. Figure 1 illustrates age, visual acuity, and straylight distributions in each cataract group.

The evaluations concerning log(s)-logMAR-related analyses were based on 776 total observations, with mean visual acuity of 0.02 ± 0.18 log units (range −0.30 to 0.70 log units) and mean straylight of 1.23 ± 0.22 log units (range 0.61 to 2.09 log units). The total number of cataract eyes was 725 for evaluations concerning log(s)-age-related analyses with a mean age of 63 ± 9 years (range 44 to 85 years of age). Figures 2 and 3 show the log(s)-age and log(s)-logMAR linear regressions for studies comprising the required data.

3.2. Effect of Cataract Morphology on Straylight. Straylight varied as a function of cataract morphology (Table 3); it was significantly higher in the three cataract groups (1.22 ± 0.20 log units in nuclear cataract, 1.26 ± 0.23 log units in cortical cataract, and 1.48 ± 0.34 log units in PSC) compared to the control group (1.12 ± 0.16 log units, $P < 0.05$). In addition, in all cataracts combined, straylight was significantly increased (1.26 ± 0.12 log units) relative to the control group ($P < 0.05$).

3.3. Correlation with Age. Straylight showed the highest correlation with age in Congdon et al.'s nuclear group ($R^2 = 0.36$, $P < 0.05$), and it showed no to a very weak correlation in several other groups (Table 3). Figure 1 shows phakic normative curves for each type of cataract; the data were derived from 574 eyes of nuclear, 93 of cortical, and 58 eyes of PSC. Overall, cortical cataract showed the highest correlation between log(s) and age ($R^2 = 0.22$, $P < 0.05$), and the overall PSC showed the lowest correlation between the two variables ($R^2 = 0.11$, $P < 0.05$) (Table 4). Figure 2 shows reference curves for cataracts and control group. The overall relationships read as

$$\text{straylight value} = 0.009 \times \text{age} + 0.60$$
$$(\text{nuclear group}; R^2 = 0.20, P < 0.05), \quad (2)$$

$$\text{straylight value} = 0.012 \times \text{age} + 0.50$$
$$(\text{cortical group}; R^2 = 0.22, P < 0.05),$$

$$\text{straylight value} = 0.014 \times \text{age} + 0.53$$
$$(\text{PSC group}; R^2 = 0.11, P < 0.05),$$

whereas that of the control group reads

$$\text{straylight value} = 0.007 \times \text{age} + 0.68$$
$$(\text{control group}; R^2 = 0.17, P < 0.05). \quad (3)$$

Mean straylight values are displayed in Tables 2 and 3. The figures show differences in different studies.

The mean age of each group is depicted in Figure 3. Using the log(s)-age norm curve equation obtained by van den Berg et al. [23], we calculated the expected mean straylight for each cataract type of each study, overall cataract types, all cataract types combined, and control groups. The results were compared with the measured straylight values. The residuals are

TABLE 3: Overview of the analysis on the data derived from raw data or published plots of each individual study (NC: nuclear cataract; CC: cortical cataract; and PSC: posterior subcapsular cataract).

Cataract	First author (year)	Eyes (n)	Age (Y)	Mean ± SD VA (logMAR)	SL (log(s))	log(s)-age Dependency	R^2	log(s)-logMAR Dependency	R^2
NC	Filgueira (2016)	14	69 ± 18	0.10 ± 0.08	1.33 ± 0.21	log(s) = 0.008 × age + 0.75	0.02	log(s) = 0.14 × logMAR − 0.08	0.14
	Congdon (2012)	24	65 ± 10	0.22 ± 0.14	1.36 ± 0.33	log(s) = 0.019 × age + 0.12	0.36	log(s) = 0.82 × logMAR + 1.17	0.13
	Bal (2011)	23	67 ± 9	0.28 ± 0.18	1.50 ± 0.24	log(s) = 0.001 × age + 1.54	0.00	log(s) = 0.51 × logMAR + 1.36	0.14
	Nischler (2010)	512	63 ± 9	−0.05 ± 0.12	1.19 ± 0.17	log(s) = 0.008 × age + 0.65	0.21	log(s) = 0.44 × logMAR + 1.21	0.10
	de Waard (1992)	18	NA	0.39 ± 0.14	1.54 ± 0.16	NA	NA	log(s) = 0.01 × logMAR + 1.42	0.08
CC	Filgueira (2016)	NA	NA	NA	NA	NA	NA	NA	NA
	Congdon (2012)	NA	NA	NA	NA	NA	NA	NA	NA
	Bal (2011)	15	67 ± 7	0.25 ± 0.20	1.48 ± 0.29	log(s) = 0.020 × age + 0.13	0.26	log(s) = − 0.28 × logMAR + 1.55	0.04
	Nischler (2010)	78	62 ± 8	−0.06 ± 0.09	1.20 ± 0.17	log(s) = 0.008 × age + 0.69	0.17	log(s) = 0.13 × logMAR + 1.21	0.00
	de Waard (1992)	16	NA	0.24 ± 0.13	1.34 ± 0.29	NA	NA	log(s) = 1.22 × logMAR + 1.04	0.29
PSC	Filgueira (2016)	20	56 ± 5	0.03 ± 0.05	1.17 ± 0.27	log(s) = 0.013 × age + 0.42	0.06	log(s) = 0.04 × logMAR − 0.02	0.11
	Congdon (2012)	NA	NA	NA	NA	NA	NA	NA	NA
	Bal (2011)	20	64 ± 9	0.30 ± 0.22	1.79 ± 0.20	log(s) = 0.001 × age + 1.77	0.00	log(s) = 0.13 × logMAR + 1.76	0.02
	Nischler (2010)	18	61 ± 8	0.02 ± 0.11	1.30 ± 0.27	log(s) = 0.000 × age + 1.19	0.00	log(s) = 1.02 × logMAR + 1.28	0.17
	de Waard (1992)	17	NA	0.26 ± 0.18	1.67 ± 0.21	NA	NA	log(s) = 0.33 × logMAR + 1.58	0.08

TABLE 4: Overview of the analysis on collected data from individual studies for each cataract group.

Group	Number of eyes		Age (year)	Mean ± SD VA (logMAR)	SL (log(s))	log(s)-age Dependency	R^2	log(s)-logMAR Dependency	R^2
	SL-age	SL-VA							
Nuclear	573	592	63 ± 9	−0.01 ± 0.16	1.22 ± 0.20	$\log(s) = 0.009 \times age + 0.60$	0.20	$\log(s) = 0.62 \times logMAR + 1.22$	0.25
Cortical	93	109	62 ± 8	0.03 ± 0.18	1.26 ± 0.23	$\log(s) = 0.012 \times age + 0.50$	0.22	$\log(s) = 0.33 \times logMAR + 1.24$	0.13
Posterior	58	75	60 ± 8	0.15 ± 0.20	1.48 ± 0.34	$\log(s) = 0.015 \times age + 0.53$	0.11	$\log(s) = 1.03 \times logMAR + 1.32$	0.34
All cataracts	724	776	63 ± 9	0.02 ± 0.18	1.23 ± 0.22	$\log(s) = 0.009 \times age + 0.64$	0.14	$\log(s) = 0.68 \times logMAR + 1.24$	0.26
Control	1761	1761	57 ± 8	−0.07 ± 0.11	1.12 ± 0.16	$\log(s) = 0.008 \times age + 0.68$	0.17	$\log(s) = 0.25 \times logMAR + 1.14$	0.03

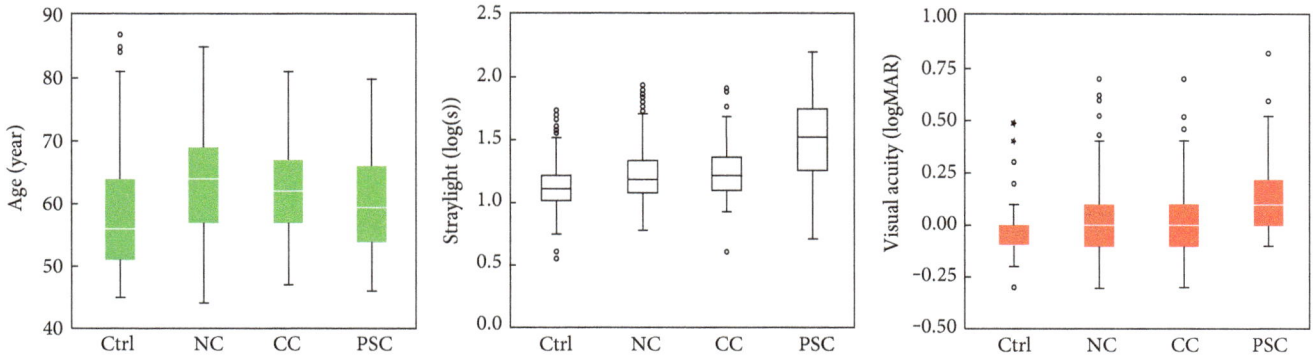

FIGURE 1: Age, intraocular straylight, and best-corrected visual acuity plotted for cataract and control groups. Straylight and visual acuity differed significantly from PSC to the other cataracts and control group. (NC: nuclear cataract; CC: cortical cataract; and PSC: posterior subcapsular cataract).

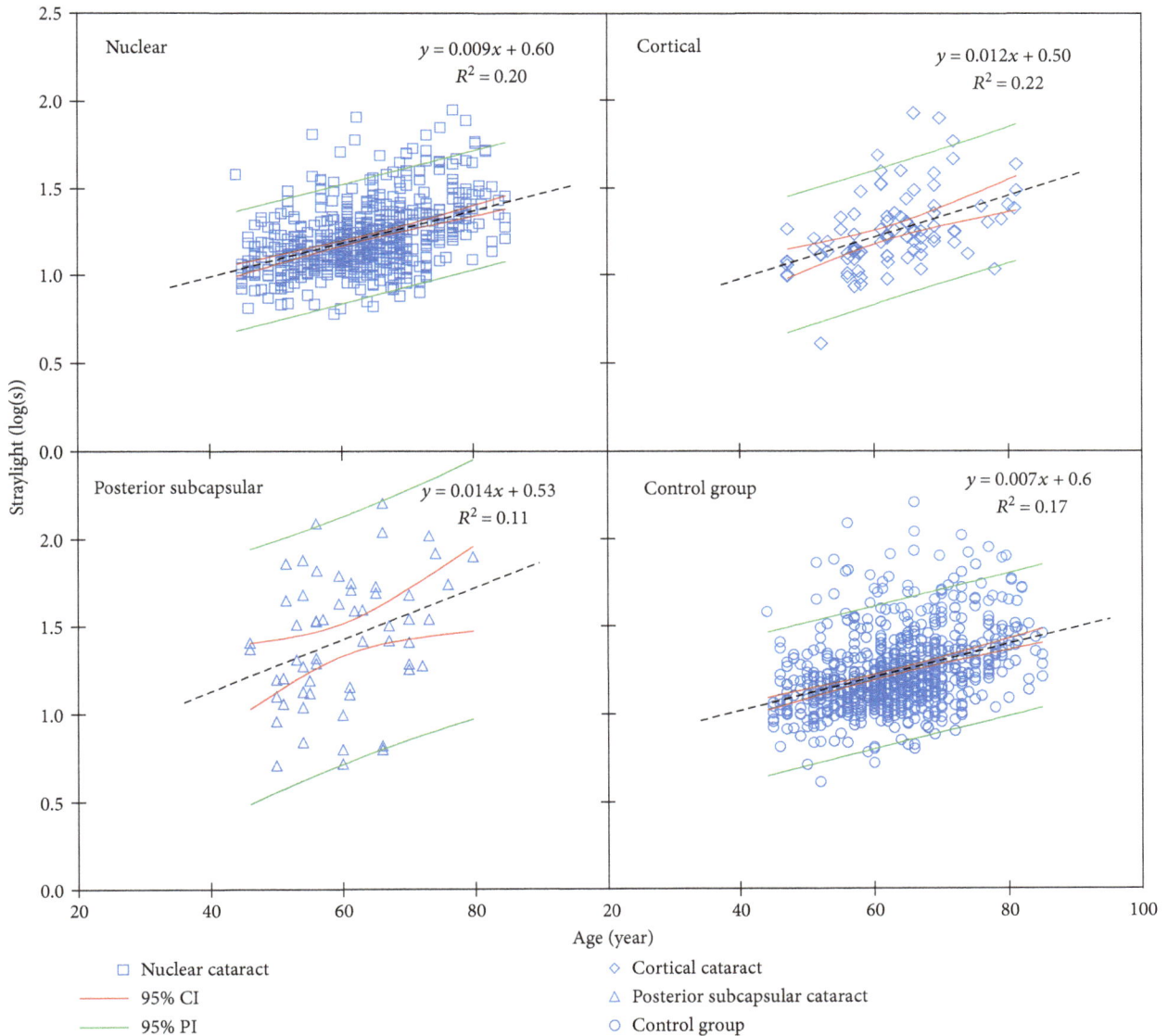

FIGURE 2: Linear models of log(s)-age dependency for nuclear cataract derived from four studies, cortical cataract derived from two studies, posterior subcapsular cataract derived from three studies and control group are plotted. Black dotted lines are the regression lines.

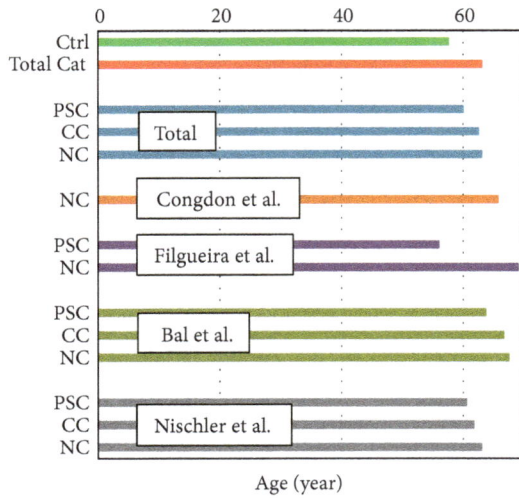

FIGURE 3: Mean age of each type of cataract in each published study. In average, patients with PSC cataract are the youngest. (Ctrl: control group; NC: nuclear cataract; Total cat: all cataract groups combined; CC: cortical cataract; and PSC: posterior subcapsular cataract).

displayed in Figure 4. We must remind the reader that not every study provided information on age (Table 1). Among three cataract groups, the mean straylight of PSC group showed the highest difference from the expected mean straylight of an age-matched phakic group; by contrast, nuclear group showed the smallest difference. The same figure shows negligible difference between measured and expected straylight in control group.

3.4. Correlation with Visual Acuity.

Straylight showed the highest correlation with logMAR visual acuity in de Waard et al.'s cortical group ($R^2 = 0.29$, $P < 0.05$) and the lowest correlation in Nischler et al.'s cortical group ($R^2 = 0.00$, $P = 0.99$). Overall, PSC showed the highest correlation between straylight and logMAR visual acuity ($R^2 = 0.34$, $P < 0.05$) and cortical cataract showed the lowest correlation, however significant, between the two variables ($R^2 = 0.13$, $P < 0.05$). The relations and correlation coefficients between log(s) and logMAR visual acuity are reported in Tables 3 and 4.

Figure 5 shows log(s)-logMAR reference curves for cataracts and control group. The overall relationships read as

$$\text{straylight value} = 0.62 \times \text{visual acuity} + 1.22$$
$$\left(\text{nuclear group}; R^2 = 0.25, P < 0.05\right),$$

$$\text{straylight value} = 0.33 \times \text{visual acuity} + 1.24$$
$$\left(\text{cortical group}; R^2 = 0.13, P < 0.05\right), \quad (4)$$

$$\text{straylight value} = 1.03 \times \text{visual acuity} + 1.34$$
$$\left(\text{PSC group}; R^2 = 0.34, P < 0.05\right),$$

whereas the norm of the control group reads as

$$\text{straylight value} = 0.25 \times \text{visual acuity} + 1.14$$
$$\left(\text{control group}; R^2 = 0.03, P < 0.05\right). \quad (5)$$

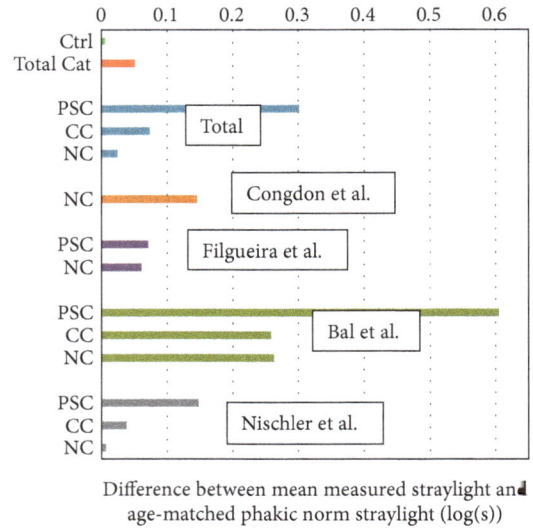

Difference between mean measured straylight and age-matched phakic norm straylight (log(s))

FIGURE 4: Differences between the mean straylight value in patients with different types of cataract for the various studies and the age-matched straylight value derived from the phakic norm curve by van den Berg et al. [23] are plotted. In all data, straylight in patients with PSC cataract showed the highest deviation from that of a noncataract (phakic) group. (Ctrl: control group; Total cat: all cataract groups combined; NC: nuclear cataract; CC: cortical cataract; and PSC: posterior subcapsular cataract).

From the above relationships, one can see that straylight varies as a function of morphology. Patients with PSC for a similar logMAR visual acuity have a higher straylight than the other cataracts and control group.

3.5. Cataract: Progression from Healthy Eyes.

We estimated the amount of progression of mean straylight and mean visual acuity from those of the control group in each individual study and cataract groups. The progression lines are demonstrated in Figure 6. Data showed that PSC in Bal et al. had the highest progression from noncataract status in terms of both straylight (ΔSL = 0.68 log units) and visual acuity (ΔVA = 0.37 log units). However, with respect to the progression of individual variables, the mean visual acuity increased the most in de Waard et al.'s nuclear group (ΔVA = 0.46 log units), whereas its mean straylight value increased (ΔSL = 0.42 log units) less than that of Bal et al.'s PSC group. The mean visual acuity deteriorated the least in Nischler et al.'s nuclear and cortical groups.

3.6. Ratio between Straylight and Age and Visual Acuity.

The ratios between straylight and age and between straylight and visual acuity are illustrated using box-and-whisker plots (Figure 7). The median of straylight parameter (s)/age (year) had the lowest value in nuclear cataract group and the highest value in PSC group, albeit with a rather more skewed distribution comparing the two other cataract groups. The differences in medians of the PSC group and the other two cataract groups were statistically significant. The median of log(s)-logMAR showed similarly lower values in nuclear and cortical groups in comparison to that of PSC group.

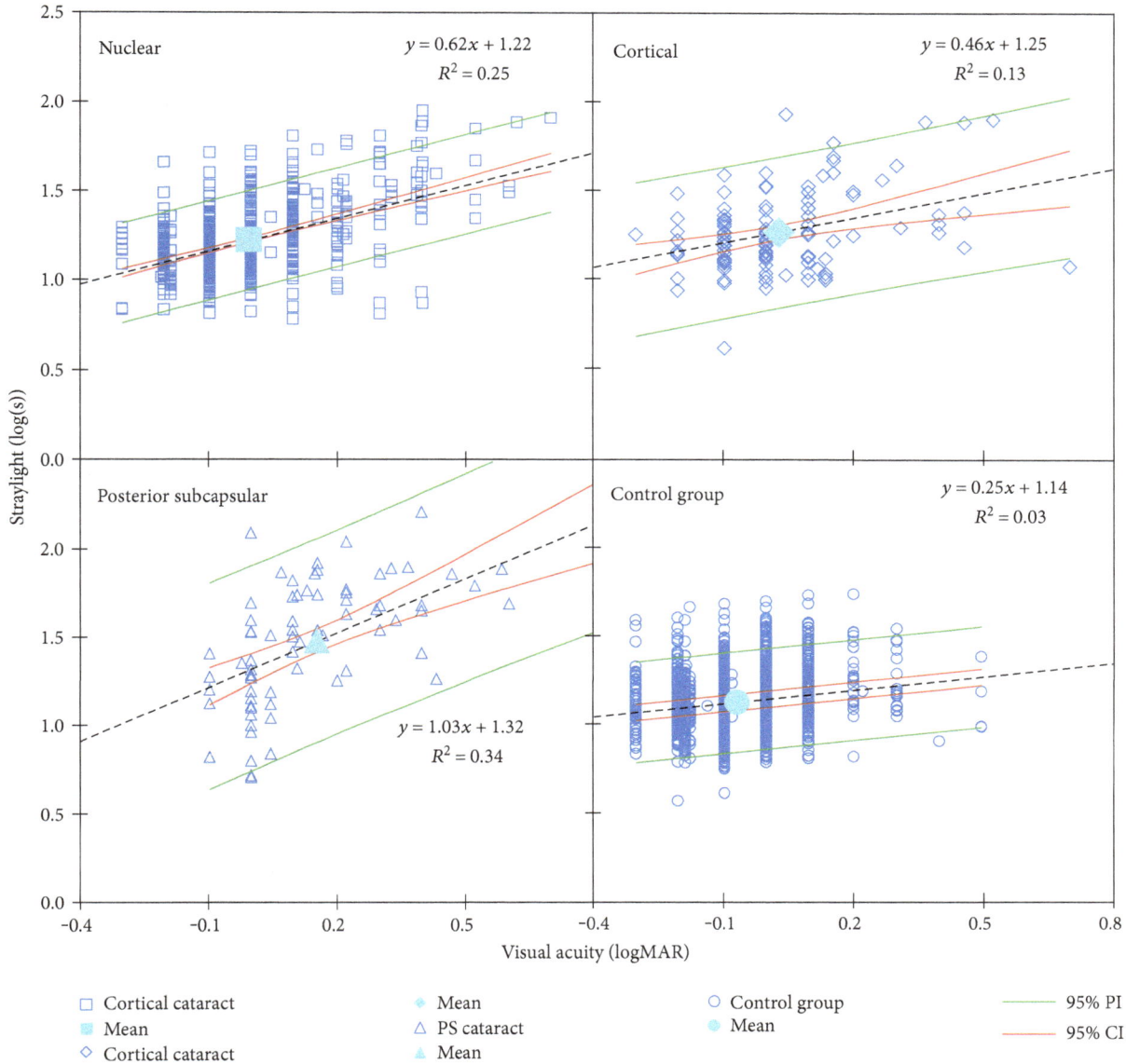

FIGURE 5: Linear models of log(s)-logMAR visual acuity dependency for nuclear cataract derived from five studies, cortical cataract derived from three studies, PSC cataract derived from four studies and control group are plotted. Black dotted lines are the regression lines.

4. Discussion

The application of the findings of this literature review is limited by the restricted range of the severity of cataracts and the difference in age between the studies. However, it is a good place to start studying the distinctive relationship between cataract morphology and visual functions. There is a strong correlation between cataract morphology, the intensity of lens opacification, and impairment of visual functions (i.e., straylight and visual acuity).

From the results, we found that PSC population was generally younger, which is in agreement with the literature [24–27] reporting that the average age of the population developing or undergoing surgery for PSC is younger than that for other types of cataract.

In the present study, the log(s)-age dependencies were obtained for cataracts of different morphologies. Among five published articles used in this literature review, four could be used for the nuclear, three for the PSC, and two for the cortical log(s)-age dependency equations (Table 1). These equations cannot be considered normative reference curves, because the different studies made a severity selection of the cataract populations. This must have influenced (weakened) the dependencies. The slopes of the dependency equations varied from one cataract group to another, but the differences were not statistically significant. The slope of the dependency function of the nuclear cataract was close to that of the control group. The reason is that Nischler et al.'s nuclear group with patients with rather good vision was remarkably larger than the rest. The differences between cataracts and control

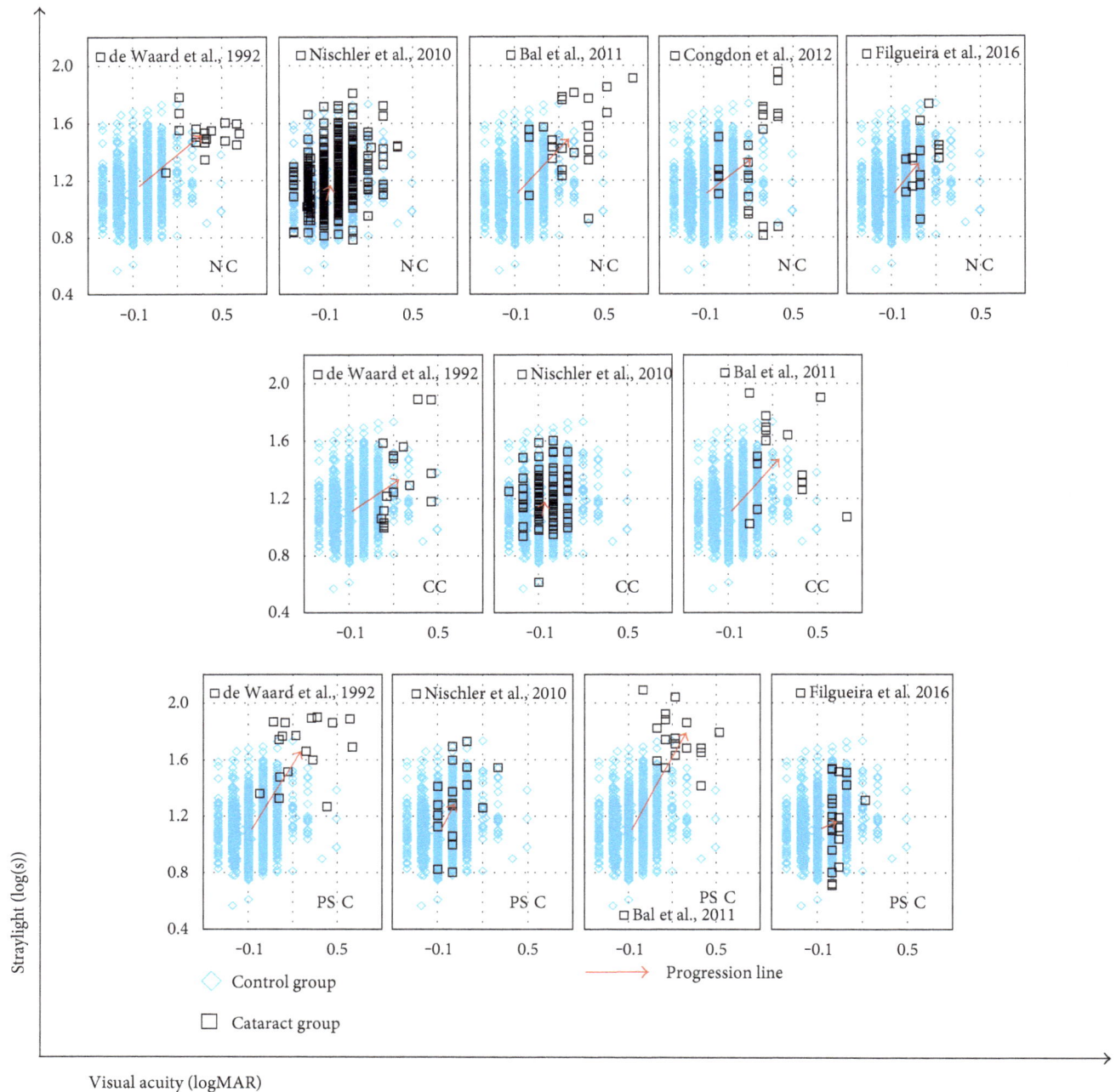

FIGURE 6: Progression of cataracts from control group is illustrated by arrows originating from mean straylight and mean visual acuity of the control group towards those of each type of cataract in each individual study. (NC: nuclear cataract; CC: cortical cataract; and PSC: posterior subcapsular cataract).

groups, as mentioned earlier, were small, with large overlap between the cataract and control populations. This points at limited validity of the LOCS cataract grading. Although LOCS serves to improve the grading and classifying slit-lamp observation, it is not precise for assessing function. As mentioned in the introduction, there is a weak relation between backscatter and forward scatter; therefore, a slit-lamp-based measurement cannot be a reliable means to quantify forward scatter. The correlation between log(s) and age also varied between cataract groups and control

group; it was the highest in cortical cataract and the lowest in PSC.

In each cataract group, the difference in the mean straylight values of individual studies and the respective dependency function was significant. This can be explained by different levels of cataract severity and significant difference in the number of eyes of the largest study and the rest. Such difference was not observed between the slopes of each study and the respective dependency functions. It appeared that the mean straylight values of the reference curves were

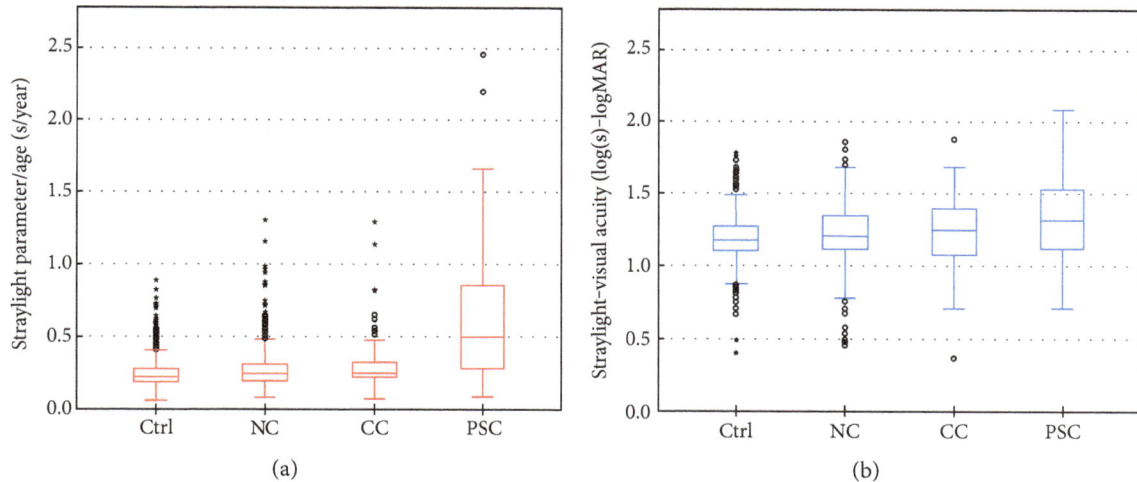

FIGURE 7: (a) Ratio between straylight parameter and age for each type of cataract: the median of such ratio is significantly higher in the PSC group. (b) The same is valid for straylight-visual acuity. Both cases suggest that straylight is highest in the patients with PSC group albeit lower and/or similar age and visual acuity than/as the other cataracts. (Ctrl: control group; NC: nuclear cataract; CC: cortical cataract; and PSC: posterior subcapsular cataract).

moderately closer to those of Nischler et al.'s nuclear and cortical groups. Nischler et al. covered the major part of the overall data in these two groups; therefore, it is no surprise that it leads the outcomes. The reason Nischler et al. had the lowest mean values in straylight and visual acuity may be due to the fact that the patients were active drivers; therefore, they had comparatively better vision than their age-equivalent peers in other studies. The lowest straylight belonged to Filgueira et al.'s PSC. This is a deviant behavior as PSC in every other study had the highest straylight value. This group's visual acuity was almost as low as that of Nischler et al. Recruiting patients with eyes at the early stage of cataract in these two studies can explain these results (Table 2). When we left out data from Nischler et al. and Filgueira et al., the difference in means of cataract groups became very small, whereas the mean straylight of PSC was approximately 0.3 log units higher than that of other cataracts. This is in agreement with the finding by Elliott et al. [28, 29] that in the advanced stages of cataracts, for patients with PSC, visual acuity alone is not an adequate assessment of visual performance and cataract management. The straylight curve established for normal phakic eyes [23] shows that straylight increases strongly with age with a logarithmic relation (to the power of 4). The change in straylight shows stable behavior in young eyes and considerably increases over 50 years of age. However, our findings showed rather linear relationship between log(s) and age. This may be related to the selection based on severity. We also found that the control group in Figure 4 shows the phakic reference norm works very well.

The correlation between log(s) and logMAR visual acuity varied from none to a moderate one in individual studies and within cataract types, but it never was strong. Overall, no type of cataract showed strong log(s)-logMAR correlation. In clinical practice, this means straylight cannot be predicted on the basis of visual acuity for any type of cataract. Figure 6 shows that, overall, in PSC group straylight deteriorated faster than

visual acuity. Some studies [30, 31] found that with increasing the severity of posterior capsule opacification (PCO), visual acuity and straylight deteriorate, albeit with different rates; the PCO severity-log(s) relation is linear, whereas the PCO severity-logMAR is curvilinear [31]. Therefore, straylight is more sensitive to the changes in PCO severity than visual acuity. Kruijt and van den Berg [32] also discussed this difference for localized processes.

Regardless of severity of cataracts, the present study supports the notion that the straylight is the highest in PSC. Fluctuations in density and discontinuous refractive index can be responsible for such amplification [33, 34]. The difference between log(s)-logMAR dependency slopes of cataracts of different morphologies and their correlation coefficients is notable. The distinction between PSC and noncataract eyes is especially remarkable. The log(s)-logMAR progression of cataracts from a control group in our study also showed that PSC deteriorated the most in terms of visual functions. Therefore, it can be inferred that patients with this type of cataract would benefit the most from surgery. However, to draw definite conclusion, further studies on the improvement of visual functions after cataract surgery considering cataract morphologies are necessary. The results presented in Figure 4 show that the age-corrected mean straylight values of Bal et al. in every cataract groups are higher than those of other studies. Unlike patients recruited in the other studies, these patients were listed for cataract surgery. When Bal et al.'s patients were excluded from analysis, PSC had the worst visual acuity; the change in visual acuity in all cataract groups was in average 0.03 log units. The changes in straylight of nuclear and cortical groups were negligible, but it decreased about 0.11 log units in PSC. Therefore, the difference in mean straylight of PSC remained remarkably higher than the other cataracts and the correlation with age decreased ($R^2 = 0.04$, $P = 0.22$). The slopes of the new reference curves remained almost unchanged. We observed no change in the new log(s)-log-MAR correlation in any cataract group, whereas the slopes changed, albeit insignificantly, with the average change of 0.06. Although the effect of excluding Bal et al.'s data on our analysis was unimportant, one needs to recognize the relatively small size of this study as an effective factor in this context.

It should be noted that correlations that were significant in one or some studies, and were not in the other(s), were in fact significant in the whole cataract group. However, this cannot be said about the whole data (different types of cataracts combined), because of different morphologies and eventually different optical dynamics.

5. Conclusion

We confirm that straylight in cataract eyes varies rather independently from age and best-corrected visual acuity. The independence of these two aspects of crystalline lens was speculated to be caused by different optical processes of remarkably different scales [3]. We found that, in accordance to the literature, to assess visual functions of cataracts, the analysis should consider cataract morphology. This becomes more crucial in PSC, where the general visual acuity might not show severe loss, but a remarkable increase of straylight above the cutoff value of 1.40 log units [35] can have negative effect on the quality of life. The norm curves obtained in this literature review serve to distinguish the particular effect of each type of cataract, from early-stage to mild, on visual impairment. However to generalize our results, scrutinize their validity in more severe cataracts, and to develop postoperative straylight improvement references, further studies are needed.

Conflicts of Interest

The Netherlands Academy of Arts and Sciences owns a patent on straylight measurement, with Dr. Thomas J. T. P. van den Berg as the inventor and licenses that to Oculus Optikgeräte GmbH for the C-Quant instrument. None of the other authors has a financial or proprietary interest in any material or method mentioned.

Acknowledgments

This research has been possible thanks to the *AGEYE Marie Curie Initial Training Network*, funded by the European Commission (FP7-PEOPLE-ITN-2013-608049). The authors thank Professor Robert Montés-Micó and Dr. Alejandro Cerviño from the University of Valencia for their cooperation and support.

References

[1] J. J. Vos, "Disability glare—a state of the art report," *CIE Journal*, vol. 3, no. 2, pp. 39–53, 1984.

[2] T. J. T. P. van den Berg, "Analysis of intraocular straylight, especially in relation to age," *Optometry and Vision Science*, vol. 72, no. 2, pp. 52–59, 1995.

[3] T. J. T. P. van den Berg, L. J. van Rijn, R. Michael et al., "Straylight effects with aging and lens extraction," *American Journal of Ophthalmology*, vol. 144, no. 3, pp. 358–363, 2007.

[4] D. Yager, T. Hage, R. Yuan, S. Mathews, and M. Katz, "The relations between contrast threshold, lens back scatter, and disability glare. Noninvasive assessment of the visual system," *OSA Technical Digest Series*, vol. 3, pp. 168–171, 1990.

[5] D. B. Elliott, S. Mitchell, and D. Whitaker, "Factors affecting light scatter in contact lens wearers," *Optometry and Vision Science*, vol. 68, no. 8, pp. 629–633, 1991.

[6] P. W. T. de Waard, J. K. Uspeerf, T. J. T. P. van den Berg, and P. T. V. A. de Jong, "Intraocular light scattering in age-related cataracts," *Investigative Ophthalmology & Visual Science*, vol. 33, no. 3, pp. 618–625, 1992.

[7] D. B. Elliott, D. Fonn, J. Flanagan, and M. Doughty, "Relative sensitivity of clinical tests to hydrophilic lens-induced corneal thickness changes," *Optometry and Vision Science*, vol. 70, no. 12, pp. 1044–1048, 1993.

[8] R. Michael, L. J. van Rijn, T. J. T. P. van den Berg et al., "Association of lens opacities, intraocular straylight, contrast sensitivity and visual acuity in European drivers," *Acta Ophthalmologica*, vol. 87, no. 6, pp. 666–671, 2009.

[9] J. E. Coppens, L. Franssen, L. J. van Rijn, and T. J. T. P. van den Berg, "Reliability of the compensation comparison stray-light measurement method," *Journal of Biomedical Optics*, vol. 11, no. 3, pp. 1–9, 2006.

[10] A. Cervino, R. Montes-Mico, and S. L. Hosking, "Performance of the compensation comparison method for retinal straylight measurement: effect of patient's age on repeatability," *The British Journal of Ophthalmology*, vol. 92, no. 6, pp. 788–791, 2008.

[11] I. Guber, L. M. Bachmann, J. Guber, F. Bochmann, A. P. Lange, and M. A. Thiel, "Reproducibility of straylight measurement by C-Quant for assessment of retinal straylight using the compensation comparison method," *Graefe's Archive for Clinical and Experimental Ophthalmology*, vol. 249, no. 9, pp. 1367–1371, 2011.

[12] D. B. Elliott and M. A. Hurst, "Simple clinical techniques to evaluate visual function in patients with early cataract," *Optometry and Vision Science*, vol. 67, no. 11, pp. 822–825, 1990.

[13] D. B. Elliott, "Evaluating visual function in cataract," *Optometry and Vision Science*, vol. 70, no. 11, pp. 896–902, 1993.

[14] R. W. Massof and G. S. Rubin, "Visual function assessment questionnaires," *Survey of Ophthalmology*, vol. 45, no. 6, pp. 531–548, 2001.

[15] G. S. Rubin, K. Bandeen-Roche, G. H. Huang et al., "The association of multiple visual impairments with self-reported visual disability: SEE project," *Investigative Ophthalmology & Visual Science*, vol. 42, no. 1, pp. 64–72, 2001.

[16] I. J. E. van der Meulen, J. Gjertsen, B. Kruijt et al., "Straylight measurements as an indication for cataract surgery," *Journal of Cataract and Refractive Surgery*, vol. 38, no. 5, pp. 840–848, 2012.

[17] D. B. Elliott, M. A. Bullimore, and I. L. Bailey, "Improving the reliability of the Pelli-Robson contrast sensitivity test," *Clinical Vision Science*, vol. 6, no. 6, pp. 471–475, 1991.

[18] G. Łabuz, N. J. Reus, and T. J. T. P. van den Berg, "Ocular straylight in the normal pseudophakic eye," *Journal of Cataract and Refractive Surgery*, vol. 41, no. 7, pp. 1406–1415, 2015.

[19] C. Nischler, R. Michael, C. Wintersteller et al., "Cataract and pseudophakia in elderly European drivers," *European Journal of Ophthalmology*, vol. 20, no. 5, pp. 892–901, 2010.

[20] T. Bal, T. Coeckelbergh, J. van Looveren, J. J. Rozema, and M. J. Tassignon, "Influence of cataract morphology on straylight and contrast sensitivity and its relevance to fitness to drive," *Ophthalmologica*, vol. 225, no. 2, pp. 105–111, 2011.

[21] N. Congdon, X. Yan, D. S. Friedman et al., "Visual symptoms and retinal straylight after laser peripheral iridotomy," *Ophthalmology*, vol. 119, no. 7, pp. 1375–1382, 2012.

[22] C. P. Filgueira, R. F. Sánchez, L. A. Issolio, and E. M. Colombo, "Straylight and visual quality on early nuclear and posterior subcapsular cataracts," *Current Eye Research*, vol. 41, no. 9, pp. 1209–1215, 2016.

[23] T. J. T. P. van den Berg, L. Franssen, B. Kruijt, and J. E. Coppens, "History of ocular straylight measurement: a review," *Zeitschrift für Medizinische Physik*, vol. 23, no. 1, pp. 6–20, 2013.

[24] N. A. P. Brown and A. R. Hill, "Cataract: the relation between myopia and cataract morphology," *The British Journal of Ophthalmology*, vol. 71, no. 6, pp. 405–414, 1987.

[25] I. Adamsons, B. Munoz, C. Enger, and H. R. Taylor, "Prevalence of lens opacities in surgical and general populations," *Archives of Ophthalmology*, vol. 109, no. 7, pp. 993–997, 1991.

[26] B. E. K. Klein, R. Klein, and S. E. Moss, "Incident cataract surgery: the beaver dam eye study," *Ophthalmology*, vol. 104, no. 4, pp. 573–580, 1997.

[27] J. Panchapakesan, P. Mitchell, K. Tumuluri, E. Rochtchina, S. Foran, and R. G. Cumming, "Five year incidence of cataract surgery: the Blue Mountains eye study," *The British Journal of Ophthalmology*, vol. 87, no. 2, pp. 168–172, 2003.

[28] D. B. Elliott, J. Gilchrist, and D. Whitaker, "Contrast sensitivity and glare sensitivity changes with three types of cataract morphology: are these techniques necessary in a clinical evaluation of cataract?" *Ophthalmic & Physiological Optics*, vol. 9, no. 1, pp. 25–30, 1989.

[29] T. J. T. P. van den Berg, L. Franssen, and J. E. Coppens, "Ocular media clarity and straylight," *Encyclopedia of the Eye*, vol. 3, pp. 173–183, 2010.

[30] W. R. Meacock, D. J. Spalton, J. Boyce, and J. Marshall, "The effect of posterior capsule opacification on visual function," *Investigative Ophthalmology & Visual Science*, vol. 44, no. 11, pp. 4665–4669, 2003.

[31] M. C. van Bree, T. J. van den Berg, and B. L. Zijlmans, "Posterior capsule opacification severity, assessed with straylight measurement, as main indicator of early visual function deterioration," *Ophthalmology*, vol. 120, no. 1, pp. 20–33, 2013.

[32] B. Kruijt and T. J. T. P. van den Berg, "Optical scattering measurements of laser induced damage in the intraocular lens," *PloS One*, vol. 7, no. 2, article e31764, 2012.

[33] D. Tang, D. Borchman, A. K. Schwarz et al., "Light scattering of human lens vesicles in vitro," *Experimental Eye Research*, vol. 76, no. 5, pp. 605–612, 2003.

[34] H. Pau, "Cortical and subcapsular cataracts: significance of physical forces," *Ophthalmologica*, vol. 220, no. 1, pp. 1–5, 2006.

[35] L. J. van Rijn, C. Nischler, R. Michael et al., "Prevalence of impairment of visual function in European drivers," *Acta Ophthalmologica*, vol. 89, no. 2, pp. 124–131, 2011.

6

Customized Toric Intraocular Lens Implantation in Eyes with Cataract and Corneal Astigmatism after Deep Anterior Lamellar Keratoplasty

Domenico Schiano Lomoriello [ID],[1] **Giacomo Savini** [ID],[1] **Kristian Naeser,**[2]
Rossella Maria Colabelli-Gisoldi,[3] **Valeria Bono,**[1] **and Augusto Pocobelli** [ID][3]

[1]*IRCCS Fondazione G.B. Bietti, Rome, Italy*
[2]*Regions Hospital Randers, Randers, Denmark*
[3]*Azienda Ospedaliera San Giovanni-Addolorata, Rome, Italy*

Correspondence should be addressed to Domenico Schiano Lomoriello; do.schiano@gmail.com

Academic Editor: David P. Piñero

Purpose. To investigate the effectiveness of toric intraocular lenses (IOLs) for treating corneal astigmatism in patients with cataract and previous deep anterior lamellar keratoplasty (DALK). *Setting*. San Giovanni-Addolorata Hospital, Rome, Italy. *Design*. Prospective interventional case series. *Methods*. Patients undergoing cataract surgery after DALK for keratoconus were enrolled. Total corneal astigmatism (TCA) was assessed by a rotating Scheimpflug camera combined with Placido-disk corneal topography (Sirius; CSO, Firenze, Italy). A customized toric IOL (FIL 611 T, Soleko, Rome, Italy) was implanted in all eyes. One year postoperatively, refraction was measured, the IOL position was recorded, and vectorial and nonvectorial analyses were performed to evaluate the correction of astigmatism. *Results*. Ten eyes of 10 patients were analyzed. The mean preoperative TCA magnitude was 4.92 ± 1.99 diopters (D), and the mean cylinder of the IOL was 6.18 ± 2.44. After surgery, the difference between the planned axis of orientation of the IOL and the observed axis was $\leq 10°$ in all eyes. The mean surgically induced corneal astigmatism was 0.35 D at 20°. The mean postoperative refractive astigmatism power was 1.13 ± 0.94 D; with respect to preoperative TCA, the reduction was statistically significant ($p < 0.0001$). The mean change in astigmatism power was 3.80 ± 1.60 D, corresponding to a correction of 77% of preoperative TCA power. Nine eyes out of 10 had a postoperative refractive astigmatism power $\leq 2D$. *Conclusions*. Toric IOLs can effectively correct corneal astigmatism in eyes with previous DALK. The predictability of cylinder correction is partially lowered by the variability of the surgically induced changes of TCA. This trial is registered with NCT03398109.

1. Introduction

Tissue transparency is the main factor affecting a successful outcome of corneal grafts, but a good postoperative refraction is also essential to achieve patients' satisfaction [1]. High astigmatism is the most common cause of unsatisfactory vision after keratoplasty when the transplanted cornea is transparent [1, 2]. Spectacles and contact lenses can be adopted for regular low-grade astigmatism but lead to poor vision or are not tolerated in cases with high astigmatism secondary to corneal transplantation [3]. Among surgical procedures, arcuate keratotomy reduces postkeratoplasty astigmatism, but the results of this technique are often unpredictable [3, 4]. Both photorefractive keratectomy (PRK) and laser in situ keratomileusis (LASIK) are effective, but not suitable for all patients who underwent corneal transplant, due to the risk of complications and the unreliable refractive outcomes [3, 5, 6]. Intrastromal corneal ring segments implantation could be also a viable option for effective correction of post-DALK astigmatism [7]. However, patients previously operated by penetrating keratoplasty (PK) presenting cataract can benefit of a phacoemulsification with toric intraocular lens (IOL) implants with a reduction of the postkeratoplasty astigmatism [8–15]. In the last decade, several studies showed that deep anterior lamellar keratoplasty (DALK) should be preferred to PK in patients with corneal pathology and healthy endothelium [16–21] because DALK leads to comparable visual outcomes and lower rates of intraoperative and postoperative complications. However, an extensive research on the major biomedical databases (PubMed, Scopus, ScienceDirect, Google Scholar) failed to identify studies investigating the implantation of toric IOLs after DALK, with the only exception of a case report in a patient with subluxated cataract after DALK [22]. The preoperative corneal cylinder in these eyes is often so high that standard manufactured toric IOL powers are insufficient. Therefore, the purpose of this study was to assess the efficacy of custom-made toric intraocular lens implantation in patients with simultaneous post-DALK high corneal astigmatism and cataract.

2. Methods

This study was designed as a prospective, noncomparative interventional case series. It has been approved by the institute review board and the regional ethical committee to adhere to the principles of the Declaration of Helsinki. All enrolled patients attended the corneal service of San Giovanni-Addolorata Hospital, where they had undergone DALK for keratoconus between January 2007 and December 2014. They reported a recent visual decrease in the transplanted eye due to cataract, significantly affecting the visual acuity. Corneal suture removal had been performed in all cases at least 1 year before cataract surgery. Corneal astigmatism was stable at least since 6 months before the cataract surgery in all patients.

2.1. Preoperative Examinations and Toric IOL Power Calculation. All patients underwent a comprehensive preoperative assessment that included uncorrected distance visual acuity (UDVA), distance-corrected visual acuity (DCVA), slit-lamp examination, optical biometry by means of partial coherence interferometry (Carl Zeiss IOLMaster V.5.4.1, Carl Zeiss Meditec, Jena, Germany), corneal tomography by means of a rotating Scheimpflug camera combined with a Placido-disc corneal topographer (Sirius; CSO, Firenze, Italy) and specular microscope (Perseus; CSO, Firenze, Italy). The magnitude and direction of the IOL cylinder were based on total corneal astigmatism (TCA) measurement, as calculated by the Sirius with ray-tracing over a 3 mm diameter. The instrument software uses all the traced rays to calculate the wavefront error, that is, the difference between the measured wavefront and an ideal spherical wavefront. The wavefront error, including astigmatism magnitude and axis, is then fitted using Zernike polynomials, as previously described [23]. TCA values were provided to the IOL manufacturer (Soleko S.p.A., Rome, Italy) that calculated the required IOL cylinder by means of proprietary software. The toric IOL was customized and manufactured in 0.25 D cylinder steps. The implanted toric IOL was a FIL 611 T (Soleko S.p.A., Rome, Italy), whose material is afoldable acrylate with 25% water content. The IOL has a plate-haptic design, a 6 mm optic diameter and 11.80 mm overall length.

The cylindrical correction is directly built on the posterior IOL surface ("real axis technology"), so that, once implanted in the capsular bag, the reference marks on the toric IOL have to be aligned to the 0–180° axis.

2.2. Surgical Procedure. Both DALK and cataract surgery were carried out by the same experienced surgeon (A.P.). DALK was performed with "big-bubble" technique with achievement of a big bubble in all cases [16, 17, 24, 25]. All patients received a routine phacoemulsification surgery under topical anesthesia. Limbal marks were made at 180 degree before the surgery with the patients in a sitting position focusing at distance. Phacoemulsification was performed with the Infiniti OZil (Alcon, Forth Worth, TX) through a 2.75 mm temporal clear cornea incision (CCI). All CCIs were performed as limbal as possible, avoiding the corneal graft-host junction. No sutures were applied at the end of the surgeries.

2.3. Postoperative Evaluations. At 12 months postoperatively, patients underwent UDVA and DCVA measurements, slit-lamp examination under mydriasis (in order to record the orientation of the IOL), corneal tomography, and specular microscopy. The difference between the preoperative and postoperative TCA was used to calculate the surgically induced corneal astigmatism (SICA).

2.4. Vector Analysis of Astigmatism. Vector analysis according to Naeser [26] was used to calculate the surgically induced corneal astigmatism (SICA), the difference in TCA between preoperative and postoperative measurements, and the error in refractive astigmatism (ERA), defined as the difference between the observed and the targeted postoperative refractive astigmatism. Briefly, the net astigmatism (M at α), where M is the astigmatic magnitude in diopters (D) and α is the astigmatic direction in degrees, was transformed into two polar values in units of diopters:

Meridional power = polar value along the reference meridian

$$\Phi \text{ degrees} = \text{KP}(\Phi) = M \cos(2*(\alpha - \Phi)). \tag{1}$$

Torsional power = polar value along the meridian

$$(\Phi + 45) \text{ degrees} = \text{KP}(\Phi + 45) = M \sin(2*(\alpha - \Phi)). \tag{2}$$

For calculation of SICA, the reference plane is the surgical meridian in zero degrees, reducing (1) and (2) to

Meridional power = polar value along zero degrees

$$\text{KP}(0) = M \cos(2*\alpha). \tag{3}$$

Torsional power = polar value along the meridian 45°

TABLE 1: Pre- and postoperative operative clinical data of patients.

	Sim K	TCP	TCA power (D)	Axial length (mm)	DCVA (LogMAR)	UDVA (LogMAR)
Preoperative	45.37 (±2.19); 45.09; 42.71–49.29	44.50 (±2.33); 41.52; 43.99–47.89	4.92 (±1.99); 4.47; 2.66–9.32	26.84 (±2.16); 27.09; 22.6–29.7	0.55 (±0.29); 0.45; 1.0–0.2	1.53 (±0.54); 1.65; 2.0–0.7
Postoperative	45.54 (±2.19); *43.16; 44.94–49.31	44.43 (±2.22); *41.22; 44.19–47.83	5.08 (±2.76); *4.21; 3.52–12.55	N/A	0.14 (±0.12); **0.15; 0.3–0	0.29 (±0.13); †0.3; 0.5–0

Sim K = simulated keratometry; TCP = total corneal power measured by ray-tracing; TCA = total corneal astigmatism; DCVA = distance-corrected visual acuity; UDVA = uncorrected distance visual acuity; IOL = intraocular lens. Each entity is reported as average (±SD); median; minimal value–maximal value. *Not statistically significant. ** $p = 0.0020$; † $p = 0.0039$.

$$KP (45) = M \sin (2 * \alpha). \qquad (4)$$

KP(0) is negative for a flattening and positive for a steepening of the surgical meridian along zero degrees.

KP(45) is negative for a clockwise and positive for a counterclockwise rotation of the cylinder median in relation to the horizontal meridian. Refractive data were transformed from the vertex to the corneal plane and then further to polar values. Meridional and torsional powers were reconverted to the usual net cylinder notation by means of the following general equations [26]:

$$M = \sqrt{KP(\Phi)^2 + KP(\Phi + 45)^2},$$
$$\alpha = \text{arc } \tan\left(\frac{M - KP(\Phi)}{KP(\Phi + 45)}\right) + \Phi. \qquad (5)$$

Equation (5) was used also to calculate the ERA, according to two models, as previously reported [27]:

(i) Model 1 is based on preoperative corneal measurements, mean observed SICA, observed IOL axis position, and IOL toric power at the corneal plane (as calculated by the manufacturer). In this model, the reference meridian Φ is the target TCA, defined as the vector sum of the preoperative TCA and the SICA.

(ii) Model 2 is based on postoperative corneal measurements, observed IOL axis position and IOL toric power at the corneal plane (as calculated by the manufacturer). In this model, the reference meridian Φ is the postoperative TCA.

The interpretation of ERA was identical for both models. KP(Φ) is negative for an overcorrection and positive for an undercorrection along the reference meridian. KP($\Phi + 45$) is negative for a clockwise and positive for a counterclockwise rotation of the cylinder median in relation to the reference meridian.

2.5. Statistical Analysis.
All statistical tests were performed using Instat (version 3.10 for Windows, GraphPad Software, La Jolla, CA). The Wilcoxon matched pairs signed-ranks test was used to compare the mean values. The Wilcoxon rank sum test was used to investigate the difference of one sample with respect to zero. A p value < 0.05 was considered statistically significant.

3. Results

Ten eyes of 10 patients (6 men) were enrolled. Mean age was 67.1 ± 7.3 years (range: 56 to 76 years). Cataract surgery and toric IOL implantation were carried out in all cases with no complications. The mean IOL power was 10.9 ± 7.9D (range: −1.25 to +21.5), and the mean cylinder at the IOL plane was 6.18 ± 2.44D (range: +3.25 to +11.5). The mean follow-up after cataract surgery was 15.9 ± 8.9 months (range: 7 to 30 months). Postoperatively, at the end of follow-up, the 0–180° reference marks on the IOL were oriented on average at 175.6° (range: 170–5°), and in 100% of eyes, the difference between the planned axis of orientation and the observed axis was ≤10°. The preoperative and postoperative parameters and the spherical equivalent power and cylinder power of the implanted IOL are reported in Table 1. Postoperatively, both UDVA and DCVA improved significantly with respect to the corresponding preoperative values. UDVA improved from 1.53 ± 0.54 to 0.29 ± 0.13 LogMAR ($p = 0.0039$), and DCVA improved from 0.55 ± 0.29 to 0.14 ± 0.12 LogMAR ($p = 0.002$). The postoperative refraction spherical equivalent was -0.16 ± 0.84 D.

3.1. Surgically Induced Corneal Astigmatism (SICA).
Surgery produced an average 0.27 ± 1.16 D steepening along the incision meridian and an average 0.23 ± 1.44 D counterclockwise rotation over the horizontal surgical meridian (Table 2). These values correspond to a mean SICA of 0.35 D at 20°. No statistically significant differences were found between the average preoperative and postoperative values of meridional and torsional power. Surgery had little effect on the orientation of the steepest TCA axis, since a change in axis orientation of the steepest meridian >10° was observed just in 1 eye.

3.2. Error in Refractive Astigmatism.
The absolute mean postoperative refractive astigmatism power (at the corneal plane) was 1.13 ± 0.94 D (range: 0–3 D). Compared to the preoperative TCA power 4.92 ± 1.99 D, the resulting average 3.80 ± 1.60 D reduction was statistically significant ($p < 0.002$) and allowed us to correct $77 \pm 16\%$ of the preoperative TCA magnitude (range 48.9 to 100 %). Nine eyes out of 10 had a postoperative refractive astigmatism power ≤2 D, whereas preoperatively, TCA was ≥2 D in all eyes. Calculations of ERA meridional powers revealed small

TABLE 2: Meridional and torsional power of preoperative and postoperative total corneal astigmatism and the surgically induced corneal astigmatism (SICA).

	Meridional power	Torsional power
Preoperative	-0.11 ± 3.60; 0.52; -4.87 to 4.38	-1.93 ± 3.72; -2.71; -6.70 to 3.48
Postoperative	0.16 ± 4.10; -0.32; -5.72 to 7.38	-1.70 ± 4.03: -2.38; -10.15 to 3.16
p value	0.6953	0.6953
SICA	0.27 ± 1.16; 0.28; -0.86 to $+3.00$	0.23 ± 1.44; 0.12; -2.00 to $+2.42$

SICA is defined as the difference between preoperative and postoperative total corneal astigmatism. Each entity is reported as average ($\pm$SD); median; minimal value–maximal value. All units are in diopters (D).

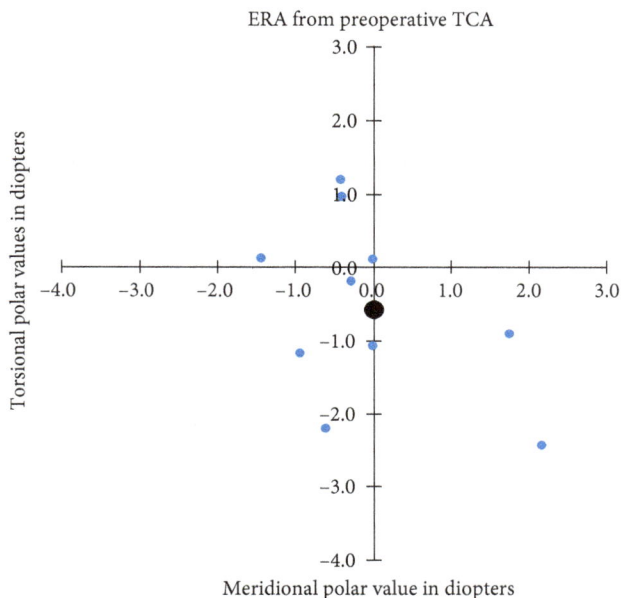

FIGURE 1: The error in refractive astigmatism (ERA) in calculations based on preoperatively measured total corneal astigmatism (TCA). *X*-axis: ERA expressed as the meridional polar value. *Y*-axis: ERA expressed as the torsional polar value. The small colored dots indicate the individual observations. The large black dots indicate the combined mean (centroid).

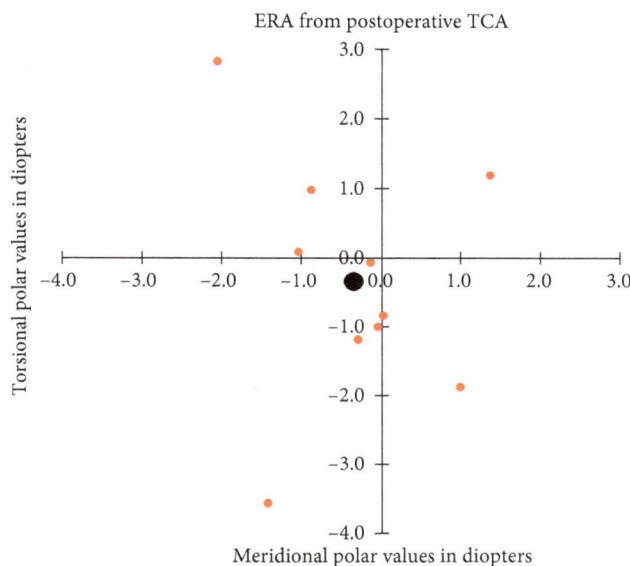

FIGURE 2: The error in refractive astigmatism (ERA) in calculations based on postoperatively measured total corneal astigmatism (TCA). *X*-axis: ERA expressed as the meridional polar value. *Y*-axis: ERA expressed as the torsional polar value. The small colored dots indicate the individual observations. The large black dots indicate the combined mean (centroid).

average overcorrections of 0.03 ($\pm$1.13) D and 0.36 ($\pm$1.04) D for measurements based on preoperative and postoperative TCA, respectively. Torsional powers disclosed average counterclockwise rotations amounting to 0.55 ± 1.22 D and 0.34 ± 1.79 D. None of these meridional and torsional average powers differed significantly from zero. Figures 1 and 2 show the distribution of individual and mean ERA based on both preoperative and postoperative TCA measurements. ERA mean absolute error (MAE) amounted to 1.43 ± 0.91 D and 1.69 ± 1.18 D for preoperative and postoperative TCA measurements, with no statistically significant difference between them. The postoperative endothelial cell reduction was 8% compared to preoperative values. No patients had postoperative corneal decompensation.

4. Discussion

Our results show that cataract extraction with toric IOL implantation is effective to reduce astigmatism and improve visual acuity in patients with previous DALK. Postoperative

improvements of UDVA, CDVA, and astigmatism were all statistically significant. Previous studies reported the effectiveness of toric IOL s implantation in eyes with previous PK [8–15]. A retrospective study, recently published on a peer-reviewed but not indexed journal, describes good outcomes for toric IOLs in eyes with previous DALK [28]. Our data confirm these results, as shown by the significant improvement of UDVA and CDVA and add some interesting findings related to vector analysis (which was not carried out by Scorcia et al.) [28]. In our sample, the refractive predictability was good, as in 90% of patients, the postoperative refractive astigmatism was within 2 D and, on average, more than 75% of astigmatism magnitude was corrected. The good outcomes can be related to two factors at least. First, the toric IOL was customized, that is, manufactured in steps of 0.25 D, according to the axial length and corneal astigmatism values that we supplied preoperatively. Moreover, the cylinder power of the IOL could be manufactured to correct as many as more than 9 D, which is not possible with standard toric IOLs. Second, calculations were based on TCA rather than on KA, as the former has been shown to provide more accurate results [29]. Vector analysis showed that using both preoperative and postoperative TCA leads to a good predictability in the refractive outcome, as the average ERA was close to zero in both cases. The ERA standard deviations for meridional (±1.13D) and torsional ($\pm$D) powers should be compared to the approximate ± 0.60 D values for normal eyes [29]. The relatively large variability may depend on a lower repeatability of TCA measurements in eyes with irregular astigmatism. On the other hand, the predictability of astigmatism correction in these eyes can be reduced due to any irregular component of corneal astigmatism, which cannot be corrected by toric IOLs and by the variable SICA induced by the incision. In this regard, although vector analysis revealed a minimal average SICA (just 0.35 D at 20°), we should consider that this value is misleading, as opposite astigmatism is cancelled out by vector analysis. A more realistic value is provided by the range of the meridional (from -0.86 to $+3.00$ D) and torsional (from -2.00 to $+2.42$ D) power changes in corneal astigmatism, which highlight the risk of TCA changes induced by the incision. The SICA standard deviations for meridional and torsional power in normal eyes were recently reported as ± 0.40 D and ± 0.48 D [29], which is far less than the similar values of ± 1.16 D and ± 1.44 D in the present series. Usually, surgery induces a corneal flattening along the surgical meridian and a compensatory steepening along its orthogonal meridian, the so-called coupling effect [26]. In the present study, a 0.27 D steepening was observed. This average result was influenced by a 3.0 D corneal steepening in a single eye with a preoperative TCA of 9.32 D. However, corneal biomechanics are obviously changed after DALK surgery, which may explain the absence of the normal average flattening. We also found a good rotational stability of the toric IOL, since in no case the misalignment of the main axis of the IOL with respect to the 0–180° axis was higher than 10° at the last follow-up. These results are in good agreement with previous studies on toric IOLs only in eyes with PK [11, 12]. As a secondary outcome, we observed that all surgeries were safe and well tolerated by the corneal endothelium. During the follow-up period, there were no postoperative complications of the grafts. No episodes of immune-mediated rejection or other complications potentially compromising the VA were recorded [30].

Readers may be concerned about the mean age of our sample (67.1 ± 7.3 years), as this means that our patients did not undergo DALK in their 20s or 30s, as it usually happens, but in their 50s or 60s. The surgical indication at this age was mainly due to contact lens intolerance or progressive visual impairment.

This study has some limitations that warrant further investigations. First, the sample size was small. Second, we compared the preoperative TCA to the postoperative refractive astigmatism in order to evaluate the reduction of the astigmatism magnitude. This is not an ideal method because it compares values obtained from different measurements (Scheimpflug imaging of the cornea versus refraction). However, due to the presence of cataract, the measurement of the preoperative refractive astigmatism would not be reliable, so that total corneal astigmatism seems to be the best parameter for comparisons. In conclusion, our results suggest that toric IOL implantation after cataract surgery in patients previously treated with DALK represents a safe and effective procedure for the correction of astigmatism.

Conflicts of Interest

The authors declare that there are no conflicts of interest regarding the publication of this paper.

Acknowledgments

This study was supported by the Italian Ministry of Health and Fondazione Roma.

References

[1] A. Vail, S. M. Gore, B. A. Bradley, D. L. Easty, C. A. Rogers, and W. J. Armitage, "Conclusions of the corneal transplant follow up study," *British Journal of Ophthalmology*, vol. 81, no. 8, pp. 631–636, 1997.

[2] P. S. Binder, "The effect of suture removal on postkeratoplasty astigmatism," *American Journal of Ophthalmology*, vol. 105, no. 6, pp. 637–645, 1988.

[3] S. Feizi and M. Zare, "Current approaches for management of postpenetrating keratoplasty astigmatism," *Journal of Ophthalmology*, vol. 2011, Article ID 708736, 8 pages, 2011.

[4] M. R. Mandel, M. B. Shapiro, and J. H. Krachmer, "Relaxing incisions with augmentation sutures for the correction of postkeratoplasty astigmatism," *American Journal of Ophthalmology*, vol. 103, no. 3, pp. 441–447, 1987.

[5] K. Bilgihan, S. C. Ozdek, F. Akata, and B. Hasanreisoglu, "Photorefractive keratectomy for post-penetrating keratoplasty myopia and astigmatism," *Journal of Cataract & Refractive Surgery*, vol. 26, no. 11, pp. 1590–1595, 2000.

[6] K. Buzard, J.-L. Febbraro, and B. R. Fundingsland, "Laser in situ keratomileusis for the correction of residual ametropia after penetrating keratoplasty," *Journal of Cataract &Refractive Surgery*, vol. 30, no. 5, pp. 1006–1013, 2004.

[7] J. C. D. Arantes, S. Coscarelli, P. Ferrara, L. P. N. Araújo, M. Ávila, and L. Torquetti, "Intrastromal corneal ring segments for astigmatism correction after deep anterior lamellar keratoplasty," *Journal of Ophthalmology*, vol. 2017, Article ID 8689017, 7 pages, 2017.

[8] M. Wade, R. F. Steinert, S. Garg, M. Farid, and R. Gaster, "Results of toric intraocular lenses for post-penetrating keratoplasty astigmatism," *Ophthalmology*, vol. 121, no. 3, pp. 771–777, 2014.

[9] N. Visser, R. Ruíz-Mesa, F. Pastor, N. J. C. Bauer, R. M. M. A. Nuijts, and R. Montés-Micó, "Cataract surgery with toric intraocular lens implantation in patients with high corneal astigmatism," *Journal of Cataract and Refractive Surgery*, vol. 37, no. 8, pp. 1403–1410, 2011.

[10] S. Srinivasan, D. S. J. Ting, and D. A. M. Lyall, "Implantation of a customized toric intraocular lens for correction of postkeratoplasty astigmatism," *Eye*, vol. 27, no. 4, article 531537, 2013.

[11] C. M. Stewart and J. C. McAlister, "Comparison of grafted and non-grafted patients with corneal astigmatism undergoing cataract extraction with a toric intraocular lens implant," *Clinical &Experimental Ophthalmology*, vol. 38, no. 8, pp. 747–757, 2010.

[12] U. De Sanctis, C. Eandi, and F. Grignolo, "Phacoemulsification and customized toric intraocular lens implantation in eyes with cataract and high astigmatism after penetrating keratoplasty," *Journal of Cataract and Refractive Surgery*, vol. 37, no. 4, pp. 781–785, 2011.

[13] D. Lockington, E. Wang, D. V. Patel, S. P. Moore, and C. N. J. McGhee, "Effectiveness of cataract phacoemulsification with toric intraocular lenses in addressing astigmatism after keratoplasty," *Journal of Cataract Refractive Surgery*, vol. 40, no. 12, pp. 2044–2049, 2014.

[14] I. Klftuoglu, Y. A. Akova, S. Egrilmez, and S. G. Yilmaz, "The results of toric intraocular lens implantation in patients with cataract and high astigmatism after penetrating keratoplasty," *C.* vol. 42, no. 2, pp. e8–e11, 2016.

[15] L. Kessel, J. Andresen, B. Tendal, D. Erngaard, P. Flesner, and J. Hjortdal, "Toricintraocular lenses in the correction of astigmatism during cataract surgery: a systematic review and meta-analysis," *Ophthalmology*, vol. 123, no. 2, pp. 275–286, 2016.

[16] M. Anwar, "Indication to deep anterior lamellar keratoplasty," in *Cornea, Surgery of the Cornea and Conjunctiva*, Elsevier Inc., New York, NY, USA, 2013.

[17] M. Anwar and K. D. Teichmann, "Big-bubble technique to bare descemet's membrane in anterior lamellar keratoplasty," *Journal of Cataract &Refractive Surgery*, vol. 28, no. 3, pp. 398–403, 2002.

[18] V. M. Borderie, A. Werthel, O. Touzeau, C. Allouch, S. Boutboul, and L. Laroche, "Comparison of techniques used for removing the recipient stroma in anterior lamellar keratoplasty," *Archives of Ophthalmology*, vol. 126, no. 1, pp. 31–37, 2008.

[19] S. L. Watson, A. Ramsay, J. K. G. Dart, C. Bunce, and E. Craig, "Comparison of deep lamellar keratoplasty and penetrating keratoplasty in patients with keratoconus," *Ophthalmology*, vol. 111, no. 9, pp. 1676–1682, 2004.

[20] R. Macintyre, S.-P. Chow, E. Chan, and A. Poon, "Long-term outcomes of deep anterior lamellar keratoplasty versus penetrating keratoplasty in Australian keratoconus patients," *Cornea*, vol. 33, no. 1, pp. 6–9, 2014.

[21] J. H. Krumeich, A. Knlle, and B. M. Krumeich, "deep anterior lamellar (dalk) vs. penetrating keratoplasty (pkp): a clinical and statistical analysis," *Klinische Monatsblatter fur Augenheilkunde*, vol. 225, no. 7, pp. 637–648, 2008.

[22] A. Kandar, "Combined special capsular tension ring and toriciol implantation for management of post-dalk high regular astigmatism with subluxated traumatic cataract," *Indian Journal of Ophthalmology*, vol. 62, no. 7, pp. 819–822, 2014.

[23] G. Savini, F. Versaci, G. Vestri, P. Ducoli, and K. Nr, "Influence of posterior corneal astigmatism on total corneal astigmatism in eyes with moderate to high astigmatism," *Journal of Cataract and Refractive Surgery*, vol. 40, no. 10, pp. 1645–1653, 2014.

[24] N. Ardjomand, S. Hau, J. C. McAlister et al., "Quality of vision and graft thickness in deep anterior lamellar and penetrating corneal allografts," *American Journal of Ophthalmology*, vol. 143, no. 2, pp. 228–235, 2007.

[25] D. Schiano-Lomoriello, R. Annamaria Colabelli-Gisoldi, M. Nubile et al., "Descemetic and predescemetic dalk in keratoconus patients: a clinical and confocal perspective study," *BioMed Research International*, vol. 2014, Article ID 123156, 7 pages, 2014.

[26] K. Naeser, "Assessment and statistics of surgically induced astigmatism," *Actaophthalmologica*, vol. 86, no. 3, p. 349, 2008.

[27] G. Savini, K. Naeser, D. Schiano-Lomoriello, and P. Ducoli, "Optimized keratometry and total corneal astigmatism for toric intraocular lens calculation," *Journal of Cataract & Refractive Surgery*, vol. 43, no. 9, pp. 1140–1148, 2017.

[28] V. Scorcia, A. Lucisano, V. Savoca Corona, V. De Luca, A. Carnevali, and M. Busin, "Deep anterior lamellar keratoplasty followed by toric lens implantation for the treatment of concomitant anterior stromal diseases and cataract," *Ophthalmology at Point of Care*, vol. 1, no. 1, article oapoc.0000008, 2017.

[29] G. Savini and K. Naeser, "An analysis of the factors influencing the residual refractive astigmatism after cataract surgery with toric intraocular lenses," *Investigative Ophthalmology Visual Science*, vol. 56, no. 2, pp. 827–835, 2015.

[30] B. Acar, C. Utine, S. Acar, and F. Ciftci, "Endothelial cell loss after phacoemulsification in eyes with previous penetrating keratoplasty, previous deep anterior lamellar keratoplasty, or no previous surgery," *Journal of Cataract and Refractive Surgery*, vol. 37, no. 11, pp. 2013–2017, 2011.

7

Continuation of Aspirin Therapy before Cataract Surgery with Different Incisions: Safe or Not?

Qingjian Li, Yiwen Qian, Yu Zhang, Gaoyuan Sun, Xian Zhou, and Zhiliang Wang ⓘ

Department of Ophthalmology, Huashan Hospital, Fudan University, Shanghai, China

Correspondence should be addressed to Zhiliang Wang; ophwzl@163.com

Qingjian Li and Yiwen Qian contributed equally to this work.

Academic Editor: Victoria W. Y. Wong

Purpose. To assess whether to continue aspirin therapy while having uncomplicated phacoemulsification cataract surgery with different incisions. *Methods.* Consecutive patients having cataract surgery under topical anesthesia with different incisions between May 2016 and August 2017 were followed. 236 eyes of 166 patients on routine aspirin therapy were randomized into 2 groups: continuation group, 112 eyes; discontinuation group, 124 eyes. 121 eyes of 94 patients on no routine anticoagulant therapy were used as the control group. Patients were examined 1 day preoperatively and 1 day and 7 days postoperatively. Intraoperative and postoperative complications were recorded. *Results.* Statistically, there was no significant difference about postoperative BCVA among three groups. A higher incidence of subconjunctival hemorrhage was shown in the continuation group than in the discontinuation group and the control group (17.0% versus 8.1%, $p = 0.038$; 17.0% versus 7.4%, $p = 0.025$, resp.). Although corneal edema was greater in clear corneal incision cases than that of scleral tunnel incision cases (22.5% versus 12.0%, $p = 0.009$), subconjunctival hemorrhage was greater in scleral tunnel incision cases (14.9% versus 6.6%, $p = 0.011$). Subgroup analyses revealed that patients of scleral tunnel incision who continued taking aspirin had a higher incidence of subconjunctival hemorrhage compared with those who discontinued (25.5% versus 10.9%, $p = 0.038$), but no same conclusion in clear corneal incision cases (8.8% versus 5.0%, $p = 0.483$). *Conclusions.* The outcomes indicated that phacoemulsification cataract surgery under topical anesthesia could be safely performed without ceasing systemic aspirin therapy. Clear corneal incision could be a better choice in patients treated with aspirin.

1. Introduction

Aspirin has been the cornerstone of preventing thromboembolic complications in patients with cerebrovascular, coronary artery, and peripheral vascular diseases. It is a weak anticoagulant and acts chiefly through the passivation of platelet cyclooxygenase 1 and suppression of thromboxane A2 production. This regimen has significantly reduced risks for morbidity and mortality due to vascular events. The potential benefit of aspirin and the low rate of adverse effects have made aspirin intaking fashionable in the elderly population [1–5]. Cataract surgery is one of the most common surgeries performed in elderly patients [6]. It is estimated that more than 20% of patients routinely took aspirin before cataract surgery [7, 8]. Patients receiving long-term antiplatelet therapy face a significant clinical challenge when they need a cataract surgery. If antiplatelet therapy is suspended, there is a risk for vascular events; however, continuation of aspirin treatment may be closely associated with serious perioperative bleeding complications [9, 10]. Hence, there is an issue of whether the risk of thromboembolic events associated with temporarily ceasing antiplatelet treatment before surgery outweighs the advantages of fewer hemorrhagic events. However, at present, there is no clear consistent recommendation in these cases before cataract surgery.

This prospective randomized study was undertaken to compare the incidence of intraoperative and postoperative complications in patients continuing aspirin therapy and those ceasing it while having phacoemulsification cataract surgery with different incisions.

2. Methods

2.1. Patients. This prospective randomized study included consecutive patients who had phacoemulsification cataract surgery under topical anesthesia with different incisions between May 2016 and August 2017 at Huashan Hospital, Fudan University, Shanghai, China. Two hundred thirty-six eyes of 166 patients on routine aspirin therapy were randomized into 2 groups: the continuation group, aspirin continued up to the time of surgery, 112 eyes; the discontinuation group, aspirin discontinued for 3 to 7 days before surgery till 1 day after surgery, 124 eyes. One hundred twenty-one eyes of 94 patients on no routine anticoagulant therapy were used as the control group. The study protocols were accepted by the Institutional Review Board of Huashan Hospital affiliated to Fudan University and performed in accordance with the tenets of the Declaration of Helsinki. Written informed consent was gained from each participant.

2.2. Exclusion Criteria. Ocular exclusion criteria were previous operation in the same eye, having phacoemulsification cataract surgery combined with other surgeries (e.g., trabeculectomy or pars plana vitrectomy), pupil dilating to be short of 4.0 mm, nuclear hardness over grade IV, uncontrolled glaucoma, floppy iris syndrome, and existence of pathological vessels in the operative eye (e.g., iris neovascularization or proliferative diabetic retinopathy). Systemic exclusion criteria were severe renal failure, fasting glucose > 9 mmol/L, and blood pressure > 170/90 mmHg. The patients on other kinds of antiplatelets and/or anticoagulants were excluded.

2.3. Data Collection. All eligible patients had a complete preoperative evaluation including ocular and systemic examination. The ophthalmologic evaluation included slit-lamp biomicroscopy, best-corrected visual acuity (BCVA), intraocular pressure (IOP), and funduscopic examination. The BCVA was converted to the logMAR value, which was used in all statistical analyses. IOP elevation and hypotony were defined as IOPs over 30 mmHg and less than 9 mmHg, respectively [11, 12]. The systemic evaluation included blood, electrocardiogram, and blood pressure. After surgery, the patients were followed up at 1 day and 7 days. All intraoperative and postoperative complications were recorded. Special concern was given to evidence of hemorrhagic complications.

2.4. Surgical Technique. Three hundred fifty-seven cases of phacoemulsification cataract surgery through different incisions were performed by 1 of 8 skilled surgeons at the same institution. Compound tropicamide eye drop which contained tropicamide (0.5%) and phenylephrine hydrochloride (0.5%) was used as preoperative mydriatic regularly. Topical anesthesia of oxybuprocaine hydrochloride (20 ml: 80 mg) was used 3 times before cataract surgery. Different incisions were applied according to surgeon's preference. Five surgeons performed through clear corneal incision, while three surgeons preferred scleral tunnel incision. In the scleral tunnel incision cases, after a conjunctival incision at 10:30, cauterization was applied to coagulate conjunctival and episcleral vessels. All surgeons did not know whether the patient was taking aspirin up to the time of surgery or had discontinued the medication some days earlier.

2.5. Statistical Analysis. SPSS for Windows Version 19.0 (SPSS, Inc., Chicago, IL, USA) was applied for all statistical analysis. Random number table was used for randomization. A two-tailed p value < 0.05 was considered statistically significant. The Kolmogorov–Smirnov test was applied to analyze the distribution of continuous variables. Continuous variables were expressed as mean ± standard deviation (SD) for normally distributed data and median (interquartile range (IQR)) for nonnormally distributed data. Categorical variables were expressed as absolute numbers and percentages. Student's t-test was applied for normally distributed data, and the Wilcoxon rank sum test was applied for nonnormally distributed data. The chi-square test was used to compare categorical variables between the continuation group and discontinuation group. When small numbers revealed that the chi-square test might be invalid, the Fisher exact test was applied.

3. Results

Phacoemulsification cataract surgery under topical anesthesia was performed in 357 eyes of 260 patients. One hundred sixty-six patients took aspirin preoperatively on a daily basis. Table 1 characterizes demographic features. The dosage of aspirin intake was 100 mg/day routinely. Table 2 characterizes systemic indication for antiplatelet therapy. The most common systemic clinical indication for aspirin therapy was thromboembolic disease (cerebral infarction, myocardial infarction, venous thrombosis, etc.), which accounted for 70.3% of patients in our study. Other less common indications, which accounted for an additional 10.6%, included atrial fibrillation, mechanical mitral, coronary artery bypass graft, cardiac pacemaker, and dilated cardiomyopathy. But 19.1% of the patients presented no certain systemic clinical indications for aspirin therapy on a daily basis. The three groups were equally distributed in sex, age, BCVA, IOP, types of incision, surgeons, and the proportions of patients having surgery to both eyes. Statistical analysis showed no significant differences between the continuation group and discontinuation group in duration of aspirin intake and systemic indication for antiplatelet therapy.

Table 3 characterizes the postoperative BCVA and IOP in three groups, and there was no statistic difference among them. One day postoperatively, BCVA was improved from 0.58 ± 0.19 to 0.42 ± 0.39 (in the continuation group), 0.61 ± 0.18 to 0.45 ± 0.39 (in the discontinuation group), and 0.62 ± 0.17 to 0.47 ± 0.45 (in the control group), respectively. And one week postoperatively, BCVA was improved to 0.24 ± 0.19 (in the continuation group), 0.27 ± 0.21 (in the discontinuation group), and 0.27 ± 0.20 (in the control group), respectively.

Table 4 characterizes the hemorrhagic and non-hemorrhagic complications noted in the three groups. None of the patients suffered from thromboembolic events in our study during the follow-up period. No surgery was canceled or postponed because of bleeding complications. Subconjunctival hemorrhage was the most frequent hemorrhagic complication. There was a higher incidence of subconjunctival

TABLE 1: Demographic characteristics.

Parameter	Continuation group	Discontinuation group	Control group	p value
Patients, n	81	85	94	—
Eye, n	112	124	121	—
Sex, n				0.223^a
Male	46	39	42	
Female	35	46	52	
Age, year				0.193^b
Mean ± SD	75.2 ± 8.6	76.3 ± 7.3	74.5 ± 8.0	
Range	50–93	55–90	58–89	
BCVA, logMAR				0.165^b
Mean ± SD	0.58 ± 0.19	0.61 ± 0.18	0.62 ± 0.17	
IOP, mmHg				0.210^b
Mean ± SD	15.9 ± 2.6	15.2 ± 2.6	15.6 ± 2.9	
Aspirin duration, month				0.119^c
Median (IQR)	60 (24–96)	60 (36–120)	—	
Type of incision, n				0.706^a
Corneal incision	57	60	65	
Scleral incision	55	64	56	

BCVA = best-corrected visual acuity; IOP = intraocular pressure; [a]chi-square test; [b]Student's t-test; [c]Wilcoxon rank sum test.

TABLE 2: Systemic indication for antiplatelet therapy.

Systemic indication for antiplatelet therapy	Eyes, n (%)		p value
	Continuation group ($n = 112$)	Discontinuation group ($n = 124$)	
Thromboembolic disease	84 (75.0)	82 (66.1)	0.136^a
Atrial fibrillation	4 (3.6)	7 (5.6)	0.450^a
Mechanical mitral	1 (0.9)	4 (3.2)	0.373^d
Coronary artery bypass graft	1 (0.9)	3 (2.4)	0.624^d
Cardiac pacemaker	1 (0.9)	2 (1.6)	1.000^d
Dilated cardiomyopathy	1 (0.9)	1 (0.9)	1.000^d
Precaution	20 (17.8)	25 (20.2)	0.653^a

Precaution = patients without certain systemic clinical indication; [a]chi-square test; [d]Fisher's exact test.

TABLE 3: Postoperative BCVA and IOP by group.

Parameter	Continuation group ($n = 112$)	Discontinuation group ($n = 124$)	Control group ($n = 121$)	p value
One day postoperative				
BCVA, logMAR	0.42 ± 0.39	0.45 ± 0.39	0.47 ± 0.45	0.598^b
IOP, mmHg	17.5 ± 4.5	18.0 ± 5.0	17.6 ± 4.9	0.729^b
One week postoperative				
BCVA, logMAR	0.24 ± 0.19	0.28 ± 0.21	0.27 ± 0.20	0.425^b
IOP, mmHg	16.2 ± 2.8	16.1 ± 3.0	15.8 ± 3.0	0.531^b

[b]Student's t-test.

TABLE 4: Incidence of complications by group.

Complication	Eyes, n (%)			p value
	Continuation group ($n = 112$)	Discontinuation group ($n = 124$)	Control group ($n = 121$)	
Hemorrhagic				
Subconjunctival hemorrhagic	19 (17.0)	10 (8.1)	9 (7.4)	0.032^{a*}
Hyphema	1 (0.9)	0 (0)	0 (0)	0.334^d
Nonhemorrhagic				
Corneal edema	21 (18.8)	22 (17.7)	19 (15.7)	0.821^a
Posterior capsule rupture	1 (0.9)	1 (0.8)	2 (1.7)	0.730^d
Hypotony (<9 mmHg)	1 (0.9)	3 (2.4)	4 (3.3)	0.455^d
IOP elevation (>30 mmHg)	3 (2.7)	6 (4.8)	2 (1.7)	0.338^d

* $p < 0.05$; [a]chi-square test; [d]Fisher's exact test.

Continuation of Aspirin Therapy before Cataract Surgery with Different Incisions: Safe...

49

TABLE 5: Incidence of complications in scleral tunnel incision cases.

Complication	Eyes, n (%)			p value
	Continuation group (n = 55)	Discontinuation group (n = 64)	Control group (n = 56)	
Hemorrhagic				
Subconjunctival hemorrhagic	14 (25.5)	7 (10.9)	5 (8.9)	0.027[a*]
Hyphema	0 (0)	0 (0)	0 (0)	—
Nonhemorrhagic				
Corneal edema	7 (12.7)	8 (12.5)	6 (10.7)	0.937[a]
Posterior capsule rupture	0 (0)	1 (1.6)	0 (0)	0.418[d]
Hypotony (<9 mmHg)	0 (0)	2 (3.1)	2 (3.6)	0.386[d]
IOP elevation (>30 mmHg)	1 (1.8)	4 (6.2)	0 (0)	0.105[d]

* $p < 0.05$; [a]chi-square test; [d]Fisher's exact test.

TABLE 6: Incidence of complications in clear corneal incision cases.

Complication	Eyes, n (%)			p value
	Continuation group (n = 57)	Discontinuation group (n = 60)	Control group (n = 65)	
Hemorrhagic				
Subconjunctival hemorrhagic	5 (8.8)	3 (5.0)	4 (6.2)	0.702[d]
Hyphema	1 (1.8)	0 (0)	0 (0)	0.332[d]
Nonhemorrhagic				
Corneal edema	14 (24.6)	14 (23.3)	13 (20.0)	0.821[a]
Posterior capsule rupture	1 (1.8)	0 (0)	2 (3.1)	0.401[d]
Hypotony (<9 mmHg)	1 (1.8)	1 (1.7)	2 (3.1)	0.833[d]
IOP elevation (>30 mmHg)	2 (3.5)	2 (3.3)	2 (3.1)	0.991[d]

[a]Chi-square test; [d]Fisher's exact test.

hemorrhage in the continuation group than in the discontinuation group and the control group (17.0% versus 8.1%, $p = 0.038$; 17.0% versus 7.4%, $p = 0.025$, resp.).

The incidence of subconjunctival hemorrhage was significantly greater in the scleral tunnel incision cases than in the clear corneal incision cases (14.9% versus 6.6%, $p = 0.011$). Tables 5 and 6 characterize the hemorrhagic and nonhemorrhagic complications in different incision cases. Subgroup analyses revealed that patients of scleral tunnel incision who continued taking aspirin had a higher incidence of subconjunctival hemorrhage compared with those who stopped treatment before surgery (25.5% versus 10.9%, $p = 0.038$), but there was no same conclusion in the clear corneal incision cases (8.8% versus 5.0%, $p = 0.483$, Fisher's exact test). No patient requested additional clinic visits because of the subconjunctival hemorrhage.

Corneal edema was the most frequent nonhemorrhagic complication. We found no statistical difference of nonhemorrhagic complication, such as corneal edema, elevated IOP hypotony, and posterior capsule rupture among the continuation group, discontinuation group, and control group. The incidence of corneal edema was significantly greater in the clear corneal incision cases than in the scleral tunnel incision cases (22.5% versus 12.0%, $p = 0.009$), but this complication faded away spontaneously within a week without clinical consequences.

Another common postoperative nonhemorrhage complication was elevated IOP or hypotony. We found no statistic difference of elevated IOP or hypotony among the continuation group, discontinuation group, and control group. And 78.9% (15/19) of disordered IOP returned to normal within 7 days.

In the continuation group, one patient had an intraoperative posterior capsule rupture and received secondary implantation of intraocular lens (IOL) without clinical consequences after one month. In the discontinuation group, a patient who had an intraoperative rupture of posterior capsule had instant implantation of IOL and maintained good visual acuity. There were no cases of choroidal/suprachoroidal hemorrhage, vitreous hemorrhage, distorted pupil, retinal detachment, or endophthalmitis.

4. Discussion

Antiplatelet therapy is continually encountered in patients desiring cataract surgery. Because of the progressive aging of the population, aspirin users are more likely to be elderly and, therefore, more likely to desire a surgical procedure. The clinical challenge is to conclude whether to continue or to interrupt antithrombotic therapy. It is considered that 10% of all patients receiving oral antiplatelet medications request interrupted treatment for surgery or an invasive procedure each year [10]. In the past studies, 25.6% of the Canadian Society of Cataract and Refractive Surgery members discontinued aspirin routinely before cataract surgery [13]. 22.5% of routine aspirin users ceased the medication during the perioperative period of cataract surgery [8]. To reduce the risk of intraoperative and postoperative hemorrhagic complications, the ophthalmologists preferred to ceasing aspirin 3 to 7 days prior to cataract surgery and interrupt use 1 to 2 days postoperatively, despite the potential risk of thromboembolic events [13–15].

For decades, whether to stop antiplatelet therapy before cataract surgery remains no decision. Recent studies showed the safety of antiplatelet medications in cataract surgery and no increase in sight-threatening complications, such as severe hemorrhage affecting visual acuity or retinal detachment. [8, 16, 17]. The American College of Chest Physicians and American Academy of Neurology advised continuous use of antiplatelets before cataract surgery [18, 19]. The cataract in the Adult Eye Preferred Practice Pattern of the American Academy of Ophthalmology gave a 1- grade recommendation that aspirin should be discontinued perioperatively only if the risk of bleeding outweighed its potential benefit [20]. Same as these clinical researches, in our experience, there was no statistic difference in postoperative BCVA among the three groups. What's more, except one case of hyphema postoperatively in the continuation group, no case of choroidal/suprachoroidal hemorrhage, vitreous hemorrhage, distorted pupil, retinal detachment, or endophthalmitis happened in patients with aspirin treatment.

We observed a higher incidence of subconjunctival hemorrhage in patients who continued aspirin therapy compared with those who stopped treatment. This complication was self-limiting without permanent sequelae. Cauterization was applied to coagulate conjunctival and episcleral vessels in the scleral incision cases, but the incidence of subconjunctival hemorrhage was significantly greater in the scleral tunnel incision cases than in the clear corneal incision cases. In 2006, the study by Kumar et al. [21] showed no difference in incidence of subconjunctival hemorrhage between the aspirin group and control group. But the primary diseases between the two groups were unbalanced and it was relatively a small sample study.

Results of the subgroup analyses showed that patients of scleral tunnel incision who continued taking aspirin had a higher incidence of subconjunctival hemorrhage compared with those who discontinued for 3 to 7 days before surgery, but there is no same conclusion in the clear corneal incision cases. This meant that aspirin would markedly increase the risk of subconjunctival hemorrhage in scleral tunnel incision cases. No patient requested additional clinic visits because of the subconjunctival hemorrhage. In a study by Kobayashi [14], patients on antiplatelets and/or anticoagulants continuously showed a higher incidence of subconjunctival hemorrhage compared with the discontinuation group (16.5% versus 10.8%, $p = 0.0309$). And the possible reason for bleeding might be the use of subtenon's anesthesia and it was out of date.

One patient who continued taking aspirin in the clear corneal incision cases had a postoperative hyphema (<2.0 mm) that resolved spontaneously in two weeks without affecting visual acuity. The possible explanation was injury of iris vessels during phacoemulsification. The happening of bleeding complication was probably coincidental.

Corneal edema was the main nonhemorrhagic complication. In our study, there was no significant difference in nonhemorrhagic complications among the continuation group, discontinuation group, and control group. The incidence of corneal edema was significantly greater in the clear corneal incision cases than in the scleral tunnel incision cases, but this complication faded away spontaneously within a week without clinical consequences. The possible explanation for the nonhemorrhagic complication is the excessive manipulation through the incision.

The major advantage of this study was comparisons of the incidence of intraoperative and postoperative complications among the three groups in different incision cases. The patients of scleral tunnel incision who continued taking aspirin had a higher incidence of subconjunctival hemorrhage compared with those who stopped treatment before surgery, but there was no same conclusion in the clear corneal incision cases. The patients with clear corneal incision had more chance of corneal edema but less subconjunctival hemorrhage compared to patients with scleral tunnel incision. Subconjunctival hemorrhage usually lasts for 2-3 weeks and longer in patients with aspirin treatment. But corneal edema fades away spontaneously within a week without clinical consequences. So, we hold the opinion that clear corneal incision is better than scleral tunnel incision in patients treated with aspirin.

The patients on other kinds of antiplatelets and/or anticoagulants were excluded from this study. Therefore, we believe that the results represent a true reflection of the hemorrhagic risks associated with the continuation of aspirin uncomplicated by the effect of other medicines.

This study has limitations. First, because the number of patients was relatively small, the power of analysis was not great enough to discover tiny differences that might have been existent. Second, there were certain indications for use of aspirin that put most routine users at higher risk for bleeding complications than those not on the medication. For example there was no operative history of percutaneous coronary intervention in the control group. A comparison between the continuation group and discontinuation group is likely to reduce the bias.

Although patients taking aspirin may be at higher risk for bleeding complications, the practical situation that lots of patients are advised to stop or alter antiplatelet therapy before routine cataract surgery may increase risk of vascular event. If a vascular event did occur, it was much more fearful and resulted in a higher mortality. Furthermore, the technique placing incisions in the avascular clear cornea under topical anesthesia reduces the risk of bleeding complications. A clear consistent recommendation to maintain antiplatelet therapy during phacoemulsification cataract surgery should be instituted by national and international ophthalmic societies.

5. Conclusions

The outcomes in our study indicate that phacoemulsification cataract surgery under topical anesthesia could be safely performed without ceasing systemic aspirin therapy. Clear corneal incision could be a better choice in patients treated with aspirin compared with scleral tunnel incision.

Conflicts of Interest

None of the authors has a financial or proprietary interest in any material or method mentioned.

Authors' Contributions

Zhiliang Wang, Qingjian Li, and Yiwen Qian conceived the study design. Zhiliang Wang and Yu Zhang performed the surgeries. Gaoyuan Sun and Xian Zhou analyzed and interpreted the data. Qingjian Li drafted the manuscript. All authors read and approved the final manuscript.

Acknowledgments

This work was supported by grants from the Natural Science Foundation of China (No. 81670878) and the Science and Technology Commission of Shanghai (15ZR1425400).

References

[1] C. A. Kiire, R. Mukherjee, N. Ruparelia, D. Keeling, B. Prendergast, and J. H. Norris, "Managing antiplatelet and anticoagulant drugs in patients undergoing elective ophthalmic surgery," *British Journal of Ophthalmology*, vol. 98, no. 10, pp. 1320–1324, 2014.

[2] D. A. Garcia, D. M. Witt, E. Hylek et al., "Delivery of optimized anticoagulant therapy: consensus statement from the Anticoagulation Forum," *Annals of Pharmacotherapy*, vol. 42, no. 7-8, pp. 979–988, 2008.

[3] M. Moussouttas, "Emerging therapies: clopidogrel and aspirin," *Stroke*, vol. 36, no. 4, p. 707, 2005.

[4] R. Saxena and P. Koudstaal, "Anticoagulants versus antiplatelet therapy for preventing stroke in patients with nonrheumatic atrial fibrillation and a history of stroke or transient ischemic attack," *Cochrane Database of Systematic Reviews*, no. 4, p. CD000187, 2004.

[5] J. B. Segal, R. L. McNamara, M. R. Miller et al., "Prevention of thromboembolism in atrial fibrillation. A meta-analysis of trials of anticoagulants and antiplatelet drugs," *Journal of General Internal Medicine*, vol. 15, no. 1, pp. 56–67, 2000.

[6] W. Hodge, T. Horsley, D. Albiani et al., "The consequences of waiting for cataract surgery: a systematic review," *Canadian Medical Association Journal*, vol. 176, no. 9, pp. 1285–1290, 2007.

[7] J. D. Benzimra, R. L. Johnston, P. Jaycock et al., "The Cataract National Dataset electronic multicentre audit of 55,567 operations: antiplatelet and anticoagulant medications," *Eye*, vol. 23, no. 1, pp. 10–16, 2009.

[8] J. Katz, M. A. Feldman, E. B. Bass et al., "Risks and benefits of anticoagulant and antiplatelet medication use before cataract surgery," *Ophthalmology*, vol. 110, no. 9, pp. 1784–1788, 2003.

[9] A. Grzybowski, F. J. Ascaso, K. Kupidura-Majewski, and M. Packer, "Continuation of anticoagulant and antiplatelet therapy during phacoemulsification cataract surgery," *Current Opinion in Ophthalmology*, vol. 26, no. 1, pp. 28–33, 2015.

[10] J. D. Douketis, P. B. Berger, A. S. Dunn et al., "The perioperative management of antithrombotic therapy: American College of Chest Physicians Evidence-Based Clinical Practice Guidelines (8th Edition)," *Chest*, vol. 133, no. 6, pp. 299S–339S, 2008.

[11] M. Pavlidis, N. Korber, and F. Hohn, "Surgical and functional results of 27-gauge vitrectomy combined with coaxial 1.8 mm microincision cataract surgery: a consecutive case series," *Retina*, vol. 36, no. 11, pp. 2093–2100, 2016.

[12] M. Kim, Y. S. Park, D. H. Lee, H. J. Koh, S. C. Lee, and S. S. Kim, "Comparison of surgical outcome of 23-gauge and 25-gauge microincision vitrectomy surgery for management of idiopathic epiretinal membrane in pseudophakic eyes," *Retina*, vol. 35, no. 10, pp. 2115–2120, 2015.

[13] L. Ong-Tone, E. C. Paluck, and R. D. Hart-Mitchell, "Perioperative use of warfarin and aspirin in cataract surgery by Canadian Society of Cataract and Refractive Surgery members: survey," *Journal of Cataract and Refractive Surgery*, vol. 31, no. 5, pp. 991–996, 2005.

[14] H. Kobayashi, "Evaluation of the need to discontinue antiplatelet and anticoagulant medications before cataract surgery," *Journal of Cataract and Refractive Surgery*, vol. 36, no. 7, pp. 1115–1119, 2010.

[15] E. I. Assia, T. Raskin, I. Kaiserman, Y. Rotenstreich, and F. Segev, "Effect of aspirin intake on bleeding during cataract surgery," *Journal of Cataract and Refractive Surgery*, vol. 24, no. 9, pp. 1243–1246, 1998.

[16] I. S. Barequet, D. Sachs, B. Shenkman et al., "Risk assessment of simple phacoemulsification in patients on combined anticoagulant and antiplatelet therapy," *Journal of Cataract and Refractive Surgery*, vol. 37, no. 8, pp. 1434–1438, 2011.

[17] K. Carter and K. M. Miller, "Phacoemulsification and lens implantation in patients treated with aspirin or warfarin," *Journal of Cataract and Refractive Surgery*, vol. 24, no. 10, pp. 1361–1364, 1998.

[18] M. J. Armstrong, G. Gronseth, D. C. Anderson et al., "Summary of evidence-based guideline: periprocedural management of antithrombotic medications in patients with ischemic cerebrovascular disease: report of the Guideline Development Subcommittee of the American Academy of Neurology," *Neurology*, vol. 80, no. 22, pp. 2065–2069, 2013.

[19] J. D. Douketis, A. C. Spyropoulos, F. A. Spencer et al., "Perioperative management of antithrombotic therapy: Antithrombotic Therapy and Prevention of Thrombosis, 9th ed: American College of Chest Physicians Evidence-Based Clinical Practice Guidelines," *Chest*, vol. 141, no. 4, pp. e326S–e350S, 2012.

[20] R. J. Olson, R. Braga-Mele, S. H. Chen et al., "Cataract in the adult eye preferred practice pattern(R)," *Ophthalmology*, vol. 124, no. 2, pp. P1–P119, 2017.

[21] N. Kumar, S. Jivan, P. Thomas, and H. McLure, "Sub-Tenon's anesthesia with aspirin, warfarin, and clopidogrel," *Journal of Cataract and Refractive Surgery*, vol. 32, no. 6, pp. 1022–1025, 2006.

A Novel "Slit Side View" Method to Evaluate Fluid Dynamics during Phacoemulsification

Hisaharu Suzuki ⓘ,[1] Tsutomu Igarashi ⓘ,[2] Toshihiko Shiwa,[2] and Hiroshi Takahashi[2]

[1]Department of Ophthalmology, Nippon Medical School Musashikosugi Hospital, 1-396 Kosugi-cho, Nakahara-ku, Kawasaki City, Kanagawa 211-8533, Japan
[2]Department of Ophthalmology, Nippon Medical School, 1-1-5 Sendagi, Bunkyo-ku, Tokyo 113-8603, Japan

Correspondence should be addressed to Hisaharu Suzuki; s5054@nms.ac.jp

Academic Editor: Tamer A. Macky

Due to recent technical advances in cataract surgeries, there has been a significant improvement in the safety and surgical outcomes of phacoemulsification. However, the corneal endothelium can be damaged during phacoemulsification by multiple factors. Therefore, we used a slit lamp to analyze the fluid dynamics of ophthalmic viscosurgical devices (OVDs) in the anterior chamber during phacoemulsification. In this experimental study, extracted porcine eyes were injected with OVDs stained with fluorescein through a side port of the eye and then fixed on a slit lamp microscope. After inserting a phaco tip, phacoemulsification simulation was then performed on the iris plane. Subsequent movements of OVDs in the anterior chamber were observed during the procedure by using a slit lamp microscope. Aspiration and removal of cohesive OVDs from the inside of the anterior chamber occurred within a few seconds after the ultrasonic vibration. Aspiration of dispersive OVDs occurred gradually, with some of the OVDs remaining on the side of the anterior chamber side in an irregular shape. This shape enabled the OVD to trap the air, thereby preventing the air from directly touching the corneal endothelium. Viscoadaptive OVDs remained inside the anterior chamber as a lump, with the infusion solution flowing between the corneal endothelium and the OVD, thus leading to the eventual aspiration of the OVD. Viscous dispersive OVDs remained as a lump between the corneal endothelium and the phaco tip. However, once the infusion solution flowed between the cornea and the OVD, the OVD detached from the corneal endothelium, indicating that this type would likely be aspirated and removed. This method, termed the "slit side view," enables viewing of the movement of OVDs during surgery, as well as observation of the fluid dynamics in the anterior chamber.

1. Introduction

Today, most cataract surgeries are performed by using the phacoemulsification technique. Due to recent technical advances, there has been a significant improvement in the safety and surgical outcomes of phacoemulsification. However, the corneal endothelium can be damaged during phacoemulsification by multiple factors, such as excessive duration of the phacoemulsification [1–4]. Since the introduction of Healon® (sodium hyaluronate 1.0%) in 1980, many ophthalmic viscosurgical devices (OVDs) have become available. Moreover, OVDs play an important role in endothelium protection [5, 6]. Therefore, it is important to understand the dynamics of OVDs in the anterior chamber during phacoemulsification.

The surgical microscope is an essential apparatus when performing phacoemulsification. However, when using this microscope, observations are primarily made from the front, which complicates a clinician's ability to understand the detailed positional relationships that are present inside the anterior chamber. In contrast, a slit lamp microscope is used in outpatient clinics. When using this device, the anterior chamber space can be observed in detail. Therefore, we developed an observation method that uses a slit lamp microscope to obtain a detailed understanding of the movements that occur inside the anterior chamber during surgery. The purpose of this study was to evaluate the effectiveness of using a slit lamp to observe fluid dynamics in the anterior chamber during phacoemulsification.

2. Materials and Methods

This study was conducted in accordance with the ARVO Statement for the Use of Animals in Ophthalmic and Vision Research. The ethics committee ruled that approval was not required for the study. Extracted porcine eyes obtained from a local abattoir were used for the experiment.

Fluorescein (Ayumi Pharmaceutical) was applied to each of the OVDs to facilitate visualization. For each of the OVD staining methods, a 0.7 mg fluorescein examination test paper was divided into five equal parts, with the test paper then inserted into the tip of the syringe for each of the OVDs. OVD syringes were then stored vertically for 2 days in the refrigerator, which is our novel method to enable diffusion of the fluorescein into the OVDs. All OVDs used in the study were stored and used at room temperature.

By using an operation microscope, we first injected an OVD stained with fluorescein via the side port. The volume of each OVD was 0.4 ml. Second, we created a 2.4 mm incised corneal wound, making a continuous curvilinear capsulorhexis. Third, we transferred the porcine eye to the eyeball-fixing stand that was attached to the slit lamp microscope, inserted a phaco tip, and then fixed it over the iris surface. We observed the movement and behavior of the OVD inside the anterior chamber by using the slit lamp microscope 700GL (Takagi, Nagano-ken, Japan) (Figure 1(a)). We named this procedure the "slit side view" (SSV) (Figure 1(b)).

Phacoemulsification was performed in porcine eyes with the WhiteStar Signature PRO® System (Abbott Medical Optics, Santa Ana, CA, USA). The scale of light volume in the slit lamp microscope 700GL was set to 8/20. Ultrasound (US) oscillation was applied for 90 seconds. Observation points were 3, 25, 30, and 90 seconds. Phacoemulsification was performed with 20% power of longitudinal vibration using a 30-degree Signature Laminar® 20-gauge US tip. This method was used to perform several different intraoperative evaluations. We examined several OVDs during these evaluations, with differences in movement classified according to the type of OVD used.

We examined the movements for each of the OVDs inside the anterior chamber according to its type. These OVDs included the cohesive type (Opegan Hi®; Santen, Osaka, Japan), dispersive type [Shellgan® (Santen)], viscoadaptive type [Healon5® (Abbott Medical Optics)], and viscous dispersive type [DisCoVisc® (Alcon, Fort Worth, TX, USA)] (Table 1). We also examined a soft-shell technique [7] that uses a combined cohesive (injection volume: 0.3 ml) and dispersive (0.1 ml) type of OVD. In the soft-shell technique, we used undyed cohesive OVD. After injecting the dispersive OVD, the cohesive OVD was injected deliberately under the first OVD to push it forward against the corneal endothelium. The volume of the dispersive OVD was determined as 0.1 ml because it apparently seemed enough to coat the whole area of the corneal endothelium. The second OVD was injected until the anterior chamber was filled, and the leak of the OVD was confirmed. Moreover, in this group, we recorded the dynamics of OVD during injection with the slit side view. Recording parameters included a US power output of 20%, vacuum pressure of 200 mmHg, and bottle height of 75 cm. A Signature PRO® venturi pump was used for this part of the study. In all experiments, a 20G phaco tip was used. Three porcine eyes were evaluated for each OVD group.

3. Results

The imaging of the anterior chamber during phacoemulsification was performed at 3, 25, 30, and 90 seconds. Aspiration and removal of the cohesive type of OVDs from the inside of the anterior chamber occurred within a few seconds after the creation of the ultrasonic vibration (Figure 2). Aspiration of the dispersive type of OVDs occurred gradually, with some of the OVD remaining on the side of the anterior chamber side in an irregular shape, as if the OVD had dripped down the side. This shape enabled the OVD to trap the air and prevent the air from directly touching the corneal endothelium (Figure 3). The soft-shell technique uses a combination of the dispersive and cohesive types of OVDs. During the first step of this procedure, a dispersive type of OVD was injected, followed by a cohesive type. Results clearly showed that after being pressed by the cohesive type of OVD, the dispersive type of OVD was able to further spread on the corneal endothelial surface, the anterior surface of the crystalline lens, and the iris surface (Figure 4). After the application of US, the cohesive types of OVDs were immediately aspirated. However, the dispersive types of OVDs were retained on the surface for an extended period because they were able to form a layer of various thicknesses on the surface of the corneal endothelium (Figure 5).

The next OVD studied was the viscoadaptive type. This type of OVD remained inside the anterior chamber as a lump, with the infusion solution flowing between the corneal endothelium and the OVD (Figure 6). When this occurred, the infusion solution often flowed between the corneal endothelium and the OVD from around the incised wound, thus leading to the eventual aspiration of the OVD. Typically, this type of finding cannot be readily be detected from the front by using a microscope. Furthermore, these findings suggest that, although the viscoadaptive type of OVD appeared to be effective against physical invasion of the nucleus, it may not be able to prevent microscopic invasions, such as by free radicals and cavitation.

Subsequently, the viscous dispersive type of OVD remained as a lump between the corneal endothelium and the phaco tip (Figure 7). However, once the infusion solution flowed between the cornea and the OVD, the OVD detached from the corneal endothelium, thereby indicating that it is likely that this type would be aspirated and removed. Due to the force of infusion flow, the OVD was subsequently pushed again, thereby causing the slit to close.

4. Discussion

A variety of OVDs are available for cataract and intraocular surgeries. As there are many products already on the market, the advantages and disadvantages of each of the OVDs have been previously described [8–12]. However, when dealing

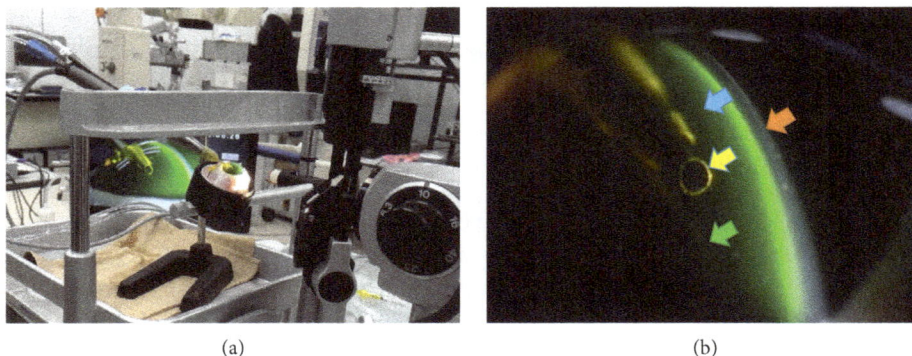

(a)   (b)

FIGURE 1: Laboratory arrangement used in the mechanical and porcine eye experiments: (a) overall picture. (b) Anatomical position in the anterior chamber: cornea (red arrow), OVD stained by fluorescein (blue arrow), US tip (yellow arrow), anterior capsule of the lens (green arrow).

TABLE 1: The viscoelastic types.

Chemical names (brand names)	Viscosity	Composition
Cohesive (Opegan Hi®)	Intrinsic viscosity 25~45 (dL/g)	1% sodium hyaluronate
Dispersive (Shellgan®)	35000~60000 mPa s (25°C, shear rate 2/s)	3% sodium hyaluronate 4% chondroitin sulfate sodium
Viscoadaptive (Healon5®)	Zero shear viscosity: about 7 million (mPa s)	23% sodium hyaluronate
Viscous dispersive (DisCoVisc®)	Viscosity (shear rate 1/s, 25°C): 75000 ± 35000 (mPa s)	1.65% sodium hyaluronate 4% chondriotin sulfate sodium

Viscosity is the commercially published data of each OVDs.

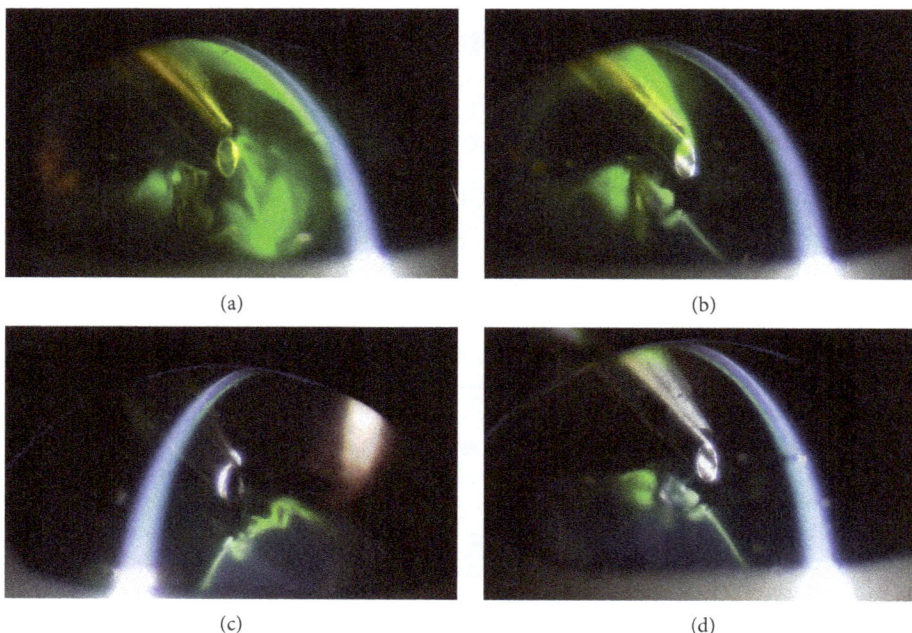

(a)   (b)

(c)   (d)

FIGURE 2: Cohesive type of ophthalmic viscosurgical devices (OVDs): (a) 3 seconds: the moment immediately after depressing the pedal of the pump. (b) 25 seconds: the OVDs are no longer washed out of the anterior chamber. (c) 30 seconds: cross-sectional view of the tip. (d) 90 seconds: the OVDs do not remain on the side of corneal endothelium.

with difficult cases, such as small pupils, corneal endothelium reduction, and shallow anterior chambers, a detailed understanding of the characteristics of these OVDs is necessary. In the eye, however, OVDs are clear and invisible. To overcome this issue, the classic method of staining an OVD with fluorescein has been used to observe dynamic

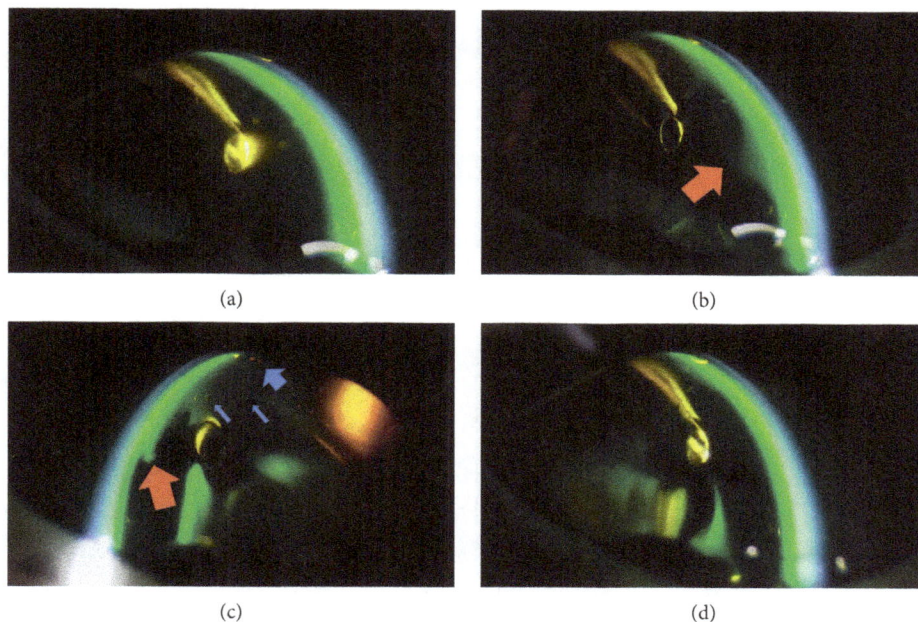

Figure 3: Dispersive type of ophthalmic viscosurgical devices (OVDs): (a) 3 seconds: OVDs remain fully on the corneal endothelium. (b) 25 seconds: the OVDs remain on the side of the anterior chamber side in an irregular shape, as if the OVDs had dripped down the side (arrow). (c) 30 seconds: cross-sectional view of the tip (red arrow indicates OVDs). Air is trapped in the OVD (blue arrow indicates airs). (d) 90 seconds: the OVDs remain on the side of the corneal endothelium.

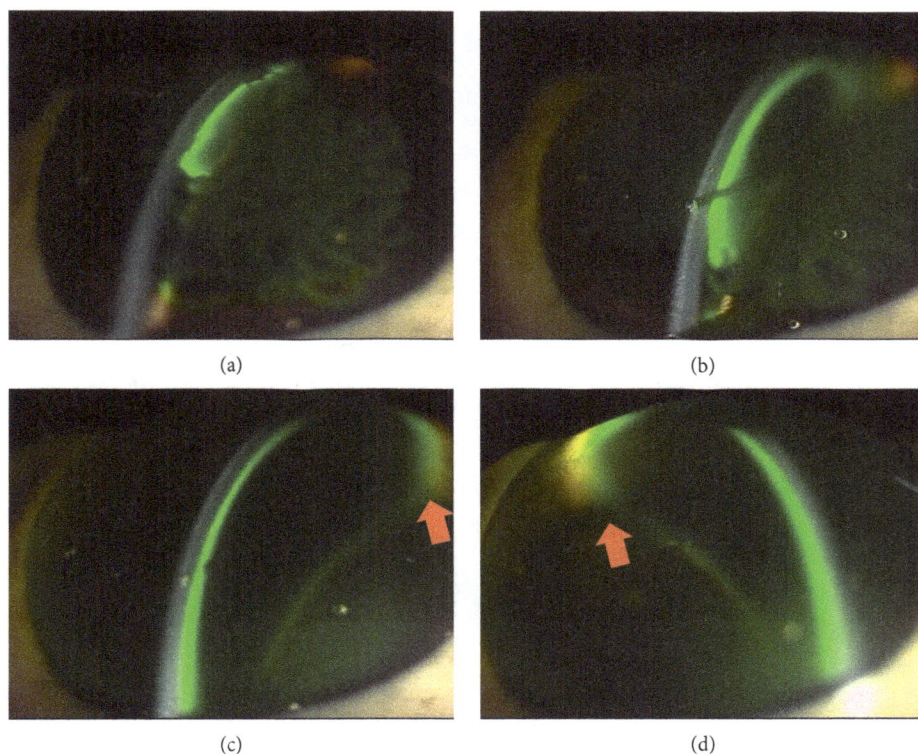

Figure 4: Creation of the soft-shell technique: (a) immediately after injecting the stained dispersive type of ophthalmic viscosurgical devices (OVDs). (b) The clear cohesive types of OVDs were then injected. (c) The dispersive types of OVDs were able to further spread on the corneal endothelial surface and on the anterior surface of the crystalline lens and the iris surface (arrow). (d) Cross-sectional view (arrow indicates OVDs).

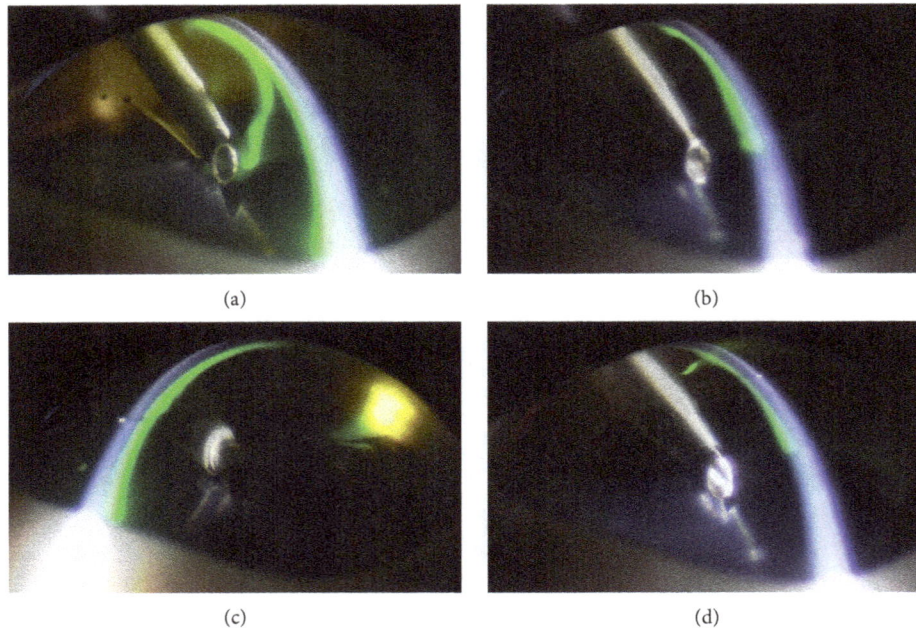

(a)

(b)

(c)

(d)

FIGURE 5: Soft-shell technique: (a) 3 seconds: after the application of ultrasound, the cohesive types of ophthalmic viscosurgical devices (OVDs) were immediately aspirated. (b) 25 seconds: the dispersive types of OVDs were retained on the surface of the corneal endothelium. (c) 30 seconds: cross-sectional view of the tip. (d) 90 seconds: dispersive types of OVDs formed a layer with a certain thickness on the surface of the corneal endothelium.

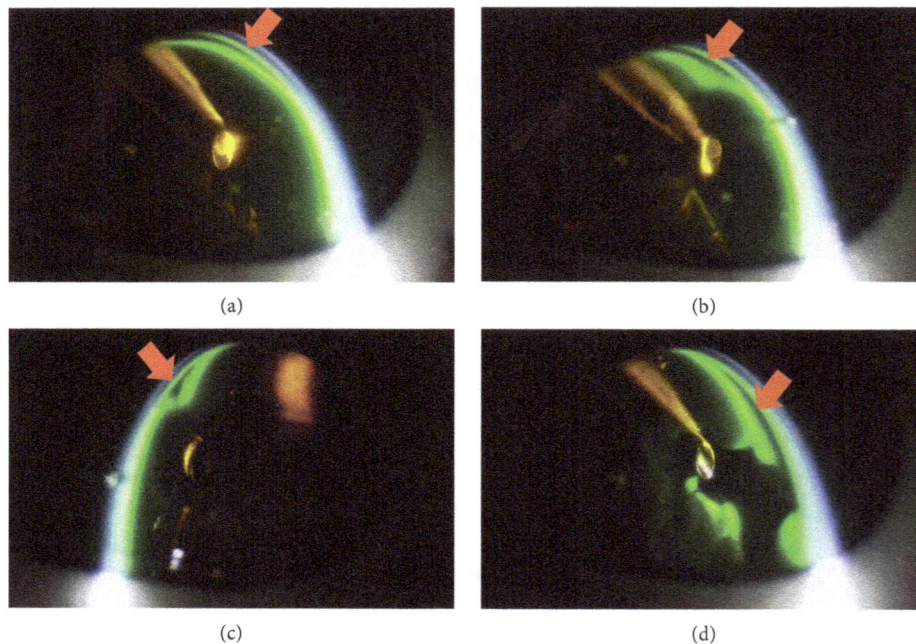

(a)

(b)

(c)

(d)

FIGURE 6: Viscoadaptive type of ophthalmic viscosurgical devices (OVDs): (a) 3 seconds: there is a clear gap between the corneal endothelium and the OVDs (arrow). (b) 25 seconds: the gap remains (arrow). (c) 30 seconds: cross-sectional view of the tip (arrow indicates gap). (d) 90 seconds: the range of the gap has expanded (arrow).

changes in clinical and experimental studies [13]. Bissen-Miyajima reported that the use of a side-view camera (Handycam, DCR-PC300K, Sony), in addition to a surgical microscope, helped to discriminate the three-dimensional movement of the stained OVDs [14]. While this method is very useful, it is difficult to observe the cross section between the corneal endothelium and the phaco tip in detail. Holmén and Lundgren have reported that the use of a surgical microscope for the anterior segment analysis system (EAS-1000, Nidek Co., Ltd.) enabled comparison of the anterior

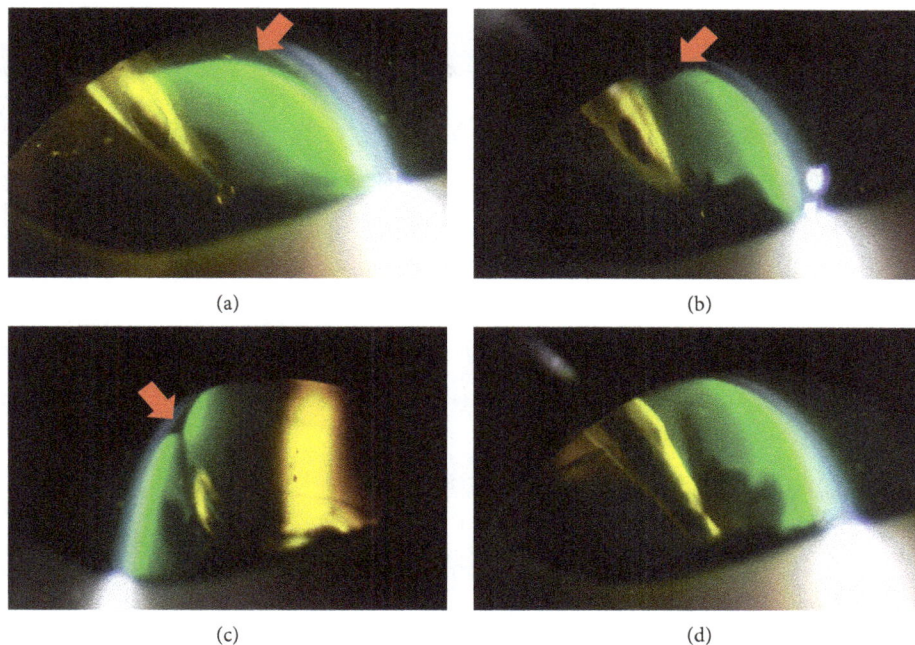

FIGURE 7: Viscous dispersive type of ophthalmic viscosurgical devices (OVDs): (a) 3 seconds: there is a clear gap between the corneal endothelium and the OVDs (arrow). (b) 25 seconds: the gap remains (arrow). (c) 30 seconds: cross-sectional view of the tip (arrow indicates gap). (d) 90 seconds: The perfusion has pressed the OVDs, and the gap is closed.

chamber depth maintenance and retention capacities of the commercially available OVDs, within a porcine cadaver eye model during simulated phacoemulsification [15]. Although results obtained by this method allow better understanding of the retention of OVDs in the anterior chamber with partial observation, it remains impossible to analyze fluid dynamics and retention of OVDs in the anterior chamber during cataract surgery. The use of our new SSV method enables better understanding of the properties and characteristics of the OVDs along with the flow of fluids; thus, these findings can be used in actual clinical situations.

In the first step of our study, we examined several OVDs to better understand their characteristics. After depressing the pedal of the phacoemulsification machine, the cohesive types of OVDs were immediately aspirated. While this result demonstrates that this type of OVD can only provide minimal corneal-endothelial protective effects, it also indicates that these OVDs can be easily removed after inserting the intraocular lens. Furthermore, these OVDs are advantageous in terms of preventing increased intraocular pressure and infections after surgery. Additionally, we discovered that the dispersive type of OVD could only be aspirated gradually, with some of the OVD remaining as an irregular shape on the side of the anterior chamber, appearing almost as if the OVD had dripped down the sides of the chamber. This sort of shape enables the OVD to trap the air (Figure 3(c)); thus, the OVD can prevent the air from directly touching the corneal endothelium. Therefore, we believe that this type of OVD could provide strong corneal endothelial protective effects. However, if the nucleus and air is trapped, then a drop in visibility may occur. For example, in clinical situations that use the dispersive type of OVD,

trapped nucleus fragments that have adhered cannot be directly removed by the tip. However, they can be detached by infusion flow, so they can be processed under conditions that have a minimal influence on the corneal endothelium. Thus, using SSV to help determine and better understand the characteristics of the OVDs is beneficial for the overall clinical procedure.

Arshinoff reported that the soft-shell technique, which uses different types of viscoelastic substances, ranging from cohesive to dispersive, can be used to protect the corneal endothelium during phacoemulsification [7]. Furthermore, Arshinoff showed that the soft-shell technique can greatly facilitate cataract surgery by using the best properties of the higher-viscosity cohesive and lower-viscosity dispersive viscoelastic agents, while eliminating the disadvantages of both. By using our SSV methodology, we were able to confirm the advantages of this technique. When performing the soft-shell technique, a dispersive type of OVD is first injected, followed by a cohesive type. In our current experiment, pressure from the cohesive type of OVD caused the dispersive type of OVD to spread on the corneal endothelial surface, the anterior surface of the crystalline lens, and even further on the iris surface. After the application of US, the cohesive types of OVDs were immediately aspirated. However, since the dispersive types of OVDs had formed a layer of various thicknesses on the surface of the corneal endothelium, it was possible to retain these OVDs over a long period of time [5]. Comparing to the dispersive OVD alone, the soft-shell technique is thought to be better in the coating effect on the corneal endothelium because in the soft-shell technique, the cohesive OVD can push the dispersive OVD equally against the corneal endothelium as shown in Figures 3 and 5. These findings appear to confirm the results of the clinical studies of Miyata et al. [16], who reported that the soft-shell technique was superior regarding protection of the corneal endothelium. In both the viscoadaptive and viscous dispersive types of OVDs, the infusion solution flowed between the corneal endothelium and the OVD. Typically, this finding cannot be readily detected from the front by the use of a normal surgical microscope. As a result, if a problem with the irrigation occurs, this may cause corneal endothelium dysfunction. Therefore, regarding protection of the corneal endothelium, this finding suggests that it is important to know the direction of the irrigation during surgery. From that point of view, similar analysis on the effect of irrigation/aspiration without US oscillation should be done in the future study.

Furthermore, it is necessary to investigate whether the direction of the infusion solution can affect the residual OVD. However, since we confirmed that these two OVDs remained in the anterior chamber as a lump, it is possible that they might serve as physical obstacles and prevent collision with the nucleus [17].

5. Conclusions

The SSV method enables us to follow the movement of OVD during surgery and to observe changes in the anterior chamber in accordance with the machine settings. Therefore, this method has the potential to serve as an outstanding evaluation technique that can be used to help perform safe ocular surgery. In this experiment, the US tip is fixed, whereas in the clinical setting, the US tip is mobile. In the next experiment, it is necessary to study the dynamics of OVD in the anterior chamber when the US tip is moved.

Disclosure

This study was presented as a video, "Observation of anterior chamber with a slit lamp microscope during cataract surgery," at these annual meetings. (1) 36th ASCRS Film Festival, Best of the Best Winner, Quality Teaching ASCRS symposium Los Angeles, California, USA, May 5–9, 2017. (2) APACRS Film Festival, Grand Prize Winner, 30th APACRS Annual Meeting Hangzhou, China, June 1–3, 2017. (3) 2017 Video Competition, 2nd Prize, Scientific Category, 35th ESCRS Annual Congress Lisbon, Portugal, October 7–11, 2017: http://player.escrs.org/video-of-the-month/observation-of-anterior-chamber-with-a-slitlamp-microscope-during-cataract-surgery.

Conflicts of Interest

The authors declare that they have no conflicts of interest.

References

[1] H. Takahashi, "Free radical development in phacoemulsification cataract surgery," *Journal of Nippon Medical School*, vol. 72, no. 1, pp. 4–12, 2005.

[2] D. M. Stănilă, A. M. Florea, A. Stănilă, and A. A. Panga, "Endothelial cells loss to the hyperopic patients during phacoemulsification," *Romanian Journal of Ophthalmology*, vol. 61, no. 4, pp. 256–260, 2017.

[3] E. K. Kim, S. M. Cristol, S. J. Kang, H. F. Edelhauser, D.-S. Yeon, and J. B. Lee, "Viscoelastic protection from endothelial damage by air bubbles," *Journal of Cataract and Refractive Surgery*, vol. 28, no. 3, pp. 531–537, 2002.

[4] P. K. Sahu, G. K. Das, S. Agrawal, S. Kumar, and N. Kumar, "Comparative evaluation of corneal endothelium in diabetic patients undergoing phacoemulsification," *Middle East African Journal of Ophthalmology*, vol. 24, no. 4, pp. 195–201, 2017.

[5] F. T. A. Kretz, I.-J. Limberger, and G. U. Auffarth, "Corneal endothelial cell coating during phacoemulsification using a new dispersive hyaluronic acid ophthalmic viscosurgical device," *Journal of Cataract and Refractive Surgery*, vol. 40, no. 11, pp. 1879–1884, 2014.

[6] H. Suzuki, K. Oki, T. Shiwa, H. Oharazawa, and H. Takahashi, "Effect of bottle height on the corneal endothelium during phacoemulsification," *Journal of Cataract and Refractive Surgery*, vol. 35, no. 11, pp. 2014–2017, 2009.

[7] S. A. Arshinoff, "Dispersive-cohesive viscoelastic soft shell technique," *Journal of Cataract and Refractive Surgery*, vol. 25, no. 2, pp. 167–173, 1999.

[8] F. H. Hengerer, H. B. Dick, T. Kohnen, and I. Conrad-Hengerer, "Assessment of intraoperative complications in intumescent cataract surgery using 2 ophthalmic viscosurgical devices and trypan blue staining," *Journal of Cataract and Refractive Surgery*, vol. 41, no. 4, pp. 714–718, 2015.

[9] T. Oshika, S. Eguchi, and K. Oki, "Clinical comparison of healon5 and healon in phacoemulsification and intraocular lens implantation; randomized multicenter study," *Journal of Cataract and Refractive Surgery*, vol. 30, no. 2, pp. 357–362, 2004.

[10] H. Suzuki, K. Oki, T. Igarashi, T. Shiwa, and H. Takahashi, "Temperature in the anterior chamber during phacoemulsification," *Journal of Cataract and Refractive Surgery*, vol. 40, no. 5, pp. 805–810, 2014.

[11] H. Suzuki, T. Igarashi, T. Shiwa, and H. Takahashi, "Efficacy of ophthalmic viscosurgical devices in preventing temperature rise at the corneal endothelium during phacoemulsification," *Current Eye Research*, vol. 41, no. 12, pp. 1548–1552, 2016.

[12] S. A. Arshinoff and R. Norman, "Tri-soft shell technique," *Journal of Cataract and Refractive Surgery*, vol. 39, no. 8, pp. 1196–1203, 2013.

[13] K. Masuda, S. Imaizumi, T. Sakaue et al., "Clinical evaluation of sodium hyaluronate containing fluorescein sodium in intraocular lens implantation," *Japanese Review of Clinical Ophthalmology*, vol. 86, pp. 320–328, 1992.

[14] H. Bissen-Miyajima, "In vitro behavior of ophthalmic viscosurgical devices during phacoemulsification," *Journal of Cataract and Refractive Surgery*, vol. 32, no. 6, pp. 1026–1031, 2006.

[15] J. J. Holmén and B. Lundgren, "Scheimpflug photography study of ophthalmic viscosurgical devices during simulated cataract surgery," *Journal of Cataract and Refractive Surgery*, vol. 29, no. 3, pp. 568–574, 2003.

[16] K. Miyata, T. Nagamoto, S. Maruoka, T. Tanabe, M. Nakahara, and S. Amano, "Efficacy and safety of the soft-shell technique

9

The Effects of Uncomplicated Cataract Surgery on Retinal Layer Thickness

Ali Kurt ⓘ **and Raşit Kılıç** ⓘ

Department of Ophthalmology, Faculty of Medicine, Ahi Evran University, Kırşehir, Turkey

Correspondence should be addressed to Ali Kurt; dralikurt@gmail.com

Academic Editor: Marcel Menke

Purpose. Our aim was to assess changes in the total retinal thickness (TRT), total retinal volume (TRV), and retinal layer thickness after uncomplicated cataract surgery. *Methods*. A total of 32 eyes of 32 patients who had undergone uncomplicated phaco-emulsification surgery and intraocular lens implantation in one eye were enrolled. Effective phacoemulsification time (EPT) and total energy (TE) were recorded. Thickness and TRV were measured using optical coherence tomography. Data were collected preoperatively and at postoperative day 1, 7, 30, 90, and 180. *Results*. The study results showed a decrease in TRT, TRV, and most retinal layer thicknesses at the first postoperative day visit and then increasing at week 1, and months 1 and 3, and then relatively decreasing at month 6 although not returning to preoperative levels. The least affected layers were the retinal pigment epithelium and outer plexiform layer. There was a positive correlation between EPT and TE and ganglion cell layer in a 1 mm circle and inner nuclear layer in a 1–3 mm circle ($p < 0.05$). *Conclusion*. The results suggest that long-term follow-up of more than 6 months is necessary after cataract surgery to see whether total retinal and segmental values return to preoperative levels. This study was registered with Australian New Zealand Clinical Trials Registry (ANZCTR): ACTRN12618000763246.

1. Introduction

Cataract is the most common preventable cause of vision loss worldwide. Pseudophakic cystoid macular edema (PCME), known as Irvine–Gass syndrome, is one of the most common complications after cataract surgery. It is generally subclinical in most cases and rarely causes vision loss. Although the incidence of clinical PCME has decreased with small incision cataract surgery and phacoemulsification (PE), it can still cause unexpected vision loss [1]. The exact pathophysiology of PCME is not fully understood but seems to be related to the inflammation triggered by surgery. The inflammatory cytokines and mediators break down the blood-retina barrier and result in increased vascular permeability and cystoid macular edema [2, 3]. Other factors such as posterior capsule rupture, vitreous loss, retained lens fragments, vitreomacular traction, and iris trauma after complicated surgery can also increase the PCME incidence [1–3].

PCME is most commonly seen 4–6 weeks after surgery [1–3]. Fundus fluorescein angiography (FFA) reveals capillary dilatation, leakage from the foveal capillaries, and developing petalloid appearance. Optical coherence tomography (OCT) is a noninvasive device which enables detection of cystic spaces, retinal thickening, and subretinal fluid. OCT also has good repeatability and reproducibility when measuring retinal layer thickness at the macula [4]. It is an excellent method for monitoring disease activity [3].

The current knowledge on the effect of postoperative inflammation on retinal cells and layers is limited. We are not aware of any study assessing the retinal segments to detect the layers that are most affected by cataract surgery with long-term follow-up. The purpose of this study was to evaluate the thickness of each retinal segment quantitatively with spectral domain (SD)-OCT before and after uncomplicated cataract surgery to gain additional information on PCME.

2. Methods

This prospective study was conducted at the Ahi Evran Training and Research Hospital between December 2016 and October 2017. The study was approved by the institutional review board and adhered to the tenets of the Declaration of Helsinki. Informed consent was obtained from all the patients. A total of 43 eyes of 43 Caucasian patients who had undergone uncomplicated cataract surgery and posterior chamber intraocular lens implantation were included. Eleven patients were excluded due to the lack of follow-up examinations, and the study was finally conducted on the 32 eyes of 32 patients. The visual acuity was evaluated with a Snellen chart, and a detailed biomicroscopic anterior and posterior segment examination was performed with pupillary dilatation. Air puff tonometry was used to measure the intraocular pressure. The axial length was measured using optical low-coherence reflectometry (Lenstar LS 900, Haag-Streit AG, Koeniz, Switzerland). Best corrected visual acuity was 2/20 and higher in all patients preoperatively.

Exclusion criteria consisted of macular pathologies, retinal vascular occlusion, history of any other ocular disorders (including uveitis, severe dry eye, eye trauma, glaucoma, and pseudoexfoliation syndrome) or surgery, any systemic disorders (such as diabetes, hypertension, asthma, or chronic obstructive pulmonary disease), systemic inflammation (inflammatory bowel disease and hepatitis B or C), the current use of any topical or systemic medication or anti-inflammatory agent, and intraoperative complications such as posterior capsular rupture, vitreous loss, iris prolapse, and low scan quality images due to dense cataract.

Cataract surgery was performed with the Infiniti PE device (Alcon Inc., Forth Worth, TX, USA) using a torsional handpiece. The stop and chop technique was used in all cases. Effective phaco time and phaco energy were recorded. Postoperatively, all patients were prescribed topical moxifloxacin and dexamethasone four times a day for three weeks and Nevanac three times a day for four weeks. The same author (AK) performed all surgeries and examinations.

2.1. OCT Scan Protocol.
All subjects underwent pupillary dilatation with 1% tropicamide and 2.5% phenylephrine hydrochloride eye drops prior to imaging. We used the SD-OCT, Spectralis (Heidelberg Engineering, Heidelberg, Germany) device with software version 6.3.3.0 in this study as it has a higher repeatability index [4]. OCT imaging was carried out using the following parameters: $20° \times 15°$ degrees $(5.9 \times 4.4\,mm)$, automatic real-time averaging of 100 frames, 19 horizontal sections at $240\,\mu m$ intervals, and 512 A-scans per B-scan. We only included images with a quality higher than 15 dB in the study. The image acquisition was followed by automatic intraretinal layer segmentation performed by the inbuilt Spectralis software to include the retinal nerve fiber layer (RNFL), ganglion cell layer (GCL), inner plexiform layer (IPL), inner nuclear layer (INL), outer plexiform layer (OPL), outer nuclear layer (ONL), retina pigment epithelium (RPE), total retinal volume (TRV), and total retina thickness (TRT) (Figure 1). Intraretinal layer thicknesses were obtained for

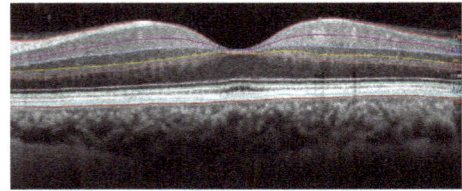

FIGURE 1: Borders of automatically segmented retinal layers on OCT images. ILM, internal limiting membrane and inner border of the RNFL layer; RNFL, outer border of the retinal nerve fiber layer; GCL, outer border of the ganglion cell layer; IPL, outer border of the inner plexiform layer; INL, outer border of the inner nuclear layer; OPL, outer border of the outer nuclear layer; ELM, external limiting membrane—outer border of the outer nuclear layer; RPE, retina pigment epithelium; BM, Bruch's membrane.

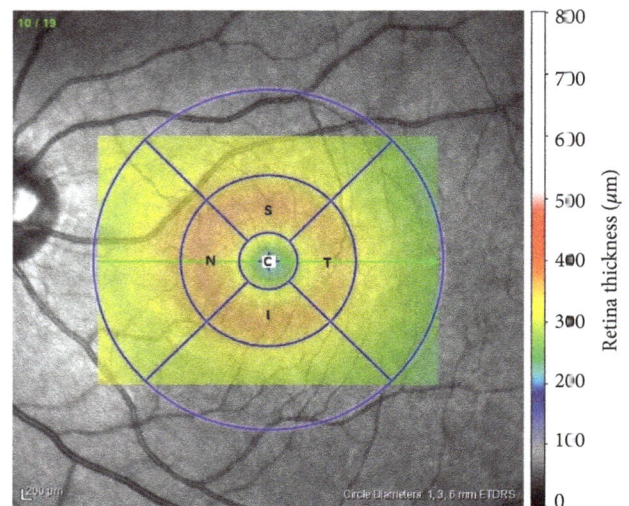

FIGURE 2: ETDRS grid for 1 mm and 1–3 mm circles on OCT images. ETDRS grid on macula. C, central 1 mm zone in macula; S, superior quadrant in 1–3 mm circle on macula; I, inferior quadrant in 1–3 mm circle on macula; T, temporal quadrant in 1–3 mm circle on macula; N, nasal quadrant in 1–3 mm circle on macula.

each ETDRS subfield at a central 1 mm circle and 1–3 mm circles that included the superior, temporal, inferior, and nasal subfields (Figure 2). The first Spectralis scan was set as a reference image, and the images during future visits were acquired with real-time image registration by follow-up mode by the ophthalmologist. The ETDRS grid was centered on the fovea manually if it was not positioned correctly automatically. We also checked the accuracy of retinal layer segmentation in every patient. The 3–6 mm subfields were not included as it exceeded the area of our imaging angle. Data were collected preoperatively and on postoperative day 1, 7 (first week), 30 (first month), 90 (third month), and 180 (sixth month). The mean thickness of the 1 mm and 1–3 mm rings was calculated and used for further statistical analysis.

2.2. Statistical Analysis.
The IBM SPSS version 20.0 (IBM Corporation, Armonk, NY, USA) software was used for statistical analyses. Measured data were described as the

TABLE 1: Thickness of macula TRT, TRV, and retinal layers with at the ETDRS circle of 1 and 3 millimeters.

		Preoperative	Postoperative day 1	Postoperative week 1	Postoperative month 1	Postoperative month 3	Postoperative month 6	p
TRT	1 mm circle	276.63 ± 27.36	272.14 ± 26.12*	274.85 ± 26.74	279.81 ± 25.80	280.65 ± 26.82*	277.85 ± 26.22	<0.001
	3 mm circle	332.25 ± 14.66	327.27 ± 13.78*	332.81 ± 13.99	337.31 ± 13.21*	337.95 ± 14.24*	337.01 ± 14.59*	<0.001
TRV	1 mm circle	0.2167 ± 0.0215	0.2143 ± 0.0201	0.2167 ± 0.0203	0.2205 ± 0.0201*	0.2214 ± 0.0208*	0.2186 ± 0.0206	<0.001
	3 mm circle	0.5237 ± 0.0241	0.5170 ± 0.0240*	0.5252 ± 0.0231	0.5315 ± 0.0224*	0.5332 ± 0.0238*	0.5315 ± 0.0246*	<0.001
RPE	1 mm circle	15.15 ± 2.20	14.70 ± 1.72	15.30 ± 1.97	15.25 ± 1.86	15.20 ± 2.14	15.45 ± 2.03	0.453
	3 mm circle	14.26 ± 1.61	13.75 ± 1.81	14.02 ± 1.60	14.40 ± 1.72	14.03 ± 1.94	14.13 ± 1.39	0.042**
ONL	1 mm circle	88.32 ± 13.96	86.26 ± 14.29	91.58 ± 10.09	91.05 ± 14.20	92.26 ± 12.55	91.32 ± 13.83	<0.001***
	3 mm circle	70.13 ± 7.83	68.86 ± 7.60	71.68 ± 6.74	72.63 ± 7.87	73.85 ± 7.88*	73.31 ± 7.58*	<0.001
OPL	1 mm circle	26.26 ± 7.10	26.58 ± 6.00	23.63 ± 4.87	26.05 ± 6.38	25.74 ± 5.07	25.37 ± 6.31	0.144
	3 mm circle	32.11 ± 2.67	31.07 ± 3.07	29.51 ± 2.51*	30.20 ± 2.59	30.23 ± 2.86	29.64 ± 2.27*	0.001
INL	1 mm circle	24.16 ± 8.20	24.21 ± 9.63	23.42 ± 8.60	24.16 ± 8.40	24.21 ± 8.03	24.26 ± 9.36	0.881
	3 mm circle	40.64 ± 3.71	40.27 ± 4.33*	41.56 ± 4.10*	41.55 ± 4.63*	41.94 ± 4.52*	42.36 ± 4.73*	<0.001
IPL	1 mm circle	23.37 ± 7.41	22.26 ± 6.40	22.47 ± 7.47	23.26 ± 7.26	23.16 ± 7.82	23.47 ± 7.31	0.055
	3 mm circle	39.94 ± 3.23	39.63 ± 3.05	40.63 ± 3.41	41.05 ± 3.49*	41.05 ± 3.51*	41.48 ± 3.83*	<0.001
GCL	1 mm circle	18.58 ± 10.65	18.32 ± 10.84	18.95 ± 10.63	19.00 ± 11.23	18.95 ± 10.12	18.63 ± 11.10	0.298
	3 mm circle	47.98 ± 5.42	47.55 ± 5.30	48.93 ± 5.21	49.61 ± 5.26*	49.88 ± 5.40*	49.65 ± 5.36*	<0.001
NFL	1 mm circle	13.20 ± 2.82	13.35 ± 3.45	13.40 ± 3.53	13.45 ± 3.80	14.05 ± 4.38	13.20 ± 3.31	0.525
	3 mm circle	21.96 ± 1.62	22.13 ± 1.87	22.69 ± 1.66*	23.02 ± 1.82*	22.96 ± 1.77*	22.59 ± 1.50	<0.001

TRT, total retinal thickness; TRV, total retinal volume; RPE, retinal pigment epithelium; ONL, outer nuclear layer; OPL, outer plexiform layer; INL, inner nuclear layer; IPL, inner plexiform layer; GCL, ganglion cell layer; RNFL, retinal nerve fiber layer. *Difference with preoperative measurement statistically significant using the Bonferroni correction. **The differences between the mean RPE values were significant according to repeated measure results, but the Bonferroni test did not reveal a significant change. ***The Bonferroni test did not reveal a significant change between the preoperative and postoperative mean ONL values. However, the decrease in the mean value in the postoperative first day has resulted in a significant difference between the mean first day value and the mean 3rd month value with Bonferroni correction.

TABLE 2: The effect of EPT and TE on GCL and INL.

ETDRS circle		1st day	1st week	1st month	3rd month	6th month
1 mm circle	EPT versus GCL	$p = 0.021\ r = 0.511$	$p = 0.039\ r = 0.443$	$p = 0.038\ r = 0.467$	$p = 0.034\ r = 0.501$	$p = 0.076\ r = 0.406$
	TE versus GCL	$p = 0.026\ r = 0.495$	$p = 0.047\ r = 0.427$	$p = 0.025\ r = 0.499$	$p = 0.025\ r = 0.525$	$p = 0.078\ r = 0.403$
3 mm circle	EPT versus INL	$p = 0.027\ r = 0.494$	$p = 0.044\ r = 0.433$	$p = 0.014\ r = 0.538$	$p = 0.084\ r = 0.418$	$p = 0.025\ r = 0.500$
	TE versus INL	$p = 0.004\ r = 0.614$	$p = 0.011\ r = 0.528$	$p = 0.003\ r = 0.634$	$p = 0.027\ r = 0.520$	$p = 0.003\ r = 0.627$

EPT, effective phaco time; GCL, ganglion cell layer; TE, total energy; INL, inner nuclear layer.

arithmetic mean ± standard deviation, whereas categorical data were described as percentages (%). Normal distribution of measured data was examined by the Kolmogorov–Smirnov test. The one-way ANOVA test was used for intergroup comparison variables for repeated measures. The Bonferroni method was used to correct the p value. The relationship between EPT and TE and all thickness parameters were analyzed with the Pearson correlation analysis. A statistical level of significance was accepted at $p < 0.05$.

3. Results

The mean age of the patients consisting of 25 (78%) males and 7 (22%) females was 63.81 ± 9.0 years (range: 48–79 years). There were 20 right and 12 left eyes. The mean preoperative axial length was 23.62 ± 0.9 mm (range: 21.3–25.2 mm). The cataract type was nuclear sclerosis in 16 (50%) cases, posterior subcapsular in 12 (37.5%) cases, cortical in 3 (9.4%) cases, and cortical + posterior subcapsular in one (3.1%) case.

We found statistically significant differences in TRT and TRV in the 1 mm circle and TRT, TRV, ONL, OPL, INL, IPL GCL, and NFL in the 1–3 mm circle compared to the

preoperative values during the follow-up visits continuing for 6 months ($p < 0.05$). The study results showed a remarkable decrease in TRT, TRV, and the thickness of most retinal layers at the first day visit after surgery. However, an increase was then observed in all parameters and reached approximately the preoperative values at the first week visit. The thickest TRT and retinal layer thickness values were observed at the first and third month visits. A slight decrease, not reaching the preoperative levels, was then seen in almost all parameters at the sixth month visit. We also noticed that the least affected layers were the RPE and OPL. The results are presented in Table 1.

The mean effective phacoemulsification time and total energy were 62.46 ± 45.03 seconds and 6.41 ± 7.34, respectively. There was a positive correlation between EPT and TE and GCL in the 1 mm circle and INL in the 1–3 mm circle ($p < 0.05$ and Table 2). There was no significant correlation between EPT and TE and other retinal layers, TRT and TRV ($p > 0.05$).

4. Discussion

The main triggering factor of PCME is thought to be surgical trauma of intraocular tissues by inducing the release of inflammatory mediators although other possible mechanisms such as photic retinopathy or vitreous traction have also been implicated [5]. Inflammatory mediators (prostaglandins, cytokines, and other vascular permeability factors) are known to be released from the anterior segment of the eye after surgery and then diffuse into the vitreous cavity and retina, stimulating the breakdown of the blood-retinal barrier (BRB) and subsequent leakage of fluids across the retinal vessel wall and into the perifoveal retinal tissues, resulting in macular edema [3]. This edema usually resolves spontaneously and only about 1–3% of cases persist, corresponding to clinical PCME with persistent symptoms [6]. Although FFA used to be considered the diagnostic gold standard for PCME, OCT is now the method of choice, being a noninvasive technique for PCME evaluation and follow-up [3].

Optical coherence tomography is a useful device to detect intraretinal cysts that indicate clinical PCME and can decrease vision noninvasively after cataract surgery [3]. Assessing the retinal layers in vivo may provide more information to elucidate the pathologic processes involved in subclinical PCME. We therefore evaluated retinal layers by OCT after uncomplicated cataract surgery and presented long-term follow-up results on TRT, TRV, and retinal layer thickness according to the ETDRS grid. We noticed that the RPE and OPL were the least affected layers. In general, we observed a decrease in TRT, TRV, and most retinal layers at the first postoperative day visit. An increase was then seen in all thickness parameters and reached approximately the preoperative levels at the first week visit. The largest TRT and retinal layer thickness values were observed at the first and third month visits. At the sixth month visit, a slight decrease was seen in almost all parameters. However, this decrease did not reach preoperative thickness levels. There was a significant thickness increase in all retinal layers except RPE and OPL in the 1–3 mm circle.

Grewing and Becker measured the retinal thickness before and 0.5 hours after cataract surgery in 10 patients and reported a decrease that was not statistically significant [7]. We noticed a decrease in TRT, TRV, and the thickness of most retinal layers after the first postoperative day. Perente et al. [8] also reported a mild postoperative retinal thickness that was not statistically significant. According to the authors, the decrease observed in the first postoperative day may be related to the previous light-scattering effect of the cataract that was possibly disrupting the optical quality of the OCT imaging [8]. However, there is not enough evidence or information in the literature to fully explain the cause.

Šiško et al. [9] reported highest retinal thickness in the ETDRS grid areas one month after uncomplicated cataract surgery. They also stated mild decreasing trend in the measurements from the first month to the sixth month, without reaching preoperative levels. Most studies have reported an increase in macular thickness after uncomplicated cataract surgery [8, 10–16]. Gharbiya et al. [10] reported a significant macular thickness increase for up to six postoperative months in 40 healthy patients. Falcão et al. [11] also found increased central macular thickness postoperatively and reported this as a nonpathological change. Cagini et al. [12] found an asymptomatic postoperative

macular thickness increase at 12 weeks in 62 eyes with a follow-up period of 28 weeks. These results are all similar to ours. Gołebiewska et al. [17] reported increased retinal thickness and retinal volume during follow-up continuing for 6 months after uncomplicated cataract surgery. We observed increased retinal volume after surgery, like others.

Measuring each retinal layer separately makes it easier to see alteration in retinal structures than the TRT. It is unclear which retinal layer(s) has the most effect on increasing the retinal thickness. We found an increase in the thickness of NFL, GCL, IPL, INL, and ONL and a decrease in OPL, but these changes were only significant in the 1–3 mm circle at the postoperative sixth month follow-up when compared to the preoperative measurements. RPE thicknesses were generally stable except for the first visit, but this first-visit change was not significant. We found increased GCL thickness in the 1 mm circle and INL thickness in the 1–3 mm circle with more TE and EPT. Another study reported a statistically significant relationship between increased retinal thickness and higher perioperative phaco power [17]. However, there is no study comparing postoperative retinal layer thickness with TE and EPT values.

The INL includes the nuclei of the bipolar, horizontal, amacrine, and Muller cells. The deep capillary plexus is also in this layer. Park et al. [18] have shown that the vascular endothelial growth factor (VEGF) has a crucial role in the vitality of the amacrine and bipolar cells. Sigler et al. [19] have reported cystic changes in the INL and ONL in patients with clinical PCME. We did not find clinical PCME and therefore did not observe cystic changes in any of our patients; an increased thickness of the INL may be related to the inflammatory effects of VEGF, which is an inflammatory mediator [20]. INL thickness was also increased in relation to optic neuritis, which is an inflammatory disease in another study [21]. In the neurology literature, the use of INL as a parameter to monitor the efficacy of anti-inflammatory treatments in multiple sclerosis has been proposed [22]. The superficial capillary plexus is located in the NFL, and its hyperpermeability may have been responsible for the significantly increased thickness of the NFL and GCL in our study.

Nepafenac (Alcon Research Ltd., Fort Worth, TX USA), a topical ocular nonsteroidal anti-inflammatory drug (NSAID) used to treat the pain and inflammation associated with cataract surgery, is available as an ophthalmic suspension in concentrations of 0.1% and 0.3% [23]. Unlike other NSAIDs, nepafenac is a prodrug that is deaminated to its active metabolite (amfenac) in the ocular tissues. It is a potent inhibitor of the cyclooxygenase (COX) isoforms COX-1 and COX-2 and is distributed rapidly in both the anterior and posterior segments of the eye. It is well known that the retinal thickness increase is significantly lower in patients administered an NSAID after cataract surgery [23, 24]. It may therefore be better to avoid NSAID use when evaluating retinal layer thickness after cataract surgery.

Our study has a few limitations. First, the sample size could be larger. Second, the retinal thickness values continued to show a slight decrease at the sixth month visit, and the follow-up should therefore be longer than 6 months.

In conclusion, we presented the six-month follow-up results of TRT, TRV, and retinal layer thickness after uncomplicated cataract surgery in this study. The thickest values were observed at the first and third month visits. A slight decrease without reaching preoperative levels was found in all thickness parameters at the sixth month visit. The postoperative thickness increase was more prominent in the 1–3 mm circle than in the 1 mm circle. On the other hand, OPL was the only retinal layer with decreased thickness after surgery. These findings may be useful for understanding the pathophysiological pathways of PCME. The results suggest that long-term follow-up of more than 6 months is needed to see whether total retinal and segmental changes return to preoperative levels.

Disclosure

The authors declare that the manuscript has not been published previously nor under consideration for publication elsewhere, in whole or in part.

Conflicts of Interest

The authors declare that they have no conflicts of interest.

References

[1] L. Kessel, B. Tendal, K. J. Jørgensen et al., "Post-cataract prevention of inflammation and macular edema by steroid and nonsteroidal anti-inflammatory eye drops: a systematic review," Ophthalmology, vol. 121, no. 10, pp. 1915–1924, 2014.

[2] Y. Yonekawa and I. K. Kim, "Pseudophakic cystoid macular edema," Current Opinion in Ophthalmology, vol. 23, no. 1, pp. 26–32, 2012.

[3] C. Lobo, "Pseudophakic cystoid macular edema," Ophthalmologica, vol. 227, no. 2, pp. 61–67, 2012.

[4] I. Ctori and B. Huntjens, "Repeatability of foveal measurements using spectralis optical coherence tomography segmentation software," PLoS One, vol. 10, no. 6, Article ID e0129005, 2015.

[5] T. Yilmaz, M. Cordero-Coma, and M. J. Gallagher, "Ketorolac therapy for the prevention of acute pseudophakic cystoid macular edema: a systematic review," Eye, vol. 26, no. 2, pp. 252–258, 2012.

[6] L. D. Salomon, "Efficacy of topical flurbiprofen and indomethacin in preventing pseudophakic cystoid macular edema. Flurbiprofen—CME study group I," Journal of Cataract and Refractive Surgery, vol. 21, pp. 73–81, 1995.

[7] R. Grewing and H. Becker, "Retinal thickness immediately after cataract surgery measured by optical coherence tomography," Ophthalmic Surgery and lasers, vol. 31, pp. 215–217, 2000.

[8] I. Perente, C. A. Utine, C. Ozturker et al., "Evaluation of macular changes after uncomplicated phacoemulsification surgery by optical coherence tomography," Current Eye Research, vol. 32, no. 3, pp. 241–247, 2007.

[9] K. Šiško, N. K. Knez, and D. Pahor, "Influence of cataract surgery on macular thickness: a 6-month follow-up," Wiener klinische Wochenschrift, vol. 127, no. 5, pp. S169–S174, 2015.

[10] M. Gharbiya, F. Cruciani, G. Cuozzo, F. Parisi, P. Russo, and S. Abdolrahimzadeh, "Macular thickness changes evaluated with spectral domain optical coherence tomography after uncomplicated phacoemulsification," Eye, vol. 27, no. 5, pp. 605–611, 2013.

[11] M. S. Falcão, N. M. Gonçalves, P. Freitas-Costa et al., "Choroidal and macular thickness changes induced by cataract surgery," Clinical Ophthalmology, vol. 8, pp. 55–60, 2014.

[12] C. Cagini, T. Fiore, B. Iaccheri, F. Piccinelli, M. A. Ricci, and D. Fruttini, "Macular thickness measured by optical coherence tomography in a healthy population before and after uncomplicated cataract phacoemulsification surgery," Current Eye Research, vol. 34, no. 12, pp. 1036–1041, 2009.

[13] S. Nicholas, A. Riley, H. Patel, B. Neveldson, G. Purdie, and A. P. Wells, "Correlations between optical coherence tomography measurement of macular thickness and visual acuity after cataract extraction," Clinical and Experimental Ophthalmology, vol. 34, no. 2, pp. 124–129, 2006.

[14] B. Von Jagow, C. Ohrloff, and T. Kohnen, "Macular thickness after uneventful cataract surgery determined by optical coherence tomography," Graefe's Archive for Clinical and Experimental Ophthalmology, vol. 245, no. 12, pp. 1765–1771, 2007.

[15] Z. Biro, Z. Balla, and B. Kovacs, "Change of foveal and perifoveal thickness measured by OCT after phacoemulsification and IOL implantation," Eye, vol. 22, no. 1, pp. 8–12, 2008.

[16] T. Kusbeci, L. Eryigit, G. Yavas, and U. U. Inan, "Evaluation of cystoid macular edema using optical coherence tomography and fundus fluorescein angiography after uncomplicated phacoemulsification surgery," Current Eye Research, vol. 37, no. 4, pp. 327–333, 2012.

[17] J. Gołebiewska, D. Kęcik, M. Turczyńska, J. Moneta-Wielgoś, D. Kopacz, and K. Pihowicz-Bakoń, "Evaluation of macular thickness after uneventful phacoemulsification in selected patient populations using optical coherence tomography," Klinika Oczna, vol. 116, pp. 242–247, 2014.

[18] H. Y. Park, J. H. Kim, and C. K. Park, "Neuronal cell death in the inner retina and the influence of vascular endothelial growth factor inhibition in a diabetic rat model," American Journal of Pathology, vol. 184, no. 6, pp. 1752–1762, 2014.

[19] E. J. Sigler, J. C. Randolph, and D. F. Kiernan, "Longitudinal analysis of the structural pattern of pseudophakic cystoid macular edema using multimodal imaging," Graefe's Archive for Clinical and Experimental Ophthalmology, vol. 254, no. 1, pp. 43–51, 2016.

[20] Y. B. Shaik-Dasthagirisaheb, G. Varvara, G. Murmura et al., "Vascular endothelial growth factor (VEGF), mast cells and inflammation," International Journal of Immunopathology and Pharmacology, vol. 26, no. 2, pp. 327–335, 2013.

[21] M. Kaushik, C. Y. Wang, M. H. Barnett et al., "Inner nuclear layer thickening is inversely proportional to retinal ganglion cell loss in optic neuritis," PLoS One, vol. 8, no. 10, Article ID e78341, 2013.

[22] B. Knier, P. Schmidt, L. Aly et al., "Retinal inner nuclear layer volume reflects response to immunotherapy in multiple sclerosis," Brain, vol. 139, no. 11, pp. 2855–2863, 2016.

[23] R. P. Singh, G. Staurenghi, A. Pollack et al., "Efficacy of nepafenac ophthalmic suspension 0.1% in improving clinical outcomes following cataract surgery in patients with diabetes: an analysis of two randomized studies," Clinical Ophthalmology, vol. 11, pp. 1021–1029, 2017.

[24] J. E. Chastain, M. E. Sanders, M. A. Curtis et al., "Distribution of topical ocular nepafenac and its active metabolite amfenac to the posterior segment of the eye," Experimental Eye Research, vol. 145, pp. 58–67, 2016.

10

Lanosterol Synthase Pathway Alleviates Lens Opacity in Age-Related Cortical Cataract

Xinyue Shen,[1,2] Manhui Zhu,[1,3] Lihua Kang ⓘ,[1] Yuanyuan Tu,[1] Lele Li,[1] Rutan Zhang,[4] Bai Qin,[1] Mei Yang,[1] and Huaijin Guan ⓘ[1]

[1]*Department of Ophthalmology, Affiliated Hospital of Nantong University, Nantong, Jiangsu 226001, China*
[2]*Department of Ophthalmology, Wuxi No. 3 People's Hospital, Wuxi, Jiangsu 214041, China*
[3]*Department of Ophthalmology, Lixiang Eye Hospital of Soochow University, Suzhou 215021, China*
[4]*Department of Chemistry, Fudan University, Shanghai 200433, China*

Correspondence should be addressed to Huaijin Guan; guanhjeye@163.com

Academic Editor: Van C. Lansingh

Purpose. Lanosterol synthase (LSS) abnormity contributes to lens opacity in rats, mice, dogs, and human congenital cataract development. This study examined whether LSS pathway has a role in different subtypes of age-related cataract (ARC). *Methods.* A total of 390 patients with ARC and 88 age-matched non-ARC patients were enrolled in this study. LSS expression was analyzed by western blot and enzyme-linked immunosorbent assay (ELISA). To further examine the function of LSS, we used U18666A, an LSS inhibitor in rat lens culture system. *Results.* In lens epithelial cells (LECs), LSS expression in LECs increased with opaque degree C II, while it decreased with opaque degree C IV and C V. While in the cortex of age-related cortical cataract (ARCC), LSS expression was negatively related to opaque degree, while lanosterol level was positively correlated to opaque degree. No obvious change in both LSS and lanosterol level was found in either LECs or the cortex of age-related nuclear cataract (ARNC) and age-related posterior subcapsular cataract (ARPSC). In vitro, inhibiting LSS activity induced rat lens opacity and lanosterol effectively delayed the occurrence of lens opacity. *Conclusions.* This study indicated that LSS and lanosterol were localized in the lens of human ARC, including ARCC, ARNC, and ARPSC. LSS and lanosterol level are only correlated with opaque degree of ARCC. Furthermore, activated LSS pathway in lens is protective for lens transparency in cortical cataract.

1. Introduction

Cataract is one of the leading causes of blindness worldwide and cataract is the major cause of blindness in developing countries, including China [1, 2]. The clinical characteristic of cataract is lenticular opacity and the final visual impairment. Age-related cataract (ARC) is the most common type [3, 4]. According to different region of opacity, ARC is classified into three subtypes: age-related cortical cataract (ARCC), age-related nuclear cataract (ARNC), and age-related posterior subcapsular cataract (ARPSC) [5]. Currently, the only cure for cataract is surgical removal of the opaque lenses and substitution with transparent artificial intraocular lenses [6]. Preventing or delaying the onset of

cataracts by pharmacological interventions has been an attractive field of research in ophthalmology [7, 8].

The reason for the relative absence of cataract drugs is that the etiology for cataract remains unclear. Studies have identified multiple risk factors related to cataract formation, including genetic predisposition, aging, oxidative stress, ultraviolet (UV) light, systematic diseases, and toxic agents [9, 10]. Lipid metabolic disorders, especially cholesterol metabolic disturbance, have been proposed to be a potential factor for cataract. However, whether cholesterol is a risk or protective factor in cataract remains in debate [11–13]. Recently, researchers demonstrate that lanosterol, not cholesterol, plays a preventive role in cataract formation, inhibiting lens opacity, and reversing crystalline aggregation [14].

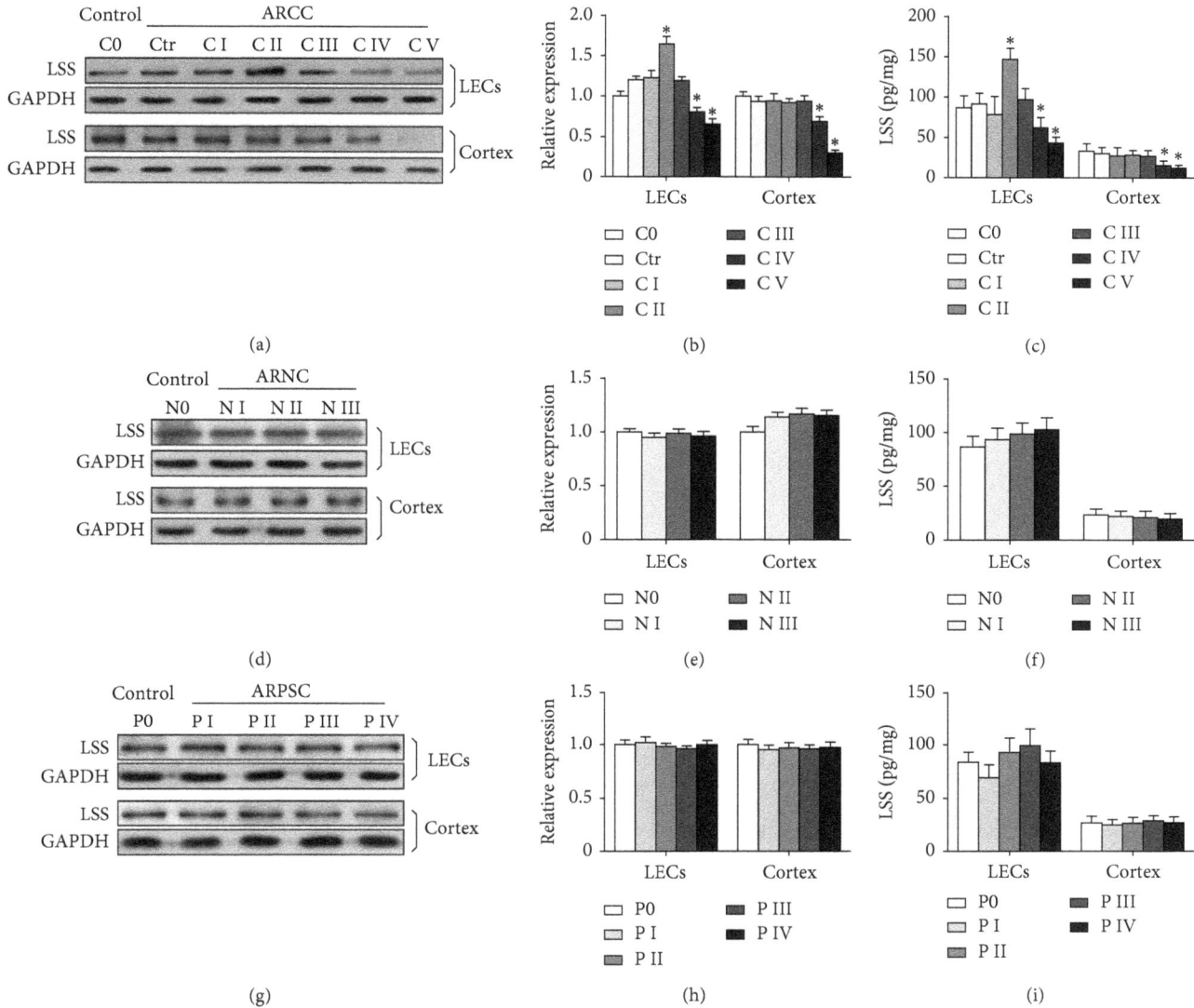

FIGURE 1: Protein levels of LSS in the human LECs and the cortex with different opaque degree from age-related cortical cataract (ARCC), age-related nuclear cataract (ARNC), age-related posterior subcapsular cataract (ARPSC). (a, d, g) LECs of control and ARCC, ARNC, ARPSC patients were processed for western blot with antibody against LSS and GAPDH ($n = 15$ for each subtype), respectively. (b, e, h) Quantification of LSS protein levels normalized to GAPDH from western blot in (a), (d), and (g), respectively. (c, f, i) LSS protein levels (pg/mg protein) in ARCC, ARNC, ARPSC patients measured by ELISA ($n = 15$ for each subtype). *$P < 0.05$.

However, the relationship between lanosterol and the subtypes of ARC is unknown.

Lanosterol is the first sterol in lipid biosynthetic pathway, which is initially converted by acetyl-CoA. The complex process of lanosterol synthesis involves several enzymes, including 3-hydroxy-3-methylglutaryl-coenzyme A (HMG-CoA) reductase, squalene epoxidase, and lanosterol synthase (LSS). LSS is a microsomal enzyme that functions as a downstream element in the lanosterol biosynthetic pathway [15], catalyzing the cyclization of the linear 2,3-monoepoxysqualene to lanosterol [15]. Inhibiting LSS activity can induce cataract in rats, dogs, and mice both in vitro and in vivo [16, 17]. Shumiya cataract rat (SCR) is a hereditary cataractous rat strain that develops cataract at approximate 11 weeks of age [18]. Lss gene

is mutated in SCR and is the major gene for cataract onset [19]. In humans, two distinct homozygous LSS missense mutations (W581R and G588S) happen in two families with extensive congenital cataracts, which impairs key catalizing functions of LSS. [14]. However, whether LSS pathway plays a role in ARC remains obscure.

In the present study, the expression of LSS, the key enzyme in the synthesis of lanosterol, in the human lens tissue was measured and the relationship between lanosterol, LSS level, and opaque degree was analyzed. Additionally, in an in vitro whole rat lens culture model, U18666A (an LSS inhibitor) was used to determine the causative effect of LSS activity on lens opacity, which may produce a novel potential strategy for the therapy of cataract.

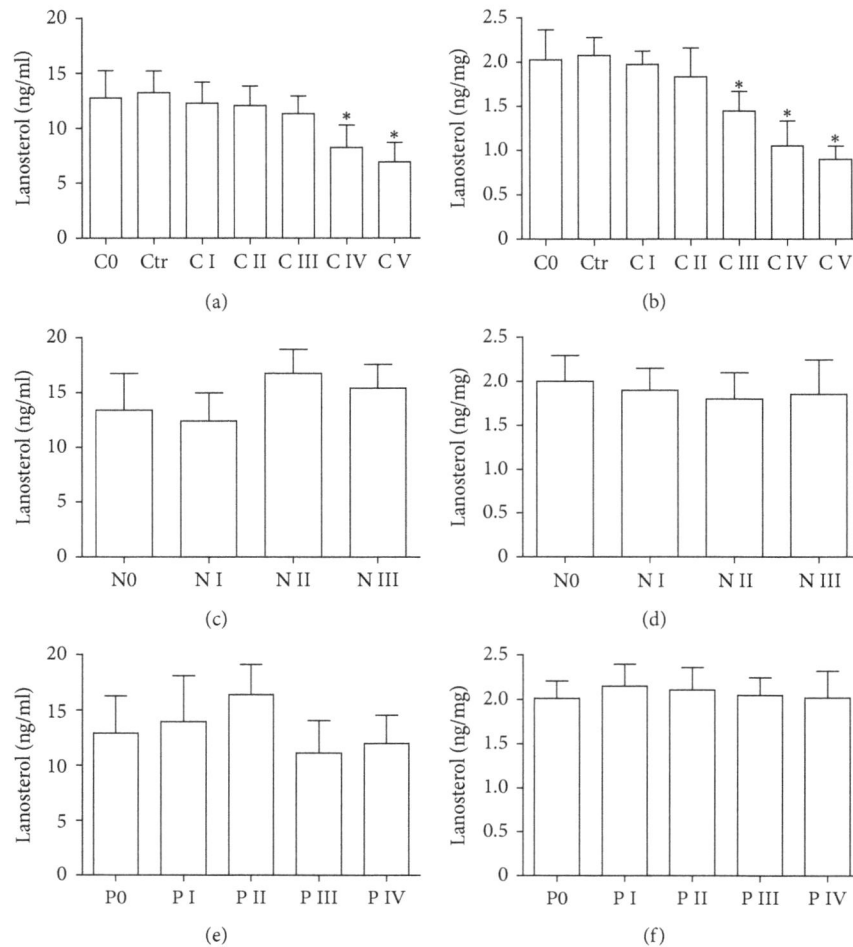

FIGURE 2: Lanosterol levels in the human LECs and cortex of different subtypes of ARC. (a, b, e). Lanosterol levels in LECs of with different opaque degree from ARCC, ARNC, and ARPSC ($n = 15$ for each subtype), respectively. (b, d, f). Lanosterol levels in cortex of with different opaque degree from ARCC, ARNC, and ARPSC ($n = 15$ for each subtype). $^*P < 0.05$.

2. Materials and methods

2.1. Human Lens Extracts.
Human lens samples including lens capsules (mainly composed of LECs) and the cortex were obtained from Department of Ophthalmology, Affiliated Hospital of Nantong University. The lens tissues from 390 patients with different subtypes of ARC during phacoemulsification were collected. The clinical diagnosis of ARC is based on criteria of the Lens Opacities Classification System II (LOCS II) [20]. We also included 88 age-matched individuals without cataract but had their lens extracted because of vitreoretinal diseases as control during extracapsular cataract extraction. Patients with the following conditions were excluded: other eye diseases such as high myopia, dislocated lens, glaucoma, uveitis, and diabetic retinopathy and systemic diseases such as hepatic dysfunction, diabetes, cancer, uncontrolled hypertension, hyperlipemia, obstructive sleep apnea, and nervous system diseases such as Alzheimer's disease. All of the extracts were preserved in −80°C until further analysis. Ethical permission was obtained from the Medical Ethics Committee of Affiliated Hospital of Nantong University (No. 2012(021)), and the informed consent was received

from all patients according to the tenets of the Declaration of Helsinki.

2.2. Rat Lens Extracts.
96 male Sprague Dawley rats (SD rats) at approximately 4 weeks of age, weighing 150–180 g with normal lens were provided from the Laboratory Animal Center of Nantong University. Rats were housed in solid bottom cages in an environmentally controlled room (20 ± 2°C, 50 ± 15% humidity) on a 12 h light/dark cycle and freely accessed standard laboratory chow and water. Before extracting lens, the rats were anesthetized by intraperitoneal injection of 80 mg/kg pentobarbital sodium. The eye globes were collected immediately after sacrifice. All experimental procedures were performed in accordance with the requirements of Animal Care and Use Committee of Nantong University.

2.3. Western Blot.
The protein of human LECs, cortex, and rat lens in each group were extracted in RIPA lysis buffer III (Sangon Biotech, China) as per the instructions. After ultrasonication, the specimens were centrifuged at 12000 rpm (15 min, 4°C), and the supernatant was collected.

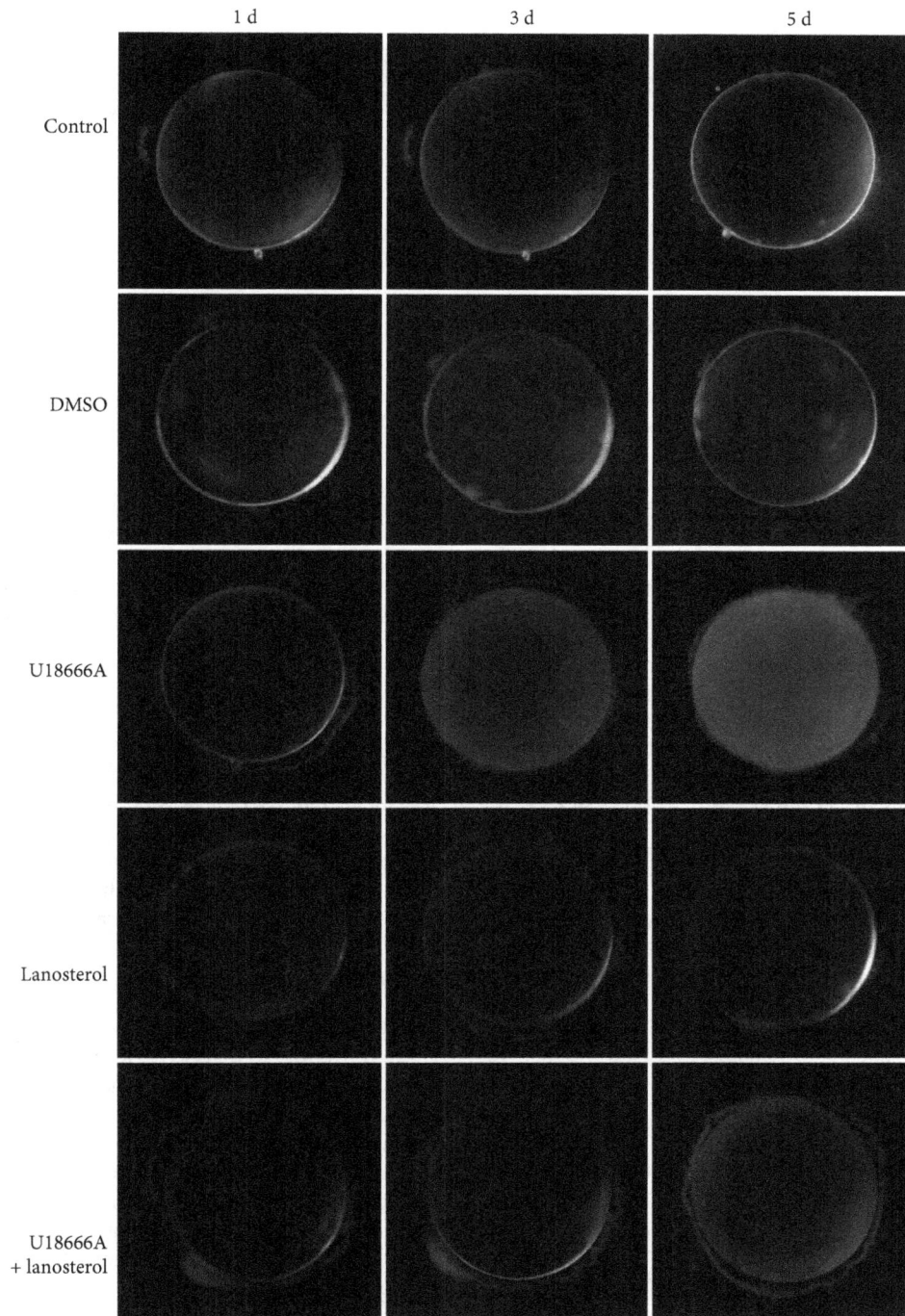

FIGURE 3: Images of the representative rat lens in each group taken in 5 days. Lens were cultured with DMSO (vehicle), 200 nM U18666A, 40 μM lanosterol, or both U18666A and lanosterol for 5 days.

Equal amounts of lysates (100 μg/lane) were separated on 10% SDS-PAGE and transferred to PVDF membranes. After blocking in 5% skimmed milk (TBST as vehicle) for 2 h, the membranes were incubated with rabbit anti-LSS antibody (1 : 500, Abcam, UK) and mouse anti-GAPDH antibody (1 : 5000, ABclonal, France) overnight at 4°C. After washing, the membranes were incubated with goat HRP-conjugated secondary antibodies (Jackson ImmunoResearch, USA). Proteins were visualized using an

ECL system (Cell Signaling, USA). Relative level of proteins was quantified with ImageJ software (National Institutes of Health, USA).

2.4. Enzyme-Linked Immunosorbent Assay (ELISA). The LSS level of human LECs and the cortex of cultured lens were quantified by ELISA using human LSS ELISA kit (QIYBO, China) according to the manufacturer's instructions. The

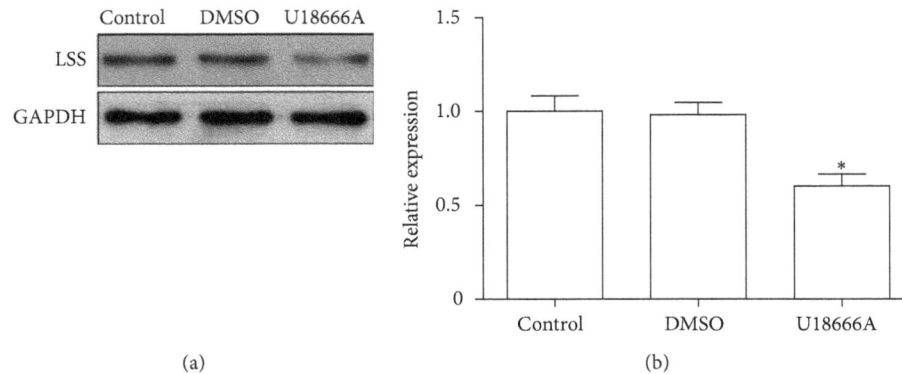

FIGURE 4: Protein levels of the LSS in rat lens in each group. (a) Rat lens were processed for western blot with antibody against LSS and GAPDH ($n = 5$). (b) Quantification of LSS protein levels normalized to GAPDH from western blot in (a). $^*P < 0.05$.

optical density was read at 450 nm wavelength using a microplate reader (ELx800, BioTek, USA).

2.5. Lens Explant Culture and Reagent.

The lenses extracted from the globes were cultured in M199 medium (Gibco, Rockville, MD) supplemented with 100 U/ml penicillin and 0.1 mg/ml streptomycin in a 75% humidified 37°C incubator with 21% O_2 and 5% CO_2 for 1 day in 24 well cell culture clusters. Lenses without opacification were then randomized into five groups with 3 lenses or more per treatment: untreated control, vehicle (DMSO) control, U18666A treatment, lanosterol treatment, and U18666A and lanosterol treatment. U18666A solution was prepared using DMSO as the solvent with the final concentration of 200 nM in culture media. Lanosterol solution was prepared using M199 medium with the final concentration of 40 μM. Final medium osmolality of each group was maintained from 295 to 310 mOsM/kg. The medium was replaced every 24 h. The opacity of lens was image analyzed at 1, 3, and 5 days. At the end of culture, the lenses were weighed and preserved in −80°C for further experiments.

2.6. Lens Transparency Assessment.

For imaging, an antibody incubation box which had been high-pressure steam disinfected was placed in vertical clean bench. To observe the transparency of lens, we sprayed 75% alcohol on vertical clean bench as much as possible. 24 well cell culture clusters were taken from incubator and placed on the antibody incubation box carefully, making sure there were no air bubbles but only 75% alcohol between the clusters and antibody incubation box. The image was captured with the Nikon D90 camera under the largest magnification. In this way, the transparency of total lens area was observed, with the black image representing transparent lens, gray image representing opaque lens.

2.7. Immunofluorescence Assay.

The cultured rat lens was fixed with chloroform fixative overnight and sugar dehydrated followed by frozen section. After permeabilization and blocking in 3% fetal bovine serum with 0.3% TritonX-100

for 30 min, the sections were incubated overnight at 4°C with IgG (negative control), anti-LSS antibody (1:500, Abcam, UK), and anti-KDEL antibody (1:250, Abcam, UK). After washing, tissue sections were incubated with FITC-conjugated (1:250) or Cy3-conjugated secondary antibody (1:1000) (Jackson ImmunoResearch) for 2 h at 37°C.

2.8. Statistical Analysis.

All data were presented as means ±SD. SPSS software (SPSS 17.0; SPSS Inc., USA) was used for statistical analysis. One-way ANOVA was used for statistical comparisons of multiple groups. The difference between two groups was determined by Student's t-test. Statistical significance was based on a P value < 0.05. Each experiment consisted of at least three replicates.

3. Results

3.1. LSS and Lanosterol Level Changes in LECs and Cortex of Human ARCC.

To detect LSS level in LECs and the cortex in human ARC tissues, western blot was performed, showing that LSS changed along with the cataract levels in LECs of human ARCC, increasing at C II and decreasing at C IV and C V. While in the cortex of human ARCC, LSS decreased with the aggravation of opaque degree (Figures 1(a) and 1(b)). Furthermore, ELISA showed that LSS had the similar change trends in different types of human ARC tissues (Figure 1(c)). However, there were no significant changes of LSS level in either LECs or the cortex of human ARNC and ARPSC (Figures 1(d)–1(i)).

Lanosterol, the catalyst of LSS, was down-regulated in LECs and the cortex of human ARCC, especially in C IV and C V groups, decreasing in LECs from C IV to C V and in the cortex from C III till C V (Figures 2(a) and 2(b)). However, lanosterol changed slightly in LECs and the cortex of human ARNC and ARPSC (Figures 2(c)–2(f)). The data were consistent with the results of LSS level, thus ARCC was chosen for subsequent experiments.

3.2. LSS Pathway Delays Lens Opacity.

To further identify the function of LSS pathway in the formation of ARCC, LSS

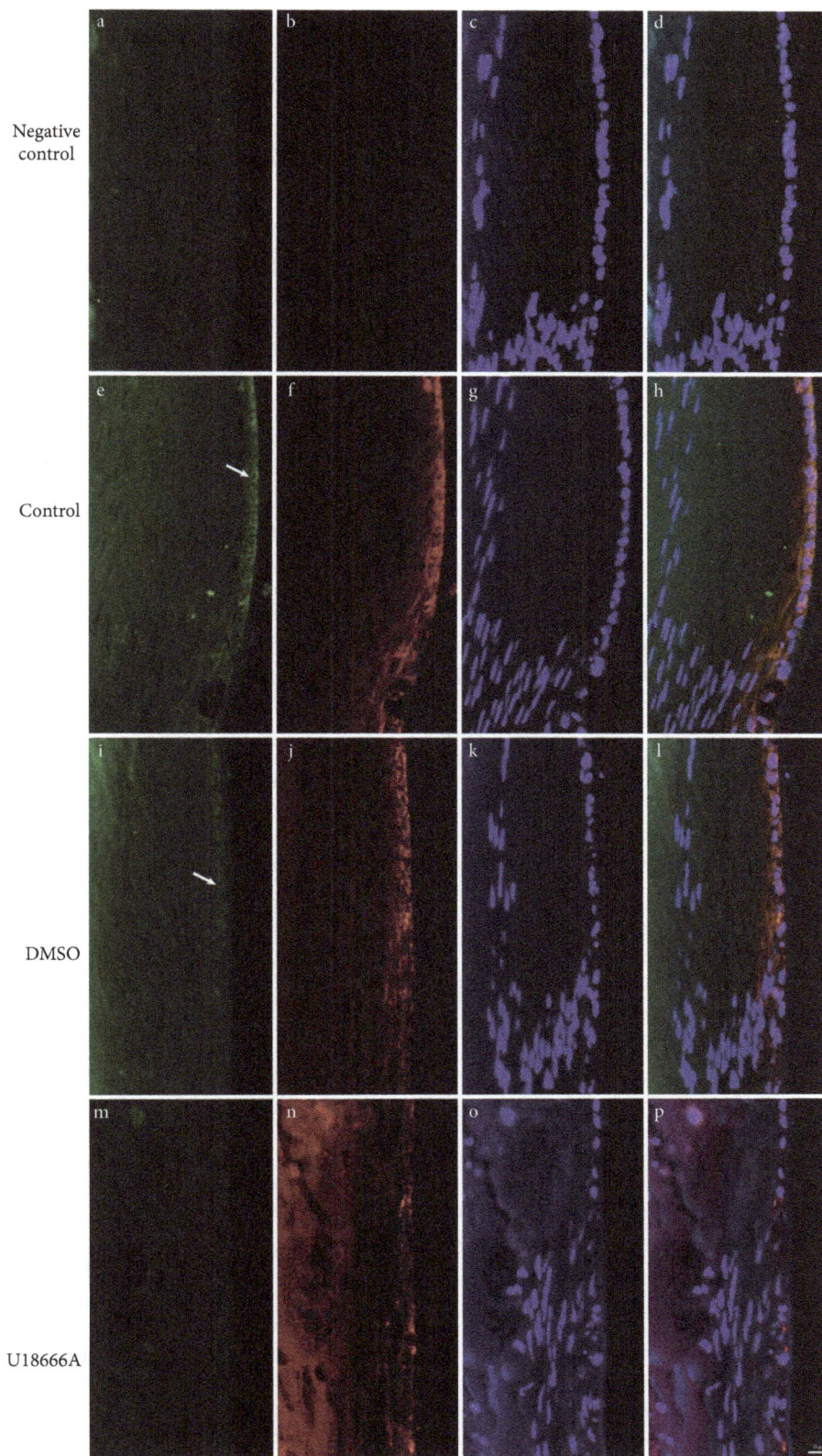

FIGURE 5: LSS localization in cultured rat lens in each group ($n = 3$). The image is shown at ×20 magnification. Black: IgG (a, b); green: LSS (e, i, m); red: KDEL (f, j, n); blue: Hoechst (c, g, k, o); black: merge (d, h, l, p). The hollow arrow shows the LSS location.

Control	DMSO	U18666A	Lanosterol	U18666A + lanosterol

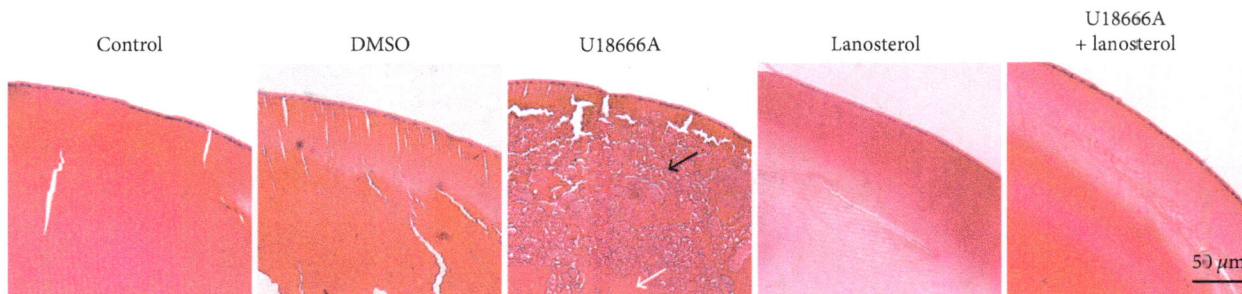

FIGURE 6: Microscopy of rat lenses treated with U18666A ($n = 3$). The image is shown at ×20 magnification. The hollow arrow shows regularly arranged fibers in nuclei. The black arrow shows fiber degeneration in the cortex.

inhibitor U18666A was used in lens culture system in vitro. U18666A treatment adversely affected the transparency of explanted rat lens within 3 d of exposure, indicated by blurring in the cortical area, while lanosterol effectively delayed the occurrence of lens opacity, but not to prevent opacity (Figure 3). After U18666A treatment, LSS expression decreased in opaque rat lens in comparison to transparent ones (Figures 4(a) and 4(b)). LSS is a membrane-associated enzyme, which is targeted to the cytoplasmic leaflet of endoplasmic reticulum (ER) [21]. Immunostaining showed colocalization of LSS with Lys-Asp-Glu-Leu (KDEL; an ER marker, ER retention sequence) [22] and the level of LSS markedly decreased after U18666A treatment (Figure 5).

Microscopy showed that there was a breakdown of structural integrity with extensive disruption in the cortical fiber cells of the opaque lens following U18666A treatment. This disrupted cortical region was completely different from nuclear region, where the fiber cells remained in order. Lens treated with lanosterol suggested slight fracture in the cortex (Figure 6).

4. Discussion

No medical treatment has any effect on cataract for its unknown etiology. Lipid metabolic disorder in cataract has recently emerged as an important field of investigation. Decreased LSS level has been observed in both SCR and human congenital cataract [14, 19], yet LSS in human ARC has not been studied. In our study, LSS expression increased when the lens was slightly opaque and then decreased when the lens were seriously opaque in LECs. In addition, LSS expression decreased in the cortex of human ARCC with the increase of damage level. In vitro, inhibiting LSS induced rat lens opacity in the cortex in 3 days. We further showed that restoring lanosterol level delayed the occurrence of opacity. These data suggest that LSS and lanosterol change with the increase of opacity of lens in ARCC, indicating that LSS pathway plays a protective role in cortical cataract.

In our study, we are unable to draw a conclusion that LSS pathway plays a protective role in human ARCC as we could not obtain the whole human lens by the process of phacoemulsification. Accordingly, we used whole rat lens to keep the complete lens structure. Recent research shows that lanosterol solution does not reverse opacification of human age-related cataractous nuclei, using human cataractous

nuclei instead of whole human ARC lens [23]. Given the different structure between the cortex and nuclei, as well as lacking the intact structure, it cannot be concluded that lanosterol cannot reverse opacification of human ARC. Therefore, whether LSS pathway plays a protective role in human ARCC needs further investigation.

Intriguingly, the change of LSS is different in LECs and the cortex. As the relatively simple cellular structure compared with other parts of the eye, LECs are the fundamental protection responsible for normal occurrence and growth of transparent lens [24]. The lens epithelium is also the initiation site for many other types of cataract [25–28]. In our study, the level of LSS increased in LECs when the opaque degree was C II with no accumulation of lanosterol and no prevention of aggravation of opacity. It is therefore reasonable to assume that LECs can synthesize more LSS without more lanosterol just as a stress response. While the mature fiber cells lose their nuclei and other cytosolic organelles during differentiation and their ability to synthesize LSS, LSS in the cortex decreases when the lens becomes opaque. Therefore, we assume that the increased LSS in LECs might fill another function rather than just being an enzyme catalyzing lanosterol synthesis [15]. Actually, apart from catalyzing lanosterol synthesis, LSS also catalyzes 24(S), 25-epoxylanosterol synthesis from 2, 3: 22, 23-diepoxysqualene, which regulates the liver X receptor, whose relationship with cataract has not been well explored.

Although risk factors accounting for ARC are varied, oxidative stress is well acknowledged. In response to oxidative stress, lens proteins including enzyme and crystallins become modified, denatured, and aggregated, contributing to cataract formation [29]. Oxidative stress alters enzymatic activities and cell proliferation. Why LSS protects lens transparency is unclear, but its role in nervous system has been extensively studied. Previous study has implied that inhibition of LSS causes secondary apoptosis in neurons due to increase in reactive oxygen species (ROS) [30]. It also observed a decreased catalase (CAT) and superoxide dismutase (SOD) activity in astrocytes after inhibiting LSS activity, which causes the dysfunction of lipid metabolism in the cerebral cortex [31, 32]. As a result, we speculate that LSS resists oxidation and after inhibiting LSS activity, oxidative stress increases and leads to dysfunctional lipid metabolism. However, our data showed no association between LSS activity and ARNC or ARPSC, which might due to other molecular mechanisms causing lens opacity in these two subtypes.

5. Conclusion

LSS and lanosterol expression change in LECs and the cortex of human ARCC. In addition, a sustained LSS pathway delays the occurrence of rat lens cortical opacity in vitro, which may make sense to clinical pharmacotherapy of cataract in the future.

Abbreviations

LSS: Lanosterol synthase
ARC: Age-related cataract
LC-MS: Liquid chromatograph-mass spectrometer
ARCC: Age-related cortical cataract
LECs: Lens epithelial cells
ARNC: Age-related nuclear cataract
ARPSC: Age-related posterior subcapsular cataract;
SCR: Shumiya cataract rat
LOCS II: Lens Opacities Classification System II
UPLC: Ultra performance liquid chromatograph
APCI: Atmospheric pressure chemical ionization source in position mode
MRM: Multiple reaction monitoring
ER: Endoplasmic reticulum.

Conflicts of Interest

The authors declare that they have no conflicts of interest.

Authors' Contributions

Xinyue Shen and Manhui Zhu contributed equally to this work.

Acknowledgments

This study was supported by the National Natural Science Foundation of China (no. 81270987) and Graduate Technology Innovation Program of Nantong University (YKC15092 and JSZZ15_0172).

References

[1] Z. Kyselova, M. Stefek, and V. Bauer, "Pharmacological prevention of diabetic cataract," *Journal of Diabetes and its Complications*, vol. 18, no. 2, pp. 129–140, 2004.

[2] Y. Wang, F. Li, G. Zhang, L. Kang, B. Qin, and H. Guan, "Altered DNA methylation and expression profiles of 8-oxoguanine DNA glycosylase 1 in lens tissue from age-related cataract patients," *Current Eye Research*, vol. 40, no. 8, pp. 815–821, 2015.

[3] B. Xu, L. Kang, G. Zhang et al., "The changes of 8-OHdG, hOGG1, APE1 and Pol beta in lenses of patients with age-related cataract," *Current Eye Research*, vol. 40, no. 4, pp. 378–385, 2015.

[4] N. Congdon, J. R. Vingerling, B. E. Klein et al., "Eye diseases prevalence research, prevalence of cataract and pseudophakia/aphakia among adults in the United States," *Archives of Ophthalmology*, vol. 122, no. 4, pp. 487–494, 2004.

[5] R. Michael and A. J. Bron, "The ageing lens and cataract: a model of normal and pathological ageing," *Philosophical Transactions of the Royal Society B: Biological Sciences*, vol. 366, no. 1568, pp. 1278–1292, 2011.

[6] H. P. Qi, S. Q. Wei, X. C. Gao et al., "Ursodeoxycholic acid prevents selenite-induced oxidative stress and alleviates cataract formation: in vitro and in vivo studies," *Molecular Vision*, vol. 18, pp. 151–160, 2012.

[7] L. N. Makley, K. A. McMenimen, B. T. DeVree et al., "Pharmacological chaperone for alpha-crystallin partially restores transparency in cataract models," *Science*, vol. 350, no. 6261, pp. 674–677, 2015.

[8] X. Yuan, D. C. Marcano, C. S. Shin et al., "Ocular drug delivery nanowafer with enhanced therapeutic efficacy," *ACS Nano*, vol. 9, no. 2, pp. 1749–1758, 2015.

[9] E. Iglesias, R. Sajnani, R. C. Levitt, C. D. Sarantopoulos, and A. Galor, "Epidemiology of persistent dry eye-like symptoms after cataract surgery," *Cornea*, vol. 37, no. 7, pp. 893–898, 2018.

[10] J. Z. Selin, B. E. Lindblad, M. Bottai, R. Morgenstern, and A. Wolk, "High-dose B-vitamin supplements and risk for age-related cataract: a population-based prospective study of men and women," *British Journal of Nutrition*, vol. 118, no. 2, pp. 154–160, 2017.

[11] M. H. Fouchet, F. Donche, C. Martin et al., "Design and evaluation of a novel series of 2,3-oxidosqualene cyclase inhibitors with low systemic exposure, relationship between pharmacokinetic properties and ocular toxicity," *Bioorganic and Medicinal Chemistry*, vol. 16, no. 11, pp. 6218–6232, 2008.

[12] C. L. Lai, W. Y. Shau, C. H. Chang, M. F. Chen, and M. S. Lai, "Statin use and cataract surgery: a nationwide retrospective cohort study in elderly ethnic Chinese patients," *Drug Safety*, vol. 36, no. 10, pp. 1017–1024, 2013.

[13] A. Vejux, M. Samadi, and G. Lizard, "Contribution of cholesterol and oxysterols in the physiopathology of cataract: implication for the development of pharmacological treatments," *Journal of Ophthalmology*, vol. 2011, Article ID 471947, 6 pages, 2011.

[14] L. Zhao, X. J. Chen, J. Zhu et al., "Lanosterol reverses protein aggregation in cataracts," *Nature*, vol. 523, no. 7562, pp. 607–611, 2015.

[15] M. W. Huff and D. E. Telford, "Lord of the rings–the mechanism for oxidosqualene:lanosterol cyclase becomes crystal clear," *Trends in Pharmacological Sciences*, vol. 26, no. 7, pp. 335–340, 2005.

[16] I. T. Pyrah, A. Kalinowski, D. Jackson et al., "Toxicologic lesions associated with two related inhibitors of oxidosqualene cyclase in the dog and mouse," *Toxicologic Pathology*, vol. 29, no. 2, pp. 174–179, 2001.

[17] R. J. Cenedella, R. Jacob, D. Borchman et al., "Direct perturbation of lens membrane structure may contribute to cataracts caused by U18666A, an oxidosqualene cyclase inhibitor," *Journal of Lipid Research*, vol. 45, no. 7, pp. 1232–1241, 2004.

[18] S. Shumiya, "Establishment of the hereditary cataract rat strain (SCR) and genetic analysis," *Laboratory Animal Science*, vol. 45, no. 6, pp. 671–673, 1995.

[19] M. Mori, G. Li, I. Abe et al., "Lanosterol synthase mutations cause cholesterol deficiency-associated cataracts in the Shumiya cataract rat," *Journal of Clinical Investigation*, vol. 116, no. 2, pp. 395–404, 2006.

[20] B. V. Magno, M. B. Datiles III, and S. M. Lasa, "Senile cataract progression studies using the Lens Opacities Classification System II," *Investigative Ophthalmology and Visual Science*, vol. 34, no. 6, pp. 2138–2141, 1993.

[21] L. Lim, V. Jackson-Lewis, L. C. Wong et al., "Lanosterol induces mitochondrial uncoupling and protects dopaminergic neurons from cell death in a model for Parkinson's disease," *Cell Death and Differentiation*, vol. 19, no. 3, pp. 416–427, 2012.

[22] D. Vaux, J. Tooze, and S. Fuller, "Identification by anti-idiotype antibodies of an intracellular membrane protein that recognizes a mammalian endoplasmic reticulum retention signal," *Nature*, vol. 345, no. 6275, pp. 495–502, 1990.

[23] P. M. Shanmugam, A. Barigali, J. Kadaskar et al., "Effect of lanosterol on human cataract nucleus," *Indian Journal of Ophthalmology*, vol. 63, no. 12, pp. 888–890, 2015.

[24] U. P. Andley, "The lens epithelium: focus on the expression and function of the alpha-crystallin chaperones," *International Journal of Biochemistry and Cell Biology*, vol. 40, no. 3, pp. 317–323, 2008.

[25] K. R. Hightower and J. P. McCready, "Effect of selenite on epithelium of cultured rabbit lens," *Investigative Ophthalmology and Visual Science*, vol. 32, no. 2, pp. 406–409, 1991.

[26] W. C. Li and A. Spector, "Lens epithelial cell apoptosis is an early event in the development of UVB-induced cataract," *Free Radical Biology and Medicine*, vol. 20, no. 3, pp. 301–311, 1996.

[27] Y. Takamura, E. Kubo, S. Tsuzuki, and Y. Akagi, "Apoptotic cell death in the lens epithelium of rat sugar cataract," *Experimental Eye Research*, vol. 77, no. 1, pp. 51–57, 2003.

[28] W. C. Li, J. R. Kuszak, K. Dunn et al., "Lens epithelial cell apoptosis appears to be a common cellular basis for non-congenital cataract development in humans and animals," *Journal of Cell Biology*, vol. 130, no. 1, pp. 169–181, 1995.

[29] V. M. Berthoud and E. C. Beyer, "Oxidative stress, lens gap junctions, and cataracts," *Antioxidants & Redox Signaling*, vol. 11, no. 2, pp. 339–353, 2009.

[30] R. J. Cenedella, "Cholesterol synthesis inhibitor U18666A and the role of sterol metabolism and trafficking in numerous pathophysiological processes," *Lipids*, vol. 44, no. 6, pp. 477–487, 2009.

[31] D. Copetti-Santos, V. Moraes, D. F. Weiler et al., "U18666A treatment results in cholesterol accumulation, reduced Na(+), K(+)-ATPase activity, and increased oxidative stress in rat cortical astrocytes," *Lipids*, vol. 50, no. 10, pp. 937–944, 2015.

[32] M. C. Medeiros, A. Mello, T. Gemelli et al., "Effect of chronic administration of the vinyl chalcogenide 3-methyl-1-phenyl-2-(phenylseleno)oct-2-en-1-one on oxidative stress in different brain areas of rats," *Neurochemical Research*, vol. 37, no. 5, pp. 928–934, 2012.

11

Bandage Lenses in the Postoperative Care for Cataract Surgery Patients: A Substitute for Eye Patch?

Hang Song,[1] Yingyu Li,[1] Yan Zhang,[2] Danna Shi,[1] and Xuemin Li [1]

[1]*Department of Ophthalmology, Peking University Third Hospital, Beijing, China*
[2]*Sino Japanese Union Hospital of Jilin University, Changchun, Jilin, China*

Correspondence should be addressed to Xuemin Li; lxmlxm66@sina.com

Academic Editor: Suphi Taneri

Purpose. To explore whether bandage lenses could be a safe and effective substitute for eye patch in the postoperative care for cataract surgery patients in terms of infection prevention, ocular impacts, and patient satisfaction. *Methods.* Patients who underwent cataract surgery were randomly divided into the eye patch group (Group A) and the bandage lens group (Group B). Bacterial culture samples were collected perioperatively from different sites. Evaluations of anterior segment condition and patient satisfaction were conducted on the first day of postoperative follow-up. *Results.* The positive rate of bacterial cultures in Group A was higher than that in Group B, but the difference was not statistically significant. Group B had significantly longer tear breakup time, higher tear meniscus height, and slightly better patient satisfaction than Group A. *Conclusion.* Bandage lenses can be used as a safe and effective substitute for eye patch in the postoperative care for cataract surgery patients. The Clinical Study registration number is ChiCTR-IOC-17012167.

1. Introduction

Endophthalmitis is one of the most severe complications after cataract surgery, which often leads to visual deprivation. There are several methods to reduce the risk of postoperative infection, such as using perioperative antibiotic eye drops [1], administering povidone-iodine 5% solution in the conjunctival sac prior to surgery [2, 3], using intracameral antibiotics [4], and prophylactic subconjunctival antibiotic injection at the conclusion of cataract surgery [3]. Wearing an eye patch for at least four hours after surgery was also considered as an effective measure to prevent bacterial contamination and protect the eyes from mechanical injury [1]. But the limitations of eye patch coverage have also become manifested [5, 6]. Research has shown that an eye patch might constrain lid closure, delay postoperative healing, increase discomfort, and is inapplicable to patients with monocular vision [6]. Given these limitations, attempts to remove postsurgical eye coverage have been made, which allow patients to gain the so-called "instant vision" [7].

A major difficulty, however, is that patients without any coverage would be subject to significantly higher discomfort and pain scores as well as significantly worse tear breakup time [8], and administering artificial tear eye drops could only partially improve the outcomes [7].

In this paper, we propose to use therapeutic contact lens to improve the current approach to "instant vision" by overcoming its side effects. Therapeutic contact lens, also known as "bandage lens," is designed to protect and facilitate the healing of a sick eye. Serving as a blanket for the cornea, bandage lens retains its moisture, promotes epithelialization [9], blocks small wound leaks, relieves suture irritation [10], and smoothens wound margin irregularities. A modified bandage lens can also act as a drug delivery system [11, 12]. It is widely used in chronic epithelial defects, corneal ulcer, chemical burns, and post cornea-related surgery. Our study aims at evaluating the efficacy of the eye patch and bandage lenses in preventing eye infections after cataract surgery and investigating their ocular impacts and patient satisfaction level.

2. Methods

2.1. Study Design. This is a prospective, randomized, and controlled experimental study. Altogether, 52 subjects (52 eyes) were recruited at the Department of Ophthalmology, Peking University Third Hospital, from September 20th to November 1st, 2017. Informed consent was obtained from all participants. The study was approved by the Institutional Review Board of Peking University Third Hospital, and all the examinations were conducted in accordance with the tenets of the Declaration of Helsinki.

All the recruited patients had age-related cataract and were recommended for phacoemulsification and intraocular lens implantation surgery after an initial assessment. They were randomly assigned to either Group A or Group B. All patients underwent the same procedure of preoperative preparation. Three days before surgery, levofloxacin eye drops were administered four times a day. One hour before surgery, a nurse sequentially conducted conjunctiva washing with 50 ml of saline solution containing tobramycin at a concentration of 16 mg/ml, lacrimal passage irrigation with 3 ml of saline solution, and mydriatic treatment for six times for each patient. Phacoemulsification and intraocular lens implantation were performed by the same ophthalmologist right after an instillation of 5% povidone-iodine into the operated eye.

After surgery, patients in Group A received subconjunctival injection of tobramycin dexamethasone, started wearing eye patches on the same day, and began using anti-inflammatory eye drops the next day. Patients in Group B were instructed to wear therapeutic silicone hydrogel contact lenses (Bausch & Lomb Pure Vision, balafilcon A, New York, USA) on the day of surgery and started using anti-inflammatory eye drops since the day of surgery. The varieties of postoperative anti-inflammatory eye drops included levofloxacin, prednisolone, and pranoprofen, which were administered for one month at a frequency of four times per day in the first week, three times per day in the second week, twice per day in the third week, and once per day in the fourth week.

2.2. Inclusion and Exclusion Criteria

2.2.1. Inclusion Criteria. The following are the various inclusion criteria:

  (1) patients who were diagnosed with age-related cataract

  (2) patients who were willing to receive phacoemulsification and intraocular lens implantation to improve their vision quality

2.2.2. Exclusion Criteria. The following are the various exclusion criteria:

  (1) patients who have received eye operation within three months

  (2) patients who have worn contact lens within two weeks

  (3) patients with recurrent inflammation or eye traumas

  (4) patients with nasolacrimal duct obstruction

  (5) patients with prior use of systemic antibiotics and/or steroids in the past week

  (6) patients with severe ocular surface disorders

2.3. Data Collection. Five bacterial culture samples were collected with a cotton swab, respectively, from conjunctiva sac swabbing before conjunctiva washing and incision site and eyelid swabbing at the end of surgery as well as on the first day after surgery. For patients who wore bandage lenses, the soft contact lenses were removed with sterile forceps without any anesthetic drops, from which an extra culture sample was obtained in addition to the abovementioned five bacterial culture samples.

Follow-up was carried out on the first day after surgery by the same doctor. After bacterial culture samples were collected, a thorough eye examination of the anterior segment was performed. Tear film breakup time (TBUT) was employed to assess the stability of tear film and was measured three times in each case, from which an average value was calculated and adopted. Tear meniscus height was recorded and graded as 1 (0.1 mm to <0.2 mm), 2 (0.2 mm to <0.4 mm), or 3 (≥0.4 mm). The results of subconjunctival hemorrhage, conjunctival congestion, corneal swelling, whole corneal staining (incision site excluded), keratic precipitates, and anterior chamber flare were all evaluated with a dichotomous scale and recorded as absent or present. The subjects' feeling of pain, initial foreign body sensation, the foreign body sensation after eye patch or bandage lens removal, tearing, and photophobia were also measured with a dichotomous scale.

2.4. Bacterial Culture and Identification. Both swabbing samples and contact lens samples were smeared onto two types of media, respectively: one contained blood, and the other chocolate agar. The blood culture media plates were incubated to identify aerobic and microaerophilic bacteria. The chocolate agar plates were incubated in an anaerobic bag to isolate anaerobic bacteria. If any bacterium was found to grow within one week, the bacterium colony would be isolated for species identification using an automatic microbiology analysis system (Biomerieux VITEK 2 Compact).

2.5. Statistical Analysis. SPSS 13.0 (SPSS, Inc., Chicago, Illinois, USA) was employed for the statistical analysis of ocular surface conditions. Independent T-test analysis was performed to compare TBUT between the two groups. The chi-square test was used to analyze the dichotomous variables. Mann–Whitney U test was employed to analyze tear meniscus height. The level of statistical significance in this study was set at 0.05.

3. Results

3.1. Safety Evaluation Based on Bacterial Culture. The positive rate of bacterial cultures in different swabs is shown in Table 1. Altogether, there were four subjects in Group A and

TABLE 1: Positive rate of bacterial cultures in different swabs.

Site and time point of swabs	Positive in Group A ($N = 25$) n (%)	Positive in Group B ($N = 27$) n (%)	P value※
Conjunctiva sac before surgery	0 (0)	0 (0)	1.000
Incision site at the end of surgery	1 (4)	0 (0)	0.481
Eyelid margin at the end of surgery	2 (8)	2 (7.4)	1.000
Incision site the first day after surgery	2 (8)	0 (0)	0.226
Eyelid margin the first day after surgery	2 (8)	0 (0)	0.226
Bandage lens culture	N/A	0 (0)	

※The result of the Fisher exact test was adopted.

TABLE 2: The distribution of positive cultures among individual subjects.

Patients with positive results	Conjunctiva sac before surgery	Incision site at the end of surgery	Eyelid margin at the end of surgery	Incision site the first day after surgery	Eyelid margin the first day after surgery	Bandage lens culture
Number 1 in Group A	(−)	Staphylococcus epidermidis	Staphylococcus epidermidis	(−)	Staphylococcus epidermidis	(−)
Number 2 in Group A	(−)	Staphylococcus epidermidis	(−)	(−)	(−)	(−)
Number 3 in Group A	(−)	(−)	Staphylococcus epidermidis	Staphylococcus epidermidis	(−)	(−)
Number 4 in Group A	(−)	(−)	Staphylococcus epidermidis	(−)	(−)	(−)
Number 1 in Group B	(−)	Staphylococcus epidermidis	(−)	(−)	(−)	(−)
Number 2 in Group B	(−)	Staphylococcus aureus	(−)	(−)	(−)	(−)

TABLE 3: Signs of the anterior segment evaluation.

Signs	Present in Group A ($N = 25$) n (%)	Present in Group B ($N = 27$) n (%)	P value※
Subconjunctival hemorrhage	4 (16)	0 (0)	0.047
Conjunctival congestion	11 (44)	11 (40.7)	1.000
Corneal swelling	15 (60)	16 (59.6)	1.000
Whole corneal staining (incision site excluded)	1 (4)	6 (22.2)	0.101
Keratic precipitates	13 (52)	18 (66.7)	0.397
Anterior chamber flare	16 (64)	23 (85.2)	0.112

※The result of the Fisher exact test was adopted.

two in Group B whose cultures had positive results, and the distribution of positive cultures among these individual subjects is shown in Table 2.

3.2. The Evaluation of Anterior Eye Segment the Day after Surgery.
On the first day after surgery, signs of the anterior segment of the operated eye were evaluated by the same doctor. Subconjunctival hemorrhage was observed at a significantly higher incidence in Group A, while conjunctival congestion, corneal swelling, whole corneal staining (incision site excluded), keratic precipitates, and anterior chamber flare showed no statistically significant difference between the two groups (Table 3). The TBUT test indicated that the tear film among patients in Group B was more stable than that in Group A (Table 4). The tear meniscus height in Group B was also significantly higher than that in Group A ($P = 0.015$, data not shown).

TABLE 4: TBUT at the first day after surgery.

TBUT (s)	Mean	SD	N	P value
Group A	4.20	2.517	25	0.015
Group B	6.48	3.867	27	

3.3. Patient Satisfaction.
Patients in neither group reported feelings of pain. Foreign body sensation was less complained in Group B than in Group A, but the variance was not statistically significant. However, foreign body sensation after coverage (eye patch or bandage lens) removal was more complained in Group B than in Group A. Complaint of tearing was nearly the same in both groups. As only the patients in Group B could see objects as soon as they finished operation, photophobia was only assessed in Group B, and two patients out of the 27 complained of it (Table 5).

TABLE 5: Subjective feelings on the first day after surgery.

Signs	Present in Group A ($N = 25$) n (%)	Present in Group B ($N = 27$) n (%)	P value[※]
Pain	0 (0%)	0 (0%)	1.000
Foreign body sensation	15 (60%)	10 (37.0%)	0.164
Foreign body sensation after coverage removal	0 (0%)	4 (14.8%)	0.112
Tearing	2 (8%)	3 (11.1%)	1.000
Photophobia	N/A	2 (7.41%)	

[※]The result of Fisher exact test was adopted.

4. Discussion

Covering the eye with an eye patch is a regular postoperative therapy for cataract surgery patients. However, the presence of secretions adhering to the eyelid is quite common when ophthalmologists take off the eye patch on the first day of postoperative follow-up. The secretions might increase the risk of infection and cause discomfort. If antibiotic ointment is administered at the conclusion of surgery, the discomfort would be more severe and the eye patch might even cause toxic anterior segment syndrome [13]. In addition, wearing an eye patch causes much inconvenience for patients with monovision, especially in outpatient surgery, after which the patient leaves the hospital immediately. Thus, it is important to explore proper substitutes for the eye patch, and in this study, we evaluated the plausibility of bandage lenses.

We developed bacterial cultures obtained from different sites and at various time points perioperatively. There was no positive culture on the first day after surgery, and the bandage lens cultures were all negative. Even though colonies of *Staphylococcus epidermidis* and *Staphylococcus aureus* were observed in the culture samples of the incision site at the end of surgery, the use of antibiotic eye drops on the day of surgery could kill the bacteria and therefore prevent infection. However, in Group A, positive cultures of *Staphylococcus epidermidis* were observed on the first day after surgery, even though none was found among those patients at the end of surgery. This might be accounted for by the bacterial contamination from the secretion of the meibomian glands [14] or conjunctiva, as an eye patch constrained the eyelid movement and blocked the process of self-scavenging. Since the etiologic agents of endophthalmitis following cataract surgery are genetically associated with bacterial flora in the conjunctiva, eyelid, and periorbital [15], immobilizing the eyelid and covering the eye may not be a good postoperative therapy to prevent infection. Although the bacterial cultures showed no statistically significant differences between these two groups, it did show a tendency that bandage lenses performed better or at least no worse than eye patch in preventing postoperative infection.

The anterior segment evaluation on the first day after surgery showed that bandage lenses played a positive role in tear film protection. Comparison of parameters like tear film breakup time and tear meniscus height implied that the tear film among patients wearing bandage lenses was more stable than those using an eye patch. Previous research has also indicated bandage lens could be a viable treatment option for the management of ocular conditions associated with dry eye diseases [16, 17]. Given that tear film is an important factor for cornea epithelial protection [18], bandage lens has its advantage over an eye patch in postsurgical cornea recovery.

Subconjunctival hemorrhage was observed at a significantly higher incidence in the eye patch group. This result could be attributed to the subconjunctival injection of tobramycin, as the operation itself might impair the microvessels and cause subconjunctival hemorrhage. In contrast, with bandage lenses, patients could use the antibiotic eye drops on the same day of surgery, thus sparing subconjunctival injection as well as the pain and subconjunctival hemorrhage it might cause.

Conjunctival congestion, corneal swelling, whole corneal staining (incision site excluded), keratic precipitates, and anterior chamber flare all showed no significant difference between the two groups. As we did these evaluations on the first day after surgery, there was not enough time for bandage lenses to produce a significantly different effect. Whether bandage lenses could improve these conditions needs further investigation.

Regarding the satisfaction levels, patients in neither group complained of feelings of pain. The results might be different if a same evaluation was conducted the second day after surgery, since the eye patch during the first day after surgery could constrain the eyelid movement and therefore prevent the massage of the incision site where epithelial cells are usually defective. With the eye covered, this pain could be neglected. Bandage lenses protect the cornea not only from potential exterior sources of injury but also from the impacts from the patient's own eyelids. The shearing effect created by the lids during the blink can inhibit reepithelialization and cause pain. Using bandage lens facilitates corneal healing in a pain-free environment.

Foreign body sensation was less complained of among patients wearing bandage lenses, though without statistical significance. However, foreign body sensation after bandage lens removal was more complained of than after eye patch removal. This, on the contrary, indicates that patients were more willing to wear bandage lenses than to wear nothing or eye patch. Only two patients out of the 27 in bandage lens group complained of photophobia, which indicated that the side effect of photophobia was at a low incidence for instant vision with bandage lenses. Besides, photophobia, which was usually reported after one week of postsurgical follow-up, might be attributed to the maladjustment to the increasing light that comes to the retina after the removal of cataract. Thus, photophobia might not be the side effect of bandage lens, but rather a common phenomenon after cataract surgery.

In this study, we removed the bandage lenses on the first day after surgery to carry out bacterial culture. In non-experimental clinical scenarios, bandage lenses could be used for longer period with improved protection for the cornea. Research has already been done with longer postoperative use of bandage lenses and showed long-term improvement in the ocular surface conditions (unpublished data).

5. Conclusion

Using bandage lens is safe and effective in protecting ocular surface and stabilizing tear film after cataract surgery and has the advantage of maintaining the "instant vision" of the operated eye, which makes it a promising substitute for eye patch coverage in the postoperative care for cataract surgery patients, especially those with monovision.

Conflicts of Interest

The authors declare that there are no conflicts of interest regarding the publication of this paper.

Authors' Contributions

Hang Song and Yingyu Li contributed equally to this work.

Acknowledgments

The authors are grateful to Dr. Wanheng Hu for his corrections to the grammar mistakes and for his helpful advice on some English expressions in this paper.

References

[1] T. Wallin, J. Parker, Y. Jin, G. Kefalopoulos, and R. J. Olson, "Cohort study of 27 cases of endophthalmitis at a single institution," *Journal of Cataract and Refractive Surgery*, vol. 31, no. 4, pp. 735–741, 2005.

[2] T. A. Ciulla, M. B. Starr, and S. Masket, "Bacterial endophthalmitis prophylaxis for cataract surgery: an evidence-based update," *Ophthalmology*, vol. 109, no. 1, pp. 13–24, 2002.

[3] M. G. Speaker and J. A. Menikoff, "Prophylaxis of endophthalmitis with topical povidone-iodine," *Ophthalmology*, vol. 98, no. 12, pp. 1769–1775, 1991.

[4] A. Haripriya, D. F. Chang, S. Namburar, A. Smita, and R. D. Ravindran, "Efficacy of intracameral moxifloxacin endophthalmitis prophylaxis at Aravind Eye Hospital," *Ophthalmology*, vol. 123, no. 2, pp. 302–308, 2016.

[5] S. Mayer, C. Wirbelauer, H. Haberle, M. Altmeyer, and D. T. Pham, "Evaluation of eye patching after cataract surgery in topical anesthesia," *Klinische Monatsblätter für Augenheilkunde*, vol. 222, no. 1, pp. 41–45, 2005.

[6] J. W. Bainbridge, J. M. Smith, G. Reddy, and J. F. Kirwan, "Is eye padding routinely necessary after uncomplicated phacoemulsification?," *Eye*, vol. 12, no. 4, pp. 637–640, 1998.

[7] E. Sipos, E. Stifter, and R. Menapace, "Patient satisfaction and postoperative pain with different postoperative therapy regimens after standardized cataract surgery: a randomized intraindividual comparison," *International Ophthalmology*, vol. 31, no. 6, pp. 453–460, 2011.

[8] E. Stifter and R. Menapace, ""Instant vision" compared with postoperative patching: clinical evaluation and patient satisfaction after bilateral cataract surgery," *American Journal of Ophthalmology*, vol. 143, no. 3, pp. 441–448, 2007.

[9] D. Chen, Y. Lian, J. Li, Y. Ma, M. Shen, and F. Lu, "Monitor corneal epithelial healing under bandage contact lens using ultrahigh-resolution optical coherence tomography after pterygium surgery," *Eye and Contact Lens*, vol. 40, no. 3, pp. 175–180, 2014.

[10] A. Mukherjee, A. Ioannides, and I. Aslanides, "Comparative evaluation of Comfilcon A and Senofilcon A bandage contact lenses after transepithelial photorefractive keratectomy," *Journal of Optometry*, vol. 8, no. 1, pp. 27–32, 2015.

[11] A. Guzman-Aranguez, B. Fonseca, G. Carracedo, A. Martin-Gil, A. Martinez-Aguila, and J. Pintor, "Dry eye treatment based on contact lens drug delivery: a review," *Eye and Contact Lens*, vol. 42, no. 5, pp. 280–288, 2016.

[12] C. M. Phan, L. Subbaraman, and L. Jones, "Contact lenses for antifungal ocular drug delivery: a review," *Expert Opinion on Drug Delivery*, vol. 11, no. 4, pp. 537–546, 2014.

[13] L. Werner, J. H. Sher, J. R. Taylor et al., "Toxic anterior segment syndrome and possible association with ointment in the anterior chamber following cataract surgery," *Journal of Cataract and Refractive Surgery*, vol. 32, no. 2, pp. 227–235, 2006.

[14] S. D. Zhang, J. N. He, T. T. Niu et al., "Effectiveness of meibomian gland massage combined with topical levofloxacin against ocular surface flora in patients before penetrating ocular surgery," *Ocular Surface*, vol. 16, no. 1, pp. 70–76, 2017.

[15] T. L. Bannerman, D. L. Rhoden, S. K. McAllister, J. M. Miller, and L. A. Wilson, "The source of coagulase-negative staphylococci in the Endophthalmitis Vitrectomy Study. A comparison of eyelid and intraocular isolates using pulsed-field gel electrophoresis," *Archives of Ophthalmology*, vol. 115, no. 3, pp. 357–361, 1997.

[16] M. S. Milner, K. A. Beckman, J. I. Luchs et al., "Dysfunctional tear syndrome: dry eye disease and associated tear film disorders-new strategies for diagnosis and treatment," *Current Opinion in Ophthalmology*, vol. 27, no. 1, pp. 3–47, 2017.

[17] J. Albietz, P. Sanfilippo, R. Troutbeck, and L. M. Lenton, "Management of filamentary keratitis associated with aqueous-deficient dry eye," *Optometry and Vision Science*, vol. 80, no. 6, pp. 420–430, 2003.

[18] J. Li, X. Zhang, Q. Zheng et al., "Comparative evaluation of silicone hydrogel contact lenses and autologous serum for management of sjogren syndrome-associated dry eye," *Cornea*, vol. 34, no. 9, pp. 1072–1078, 2015.

12

Effect of Exogenous Alpha-B Crystallin on the Structures and Functions of Trabecular Meshwork Cells

Hui Xu, Li Zhu, Yu Wang, and Yongzhen Bao (ORCID)

Department of Ophthalmology, Peking University People's Hospital, Eye diseases and Optometry Institute, Beijing Key Laboratory of Diagnosis and Therapy of Retina and Choroid Diseases, College of Optometry, Peking University Health Science Center, Beijing, China

Correspondence should be addressed to Yongzhen Bao; drbaoyz@sina.com

Academic Editor: Ciro Costagliola

Purpose. Secondary open-angle glaucoma may develop as a postoperative complication of early childhood cataract surgery. Its mechanism is poorly understood. Surgical removal of cataracts is typically incomplete, and we estimate that this disease is associated with alpha-B crystallin (CRYAB) secreted from the retained lens material. This study, for the first time, focused on the role of CRYAB in undesired changes of the structures and functions in trabecular meshwork (TM) cells. *Methods*. Cell proliferation and migration were assessed using a cell counting kit-8 (CCK8) and transwell assay analysis, respectively. Immunofluorescence (IF), quantitative real-time PCR (Rt-qPCR), and Western blot were performed to determine the effect of CRYAB on F-actin, tight junctions, and the expression of epithelial to mesenchymal transition- (EMT-) associated proteins in TM cells. *Results*. CRYAB promoted proliferation ($p < 0.0001$), migration ($p < 0.001$), and F-actin reorganization in TM cells. There were statistically significant increases in the mRNA and protein levels of zo-1, cadherin-N, and vimentin (all $p < 0.0001$) and cadherin-E decreased ($p < 0.0001$) and the mRNA level of claudin-1 increased ($p < 0.0001$) compared to those of the control group. *Conclusion*. All of the changes in structures and functions first observed in the TM cells after exposure to CRYAB resembled alterations seen in primary open-angle glaucoma, suggesting that CRYAB might be related to the pathogenesis of secondary open-angle glaucoma after congenital cataract surgery.

1. Introduction

Cataracts are a major cause of visual disability in childhood. For children with a significant disorder of visual acuity in infancy, early congenital cataract extraction combined with posterior capsule resection and preoperative vitrectomy is conducive for restoring vision and reducing amblyopia and blindness. However, in the first year after birth, lensectomy increases the incidence of postoperative secondary open-angle glaucoma [1–3], a slightly threatening complication with an incidence ranging from 6% to 58.7%, according to the variable population definition and follow-up time [4–9]. Once it occurs, treatment is difficult and prognosis is poor. The pathogenesis of this kind of glaucoma has been researched, and it has been associated with some suspected risk factors, consisting of a preexisting ocular abnormality, operation at early age, chronic postoperative inflammation, and retained lens material, and factors, including IL-4 and TGF-β in the aqueous humor of the eye [10, 11]. However, the mechanism responsible for secondary open-angle glaucoma is poorly understood to date. One study points out that the volume of trabecular cells (TM) increases as well the expression of genes and proteins related to cell morphological characteristics, inflammatory response, and ion balance regulation after TM are cocultured with lens epithelial cells (LECs), which is similar to the change in TM in primary open-angle glaucoma [12].

In addition, alpha-B crystallin (CRYAB) may play a role in the incidence of cataracts and AMD by protecting cells from apoptosis, regulating cell signals and resisting oxidative stress [13, 14]. Previous studies show that αB-crystallin promotes EMT in hepatocellular carcinoma cells [15] and plays an important role in pulmonary fibrosis [16]. Surgical removal of cataract is typically incomplete and exposes the

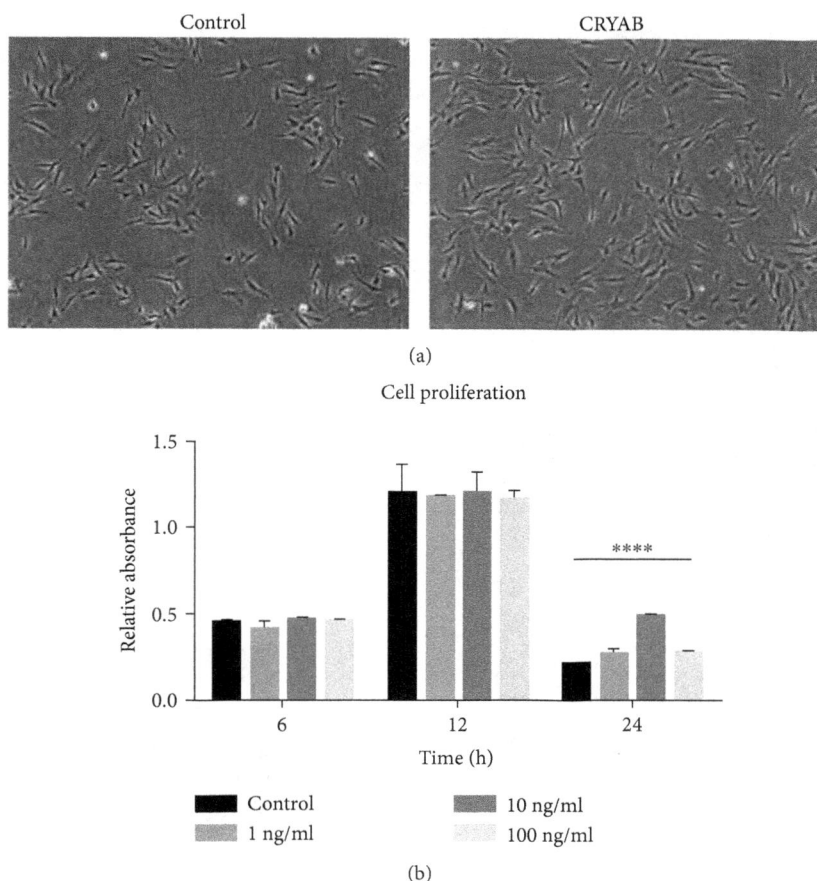

FIGURE 1: (a) Light micrographs of the TM cells treated with CRYAB (TM cells grown alone served as the control, 100x magnification). (b) CRYAB induced proliferation in TM cells. TM cell proliferation was determined with CCK8 after 6 h, 12 h, and 24 h incubation with 1 ng/ml, 10 ng/ml, and 100 ng/ml CRYAB. The 10 ng/ml CRYAB for 24 h treatment increased TM cell proliferation. $****p < 0.0001$ versus the untreated control.

internal surfaces of the equatorial and posterior lens capsule to the aqueous humor, which is covered with LECs secreting CRYAB into the aqueous humor. CRYAB likely causes the above changes in trabecular extracellular matrix and promotes epithelial to interstitial transformation, leading to the incidence of postoperative glaucoma. This prompted us to undertake this study, for the first time, to investigate whether CRYAB secreted from the retained lens material negatively affects the TM cellular structures and functions by EMT and its relation with the pathogenesis of secondary open-angle glaucoma.

2. Methods

2.1. Cell Culture. The human trabecular meshwork cell line was purchased from the American Type Culture Collection (ATCC) (Manassas, VA). The cells were maintained in T25 and were incubated with DMEM medium (Invitrogen, Carlsbad, CA) supplemented with 10% fetal bovine serum (FBS) (Invitrogen, USA), 100 units/ml penicillin, and 100 µg/ml streptomycin (Invitrogen, USA) in a tissue culture incubator at 37°C with 5% CO_2. Once they reached 80~90%

confluence, the TM cells were passaged (1 : 3~1 : 4) every 2 or 3 days.

2.2. Cell Proliferation. We inoculated the cell suspension (100 µl/well) in a 96-well plate at 37°C in 5% CO_2 after adding CRYAB at 1 ng/ml, 10 ng/ml, and 100 ng/ml. Twenty-four hours later, we added 10 µl of the CCK-8 solution to each well of the plate for one hour incubation and then measured the absorbance at 450 nm using a microplate reader.

2.3. Cell Migration. The transwells had an 8 µm pore size and were 6.5 mm in diameter (Costar; cat. no. 3422). The cells (4×10^3) were placed in the upper chamber (Costar, Cambridge, MA) with a volume of 200 µl of serum-free medium, and 10% FBS, with concentrations of crystallin (10 ng/ml), without the other test substances was placed in the bottom chamber in a volume of 600 µl per well. The cells were fixed in 4% paraformaldehyde for 20 min, stained with DAPI for 10 min and washed in PBS. The nonmigrated cells in the upper chamber were gently removed using a cotton swab. Cell migration was counted by the number of cells that moved through the filter towards the lower surface in five random fields per filter under a microscope.

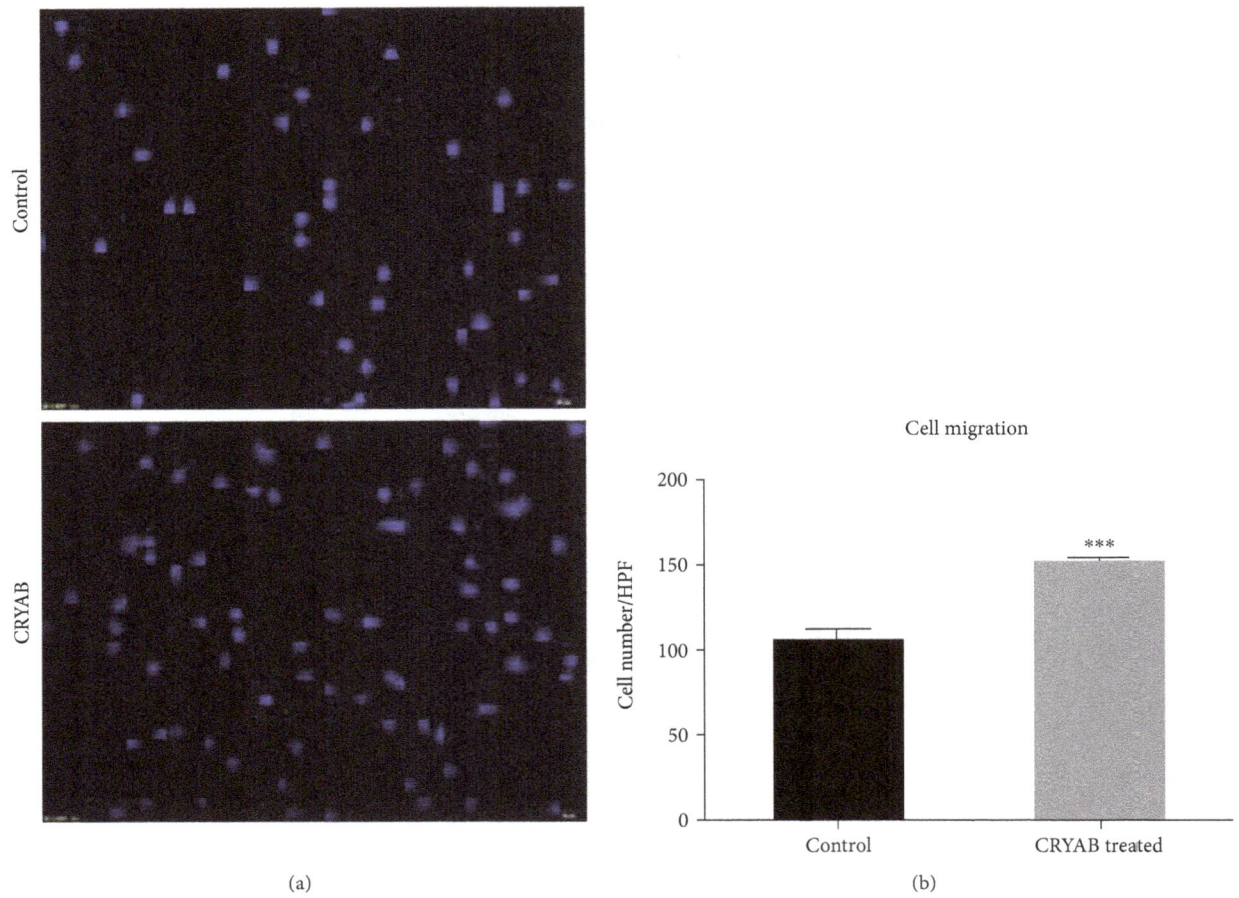

(a)

(b)

FIGURE 2: (a, b) CRYAB induced migration in TM cells. TM cell migration in response to CRYAB treatment was measured using a transwell assay (100x magnification). The amounts were assessed by the mean number of migrated cells. The number of migrated cells per high-power field (HPF) was shown. ***$p < 0.001$ versus the untreated control.

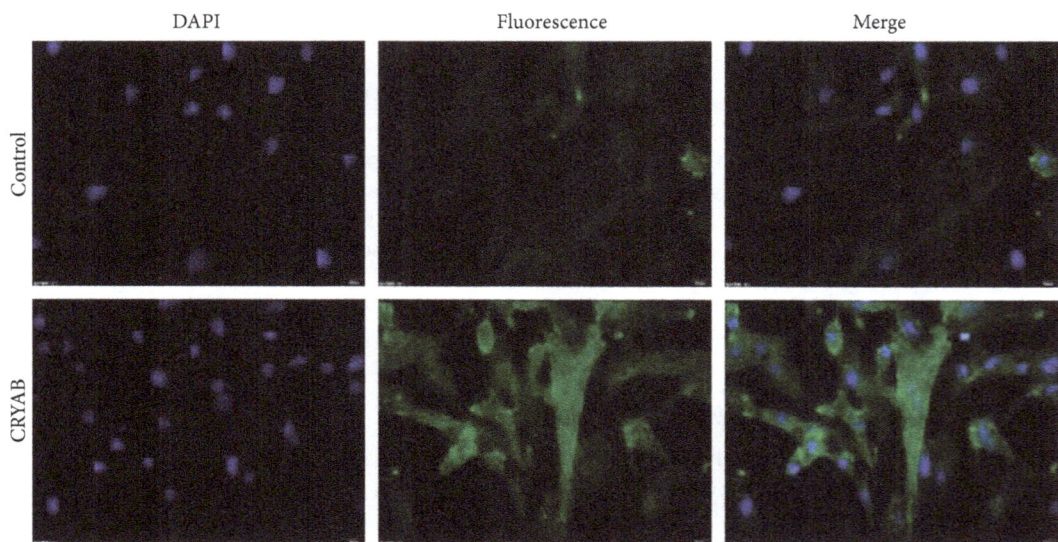

FIGURE 3: Immunofluorescence after incubation with CRYAB for 24 hours showed that F-actin protein in the CRYAB-treated TM cells irregularly accumulated inside the cell membrane.

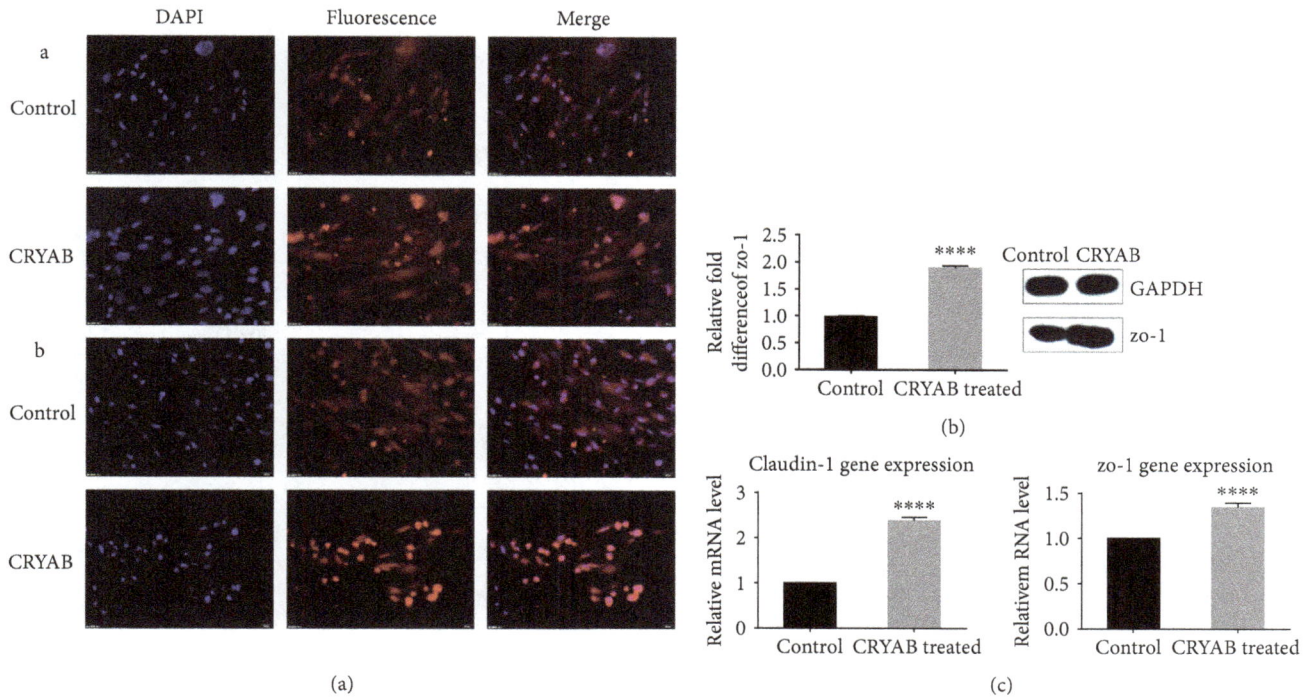

FIGURE 4: Effect of CRYAB on the expression of zo-1 and claudin-1 in TM cells. (a) Immunofluorescence manifestation of zo-1 and claudin-1. Immunofluorescence verified the upregulation of tight junction proteins (A: zo-1; B: claudin-1). (b) Western blot analysis of zo-1 expression. TM cells were exposed to 10 ng/ml CRYAB for 24 h. The expression of zo-1 increased under CRYAB conditions compared with the control. (c) Rt-qPCR analysis of zo-1 and claudin-1 mRNA expression. Compared with that of the control, the expression of zo-1 and claudin-1 was upregulated in response to CRYAB. The data represent the mean ± SD of three independent experiments. $****p < 0.0001$ versus the control.

2.4. Cytoskeleton.

The cells were fixed for 20 minutes in 4% paraformaldehyde (Sigma-Aldrich, St. Louis, MO) and were washed for 5 min in PBS 3 times. Then, they were permeabilized with 0.1% TRITON X-100 (Sigma-Aldrich) in PBS at room temperature and washed 3 times in PBS. The cells were stained with a 50 μg/ml fluorescent phalloidin conjugate solution in PBS (containing 1% DMSO from the original stock solution) for 40 minutes at room temperature in the dark and were washed 3 times with PBS to remove unbound phalloidin conjugate. The nuclei of the TM cells were stained with a 4′, 6-diamidino-2-phenylisndole (DAPI) antibody (Sigma-Aldrich). For each experimental condition, three biological repeats were performed.

2.5. Immunofluorescence.

The cells were fixed and permeabilized following the same procedure as cytoskeleton staining. Then, they were blocked with 1% BSA in PBS for 1 h and incubated with rabbit polyclonal primary antibodies against zo-1, claudin-1, cadherin-E, and cadherin-N (1 : 100 Abcam, England) and a mouse polyclonal primary antibody against vimentin (Abcam, England) overnight at 4°C. Secondary antibodies were used, including TRITC-conjugated goat anti-rabbit IgG and FITC-conjugated goat anti-mouse IgG (1 : 200 Abcam, England). They were incubated for 2 h at 37°C in a humidified atmosphere in the dark. The nuclei of the TM cells were stained with DAPI (1 : 1000; Sigma, USA). The samples were analyzed in a drop of PBS under a fluorescence microscope at this state.

2.6. RNA Extraction and Rt-qPCR.

Total RNA was obtained from the TM cells cultured in 10 ng/ml CRYAB with a Total RNA kit (Omega, USA) and was reverse transcribed into cDNA (1 μg of isolated total RNA) using a qPCR RT Kit (TOBOYO, Japan) according to the manufacturer's instructions. The RNA concentrations were quantified with a Nano instrument (NanoDrop Technologies, Wilmington, DE, USA). Rt-qPCR was carried out using a SYBR Green PCR Master Mix (TOYOBO, Japan). The system of each PCR reaction contained 4 μl of cDNA, 0.8 μl of forward and reverse primers (PCR primers were listed), and 10 μl of SYBR Green PCR Master Mix, with a final volume of 20 μl. All the PCR amplification reactions were performed on a MiniOpticon qPCR (Bio-Rad, USA). The specific primers were the following: zo-1 (forward primer (F), 5′-ACCAGTAAGTCGTCCTGATCC-3′ and reverse primer (R), 5′-TCGGCCAA ATCTTCTCACTCC-3′); claudin-1 (F, 5′-CGAGAGCTACAC GTTCACGG-3′ and R, 5′-GGGT GTCGAGG GAAAAA TAGG-3′); cadherin-E (F, 5′-AAAGG CCCATTTCCTAAAAACCT-3′ and R, 5′-TGCG TTCTCTATCCAGAGGCT-3′); cadherin-N (F, 5′-AGCC AACCTTAAC TGAGGAGT-3′ and R, 5′-GGCAAGTT GATTGGAG GGATG-3′); and vimentin (F, 5′-GACGCC ATCAACACCGAGTT-3′ and R, 5′-CTTTGTCGTTGGTT AG CTGGT-3′). The mRNA expression was normalized to the endogenous reference gene GAPDH (F, 5′-TGGA GAAAAT CTGGCACCAC-3′ and R, 5′-ACCACCCTG

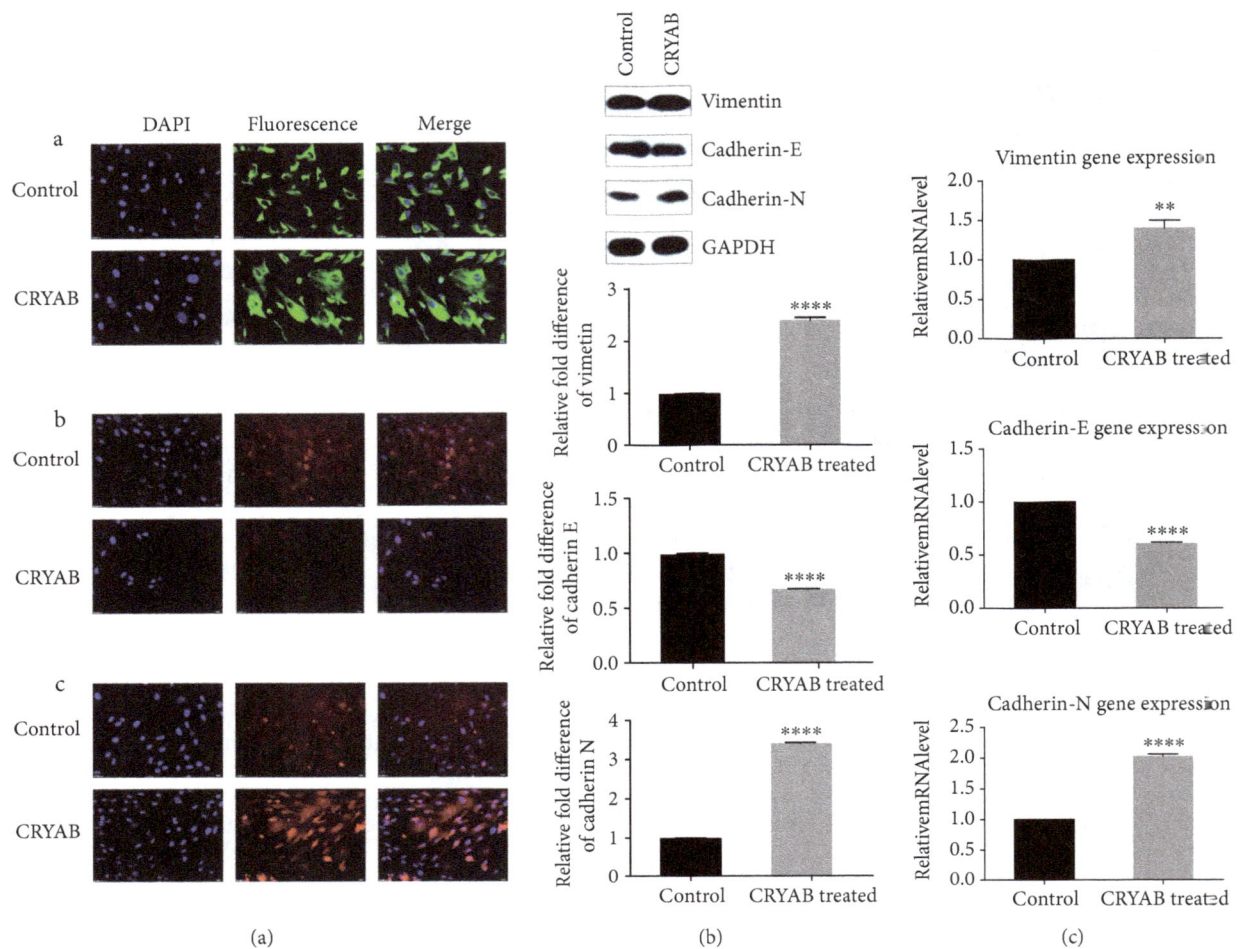

FIGURE 5: Effect of CRYAB on EMT in TM cells. (a) Immunofluorescence manifestation of vimentin, cadherin-E, and cadherin-N. Immunofluorescence verified the upregulation of vimentin and cadherin-N and the downregulation of cadherin-E (A: vimentin; B: cadherin-E; C: cadherin-N). (b) Western blot analysis of vimentin, cadherin-E, and cadherin-N expression. TM cells were exposed to 10 ng/ml CRYAB for 24 h. The expression of vimentin and cadherin-N increased, whereas cadherin-E decreased under CRYAB conditions compared with the control. (c) Real-time PCR analysis of vimentin, cadherin-E, and cadherin-N mRNA expression. Compared with the control, the expression of vimentin and cadherin-N was upregulated, while cadherin-E was downregulated in response to CRYAB. The data shown represent the mean $\pm$ SD of three independent experiments. $^{**}p < 0.01$ and $^{****}p < 0.0001$ versus the control.

TTGCTGTAGCCA A-3$'$) and was analyzed using the $2^{-\Delta\Delta Ct}$ comparative threshold method.

2.7. Protein Extraction and Western Blotting. Total protein from the TM cells was extracted using a RIPA lysis buffer (Thermo, USA). The protein concentration was detected by a bicinchoninic acid assay kit (Beyotime, China). Equal amounts of total protein (30 μg) were separated by 10% SDS-polyacrylamide gel electrophoresis and were transferred to polyvinylidene difluoride membranes (Millipore, Bedford, MA, USA) and were blocked with 5% nonfat skim milk in Tris-buffered saline supplemented with Tween 20 (TBST) for 1.5 h. The proteins were incubated with rabbit polyclonal primary antibodies against zo-1, cadherin-E, cadherin-N, vimentin, and GAPDH (1 : 1000, Cell Science Tech, USA) overnight at 4°C and were then washed and incubated in a secondary antibody conjugated to horseradish peroxidase

(1 : 2000, Cell Science Tech, USA) for 1 h at room temperature. The bands were analyzed using ImageJ software (http://imagej.nih.gov/ij/; provided in the public domain by the National Institutes of Health, Bethesda, MD, USA). GAPDH was used as the loading control.

2.8. Statistical Analysis. All the data were analyzed with the software package SPSS19.0 (SPSS Inc., Chicago, IL, USA). The statistical analysis was performed using one-way analysis of variance and a Student's *t*-test. $p < 0.01$ was considered statistically significant. The data are expressed as the means $\pm$ standard deviation (SD).

3. Result

3.1. Cell Proliferation. In the current study, we first treated the TM cells with a series of concentrations of CRYAB to induce proliferation. The protein concentration ranged from 1 to 10 ng/ml, and the total treatment time was 6 h, 12 h, and 24 h. A cell counting kit-8 was then used to assess cell proliferation by a microplate reader. At one of the tested concentrations of 10 ng/ml, CRYAB induced significant proliferation in the TM cells compared to the control condition of 1 ng/ml (Figure 1). We then chose 10 ng/ml as the protein concentration to be used in the rest of the study, as it induced a high percentage of proliferation.

3.2. Cell Migration. In the cell migration assay, the TM cells were measured in a modified Boyden chamber, in which the TM cells migrated through a porous membrane. The mean number of migrated cells in the CRYAB-treated TM cells (10 ng/ml) was significantly higher than the mean number of migrated control cells (Figures 2(a) and 2(b)).

3.3. Cytoskeleton Reorganization. The cell IF showed that F-actin in CRYAB-treated TM cells irregularly accumulated inside the cytoplasm (Figure 3).

3.4. Effect of CRYAB on Tight Junction Protein Expression. Meanwhile, the level of zo-1, with the application of CRYAB, was significantly upregulated (Figure 4(a), A). Western blot indicated results that were consistent with the IF data, showing that zo-1 was significantly regulated in the CRYAB-treated TM cells (Figure 4(b), $p < 0.0001$), and there were significant differences in the zo-1 and claudin-1 mRNA levels (Figure 4(c), $p < 0.0001$).

3.5. Effect of CRYAB on EMT. We also determined how CRYAB affected the levels of proteins related to EMT in TM. We detected traces of cadherin-N and vimentin, as shown in Figures 5(b) and 5(c), and the levels of cadherin-N and vimentin were upregulated. In contrast, cadherin-E was downregulated (all $p < 0.0001$). Additionally, the expression of cadherin-E was specifically weakened, while vimentin and cadherin-N appeared with more intense staining compared with the control group (Figures 5(a), A; 5(b); and 5(c)).

4. Discussion

The experiments presented here first show that normal TM cells resulted in changes in their function as well as in their protein and gene expression by EMT. Many of the changes resembled alternations seen in ocular tissues of patients with primary open-angle glaucoma [17–19].

We reported that CRYAB promoted the proliferation and migration of TM cells. In addition, the proliferation and migration of TM cells are associated with glaucoma. Glaucoma develops because of an imbalance between aqueous production and its outflow through the trabecular meshwork. We found that when TM cells were incubated with a variety of concentrations of CRYAB, cell proliferation and migration were significantly increased at concentrations of 10 ng/ml. Excessive proliferation and migration may obstruct drainage angle tissue accompanied by the increase of intraocular pressure (IOP). Changes in the cytoskeleton of TM cells are well studied [20–22]. The cytoskeleton is involved with cell volume, shape, and adhesion to the extracellular matrix

and to neighboring cells. CRYAB-treated TM cells present alternations in the F-actin, as we observed a major reorganization of the microfilament structure.

Tight junctions, or zo-1 and claudin-1, form a continuous barrier of fluids across the epithelium, which functions in the regulation of paracellular permeability and the maintenance of cell polarity [23]. The overexpression of tight junction proteins induces cell interaction damage as observed in glaucoma [24, 25]. Our study showed that CRYAB upregulated zo-1 at both the protein and mRNA levels, which might impair aqueous outflow by changing the connections between TM cells. However, we did not observed a change that was consistent with the mRNA in claudin-1 by means of Western blot; thus, we determined that TM cells have a post transcriptional modification process that needs to be further researched.

CRYAB seemed to trigger the expression of genes associated with EMT, then resulted in cell migration. The damage to the trabecular cells is mainly reflected in two aspects, including EMT and the deposition of extracellular matrix (ECM). EMT is mainly reflected by the gradual loss of epithelial properties. E-cadherin expression is downregulated, while mesenchymal phenotypes, such as vimentin, fibronectin, and cadherin-N expression, are upregulated [26]. We observed that TM cells treated with CRYAB had upregulated N-cadherin in addition to the loss of E-cadherin, which indicated that the TM cells acquired mesenchymal properties and displayed reduced intracellular adhesion, because E-cadherin is considered an active suppressor of invasion [27–29]. Vimentin is an intermediate filament of mesenchymal origin, which has conventional expression in TM, whereas its overexpression, as in our study, may cause TM cells to lose their epithelial properties. The acquiring of mesenchymal properties prompted the migration of the TM cells, as we observed.

Previous reports present evidence of TGF-2 in the pathogenesis of POAG [30, 31]. Moreover, TGF-2, which affects EMT, is elevated in the aqueous of patients with glaucoma [32–34]. There is convincing evidence that TGF-2 upregulates CRYAB and that the upregulation of CRYAB occurs with the up/downregulation of EMT markers [35]. In addition, a recent study suggests a direct interaction of CRYAB with beta-catenin [36], which raises the possibility of the role of CRYAB in EMT. These data suggest that CRYAB might be a target to block the secondary open-angle glaucoma. The control of inflammation after surgery provides benefits to it as well.

Overall, all the changes that the TM cells experienced after the exposure to CRYAB resembled alterations seen in primary open-angle glaucoma, which implied that CRYAB affected the TM cellular structures and functions by EMT and might be responsible for the development of secondary open-angle glaucoma. In future research, the specific mechanism should be further studied.

Conflicts of Interest

The authors declare that they have no conflicts of interest.

Acknowledgments

This work was supported by the National Natural Science Foundation of China (no. 2101000139).

References

[1] T. C. Chen, L. S. Bhatia, E. F. Halpern, and D. S. Walton, "Risk factors for the development of aphakic glaucoma after congenital cataract surgery," *Transactions of the American Ophthalmological Society*, vol. 104, pp. 241–251, 2006.

[2] W. H. Chan, S. Biswas, J. L. Ashworth, and I. C. Lloyd, "Congenital and infantile cataract: aetiology and management," *European Journal of Pediatrics*, vol. 171, no. 4, pp. 625–630, 2012.

[3] A. Churchill and J. Graw, "Clinical and experimental advances in congenital and paediatric cataracts," *Philosophical Transactions of the Royal Society B: Biological Sciences*, vol. 366, no. 1568, pp. 1234–1249, 2011.

[4] F. Ma, Q. Wang, and L. Wang, "Advances in the management of the surgical complications for congenital cataract," *Frontiers in Medicine*, vol. 6, no. 4, pp. 360–365, 2012.

[5] C. Kuhli-Hattenbach, M. Lüchtenberg, T. Kohnen, and L. O. Hattenbach, "Risk factors for complications after congenital cataract surgery without intraocular lens implantation in the first 18 months of life," *American Journal of Ophthalmology*, vol. 146, no. 1, pp. 1–7.e1, 2008.

[6] B. Urban and A. Bakunowicz-Łazarczyk, "Aphakic glaucoma after congenital cataract surgery with and without intraocular lens implantation," *Klinika Oczna*, vol. 112, no. 4–6, pp. 105–107, 2010.

[7] T. C. Chen, L. S. Bhatia, E. F. Halpern, and D. S. Walton, "Risk factors for the development of aphakic glaucoma after congenital cataract surgery," *Journal of Pediatric Ophthalmology and Strabismus*, vol. 43, no. 5, pp. 274–280, 2006.

[8] M. R. Praveen, A. R. Vasavada, S. K. Shah, M. B. Khamar, and R. H. Trivedi, "Long-term postoperative outcomes after bilateral congenital cataract surgery in eyes with microphthalmos," *Journal of Cataract and Refractive Surgery*, vol. 41, no. 9, pp. 1910–1918, 2015.

[9] B. H. Shenoy, V. Mittal, A. Gupta, V. Sachdeva, and R. Kekunnaya, "Complications and visual outcomes after secondary intraocular lens implantation in children," *American Journal of Ophthalmology*, vol. 159, no. 4, pp. 720–726.e2, 2015.

[10] R. H. Trivedi, M. E. Wilson Jr, and R. L. Golub, "Incidence and risk factors for glaucoma after pediatric cataract surgery with and without intraocular lens implantation," *Journal of AAPOS*, vol. 10, no. 2, pp. 117–123, 2006.

[11] S. Asrani, S. Freedman, V. Hasselblad et al., "Does primary intraocular lens implantation prevent "aphakic" glaucoma in children?," *Journal of AAPOS*, vol. 4, no. 1, pp. 33–39, 2000.

[12] I. Michael, M. Shmoish, D. S. Walton, and S. Levenberg, "Interactions between trabecular meshwork cells and lens epithelial cells: a possible mechanism in infantile aphakic glaucoma," *Investigative Ophthalmology & Visual Science*, vol. 49, no. 9, pp. 3981–3987, 2008.

[13] J. Yaung, M. Jin, E. Barron et al., "α-Crystallin distribution in retinal pigment epithelium and effect of gene knockouts on sensitivity to oxidative stress," *Molecular Vision*, vol. 13, pp. 566–577, 2007.

[14] U. P. Andley, "Crystallins in the eye: Function and pathology," *Progress in Retinal and Eye Research*, vol. 26, no. 1, pp. 78–98, 2007.

[15] P. S. Bellaye, G. Wettstein, O. Burgy et al., "The small heat-shock protein αB-crystallin is essential for the nuclear localization of Smad4: impact on pulmonary fibrosis," *The Journal of Pathology*, vol. 232, no. 4, pp. 458–472, 2014.

[16] R. B. Nahomi, R. Huang, S. K. Nandi et al., "Acetylation of lysine 92 improves the chaperone and anti-apoptotic activities of human αB-crystallin," *Biochemistry*, vol. 52, no. 45, pp. 8126–8138, 2013.

[17] B. Paloma, C. L. Liton, C. Pratap, D. L. Epstein, and P. Gonzalez, "Genome-wide expression profile of human trabecular meshwork cultured cells, nonglaucomatous and primary open angle glaucoma tissue," *Molecular Vision*, vol. 12, pp. 774–790, 2006.

[18] P. L. Lip, D. C. Felmeden, A. D. Blann et al., "Plasma vascular endothelial growth factor, soluble VEGF receptor FLT-1, and von Willebrand factor in glaucoma," *British Journal of Ophthalmology*, vol. 86, no. 11, pp. 1299–1302, 2002.

[19] C. H. Mitchell, J. C. Fleischhauer, W. D. Stamer, K. Peterson-Yantorno, and M. M. Civan, "Human trabecular meshwork cell volume regulation," *American Journal of Physiology Cell Physiology*, vol. 283, no. 1, pp. C315–C326, 2002.

[20] M. I. Ryder, R. N. Weinreb, J. Alvarado, and J. Polansky, "The cytoskeleton of the cultured human trabecular cell. Characterization and drug responses," *Investigative Ophthalmology & Visual Science*, vol. 29, no. 2, pp. 251–260, 1988.

[21] A. F. Clark, S. T. Miggans, K. Wilson, S. Browder, and M. D. McCartney, "Cytoskeletal changes in cultured human glaucoma trabecular meshwork cells," *Journal of Glaucoma*, vol. 4, no. 3, pp. 183–188, 1995.

[22] B. Tian, B. Geiger, D. L. Epstein, and P. L. Kaufman, "Cytoskeletal involvement in the regulation of aqueous humor outflow," *Investigative Ophthalmology & Visual Science*, vol. 41, no. 3, pp. 619–623, 2000.

[23] P. Polakis, "The oncogenic activation of β-catenin," *Current Opinion in Genetics & Development*, vol. 9, no. 1, pp. 15–21, 1999.

[24] N. Wang, S. K. Chintala, M. E. Fini, and J. S. Schuman, "Activation of a tissue-specific stress response in the aqueous outflow pathway of the eye defines the glaucoma disease phenotype," *Nature Medicine*, vol. 7, no. 3, pp. 304–309, 2001.

[25] T. Borras, "Gene expression in the trabecular meshwork and the influence of intraocular pressure," *Progress in Retinal and Eye Research*, vol. 22, no. 4, pp. 435–463, 2003.

[26] Y. Chan, "To epithelial mesenchymal transition (EMT) and its molecular mechanism," *International Journal of Genetics*, vol. 29, no. 4, pp. 290–294, 2006.

[27] H. Peinado, D. Olmeda, and A. Cano, "Snail, Zeb and bHLH factors in tumour progression: an alliance against the epithelial phenotype?," *Nature Reviews Cancer*, vol. 7, no. 6, pp. 415–428, 2007.

[28] G. Christofori, "Changing neighbours, changing behaviour: cell adhesion molecule-mediated signalling during tumour progression," *The EMBO Journal*, vol. 22, no. 10, pp. 2318–2323, 2003.

[29] A. Wodarz and R. Nusse, "Mechanisms of Wnt signaling in development," *Annual Review of Cell and Developmental Biology*, vol. 14, no. 1, pp. 59–88, 1998.

[30] M. Inatani, H. Tanihara, H. Katsuta, M. Honjo, N. Kido, and Y. Honda, "Transforming growth factor-β_2 levels in aqueous humor of glaucomatous eyes," *Graefe's Archive for Clinical and Experimental Ophthalmology*, vol. 239, no. 2, pp. 109–113, 2001.

[31] R. Fuchshofer and E. R. Tamm, "The role of TGF-β in the pathogenesis of primary open-angle glaucoma," *Cell and Tissue Research*, vol. 347, no. 1, pp. 279–290, 2012.

[32] S. Saika, Y. Okada, T. Miyamoto, Y. Ohnishi, A. Ooshima, and J. W. McAvoy, "Smad translocation and growth suppression in lens epithelial cells by endogenous TGFβ2 during wound repair," *Experimental Eye Research*, vol. 72, no. 6, pp. 679–686, 2001.

[33] N. Wallentin, K. Wickstrom, and C. Lundberg, "Effect of cataract surgery on aqueous TGF-β and lens epithelial cell proliferation," *Investigative Ophthalmology & Visual Science*, vol. 39, no. 8, pp. 1410–1418, 1998.

[34] U. Valcourt, M. Kowanetz, H. Niimi, C.-H. Heldin, and A. Moustakas, "TGF-β and the Smad signaling pathway support transcriptomic reprogramming during epithelial mesenchymal cell transition," *Molecular Biology of the Cell*, vol. 16, no. 4, pp. 1987–2002, 2005.

[35] R. B. Nahomi, M. B. Pantcheva, and R. H. Nagaraj, "αB-Crystallin is essential for the TGF-β2-mediated epithelial to mesenchymal transition of lens epithelial cells," *Biochemical Journal*, vol. 473, no. 10, pp. 1455–1469, 2016.

[36] J. G. Ghosh, A. K. Shenoy, and J. I. Clark, "Interactions between important regulatory proteins and human αB crystallin," *Biochemistry*, vol. 46, no. 21, pp. 6308–6317, 2007.

13

From Presbyopia to Cataracts: A Critical Review on Dysfunctional Lens Syndrome

Joaquín Fernández,[1,2] Manuel Rodríguez-Vallejo ⓘ,[1] Javier Martínez,[1] Ana Tauste,[1] and David P. Piñero ⓘ[3,4]

[1]Department of Ophthalmology (Qvision), Vithas Virgen del Mar Hospital, 04120 Almería, Spain
[2]Department of Ophthalmology, Torrecárdenas Hospital Complex, 04009 Almería, Spain
[3]Department of Optics, Pharmacology and Anatomy, University of Alicante, Alicante, Spain
[4]Department of Ophthalmology (OFTALMAR), Vithas Medimar International Hospital, Alicante, Spain

Correspondence should be addressed to David P. Piñero; david.pinyero@ua.es

Academic Editor: Antonio Queiros

Dysfunctional lens syndrome (DLS) is a term coined to describe the natural aging changes in the crystalline lens. Different alterations in the refractive properties and transparency of the lens are produced during the development of presbyopia and cataract, such as changes in internal high order aberrations or an increase in ocular forward scattering, with a potentially significant impact on clinical measures, including visual acuity and contrast sensitivity. Objective technologies have emerged to solve the limits of current methods for the grading of the lens aging, which have been linked to the DLS term. However, there is still not a gold standard or evidence-based clinical guidelines around these new technologies despite multiple research studies have correlated their results with conventional methods such as visual acuity or the lens opacification system (LOCS), with more scientific background around the ocular scattering index (OSI) and Scheimpflug densitometry. In either case, DLS is not a new evidence-based concept that leads to new knowledge about crystalline lens aging but it is a nomenclature change of two existing terms, presbyopia and cataracts. Therefore, this term should be used with caution in the scientific peer-reviewed literature.

1. Introduction

Dysfunctional lens syndrome (DLS) describes the natural lens changes in the crystalline lens and has been helpful in educating patients, staff, and doctors about these changes for years [1]. The crystalline lens aging from presbyopia to cataracts is coined in a single term which includes three stages. The stage 1 has been popularly suggested [1, 2] from 42 to 50 years old and corresponds to the term of presbyopia, when accommodation has been lost but light scatter remains relatively limited. In the stages 2 (50 to 65 years old) and 3 (65 or older), the ocular scatter increases and a lens replacement-based procedure may be warranted [1, 2]. These ranges of age used in clinical practice can be questionable since there is broad agreement among different authors that from the age of 30–40 years there is typically a slow drift towards hyperopia [3]. Presbyopia can, therefore, start before the age of forty and the light can scatter

after sixty [4]. The DLS, therefore, is not a new evidence-based concept that leads to new knowledge about crystalline lens aging, but it is a nomenclature change of two existing terms, presbyopia and cataracts. It results from the new treatments and diagnosis tools in the modern refractive cataract patients [5]. The aim of the creation of this concept was to facilitate the comprehension of lens aging for patients, and it has sense as nowadays the treatment of Stage 1 (presbyopia) is based on a combination of guidelines for refractive error [6] and cataract [7] treatment. Therefore, it seems coherent to talk about DLS in the adult eye-preferred practice pattern instead of cataract if also presbyopia treatment is considered [7]. The main aim of the current article is to review the current evidence around the new diagnostic tools that might lead to a future change of paradigm linked to the DLS term that may serve to improve the decision criteria for the current alternatives to the treatment of presbyopia and cataracts.

2. Aging of the Crystalline Lens

2.1. Physiology of the Lens. Different alterations in the refractive properties and transparency of the lens are produced during the development of presbyopia and cataract. Although it is not well understood how lens cellular structure and function initiate changes in refraction and transparency, a common underlying mechanism in the pathology of cortical and nuclear cataract can be attributed to the failure of the microcirculation system to regulate cell volume in the lens cortex, or deliver antioxidants [8], such as the Glutathione [9, 10], to the lens nucleus [11]. Donaldson et al. [11] rigorously described the physiological optics of the crystalline lens and the development of cataract, suggesting future possible treatments based on functionality changes at the cellular level. Therefore, we recommend reading the work of Donaldson et al. [11] for a better knowledge of the physiology of the lens aging and these potential promising future treatments.

2.2. Internal Aberrations. The internal aberration variations with age have led to some controversies for years as was pointed out by Smith et al. [12]. It is agreed that the relaxed lens has a negative spherical aberration (SA) value close to the positive value of the corneal surface [12], exhibiting then a balanced compensation up to around 45 years of age [13]. Alió et al. [14] and Amano et al. [15] reported an increase with age of coma and positive SA attributed to the crystalline lens. The negative spherical aberration of the lens can be partly explained by the inherent Gradient of Refractive Index (GRIN) [16–19], and the decrease of internal negative SA with age by the increase of the refractive index of the plateau (nuclear) region of the lens in old people that has a size reaching a maximum value at 60 years old [20]. These results are in agreement with Sachdev et al. [21] and Rocha et al. [22] who evaluated the level of high order aberrations (HOAs) in eyes with cortical and nuclear cataracts. On the contrast, Lee et al. [23, 24], Wu et al. [25], and Faria-Correia et al. [26], conversely to previous authors, reported that negative internal SA was increased in nuclear cataract as well as Kuroda et al. [27] and Zhu et al. [28] who also suggested that the opposite happens in cortical cataracts, with an increase of the positive total SA measured with Hartman–Sack aberrometers. This was attributed to the fact that wavefront in the central pupillary area relatively delays in nuclear cataracts and relatively advances in normal subjects and cortical cataract [27]. The hypothesis surrounding these findings are opposite to the GRIN changes with age, but the authors explain this by a major increase of refractive index in the nucleus comparing to the surrounding which means that for nuclear cataracts, the plateau tendency might be not presented.

2.3. Scattering. Light is scattered when enters into the eye due to optical imperfections or lack of transparency from the optical media and is the main cause of glare perception [29]. The scattering should not be confused with optical aberrations, while optical aberrations deflect light in small angles ($<1°$), light scatter produces straylight over large angles ($>1°$) [30]. There are two methods for the assessment of light scattering, the light scattered into the retina (forward scattering) or the light scattered backward (backward-scattering). The slit-lamp evaluation of lens opacities is based on backward-scattering; however, it is important to note that backward-scattering represents light that not reaches the retina, and the light that reaches the retina cannot be derived from this backward-scattering [31]. First, studies assessing backward-scattering which implied the human lens were published in the mid-seventies [32] and were aimed at characterizing the molecular changes associated with the early stages of cataractogenesis [33]. A clinical device based on this measure was developed in 2008 and the term dynamic light scattering was coined for referring to the measurement of scattering due to light-particle interaction as a function of time [34, 35]. However, dynamic light scattering is focused on measuring changes in molecules, such as α-crystallin [36], whose decrease has been related to the risk of developing cataract instead of understanding the implication of the scattering on the visual function.

2.4. The Impact of Age-Related Optical Changes on Visual Performance. Besides the numerical increase of internal aberrations or scattering, the clinical significance of these parameters is determined by their influence on the visual performance. Despite internal aberrations are increased with age, it is important to note that this increase does not necessarily have a clinically significant influence on visual performance as there are also changes occurring in pupil size with age [37]. Thus, even though there is a variation of spherical aberration with age, this variation does not deteriorate visual performance in eyes with small pupils [38]. Furthermore, neural changes in the aging visual pathways, in agreement for *P* pathways and controversial for *M* [39], can have a role on the decrease on visual performance, but the role seems to be less relevant when compared against the influence of the optical properties of the ageing eye [40]. Then, it is reasonable to conduct estimations of the affected visual performance with objective systems despite not considering the neural processing. Moreover, the prediction of the possible visual performance achievable after surgery is not possible until a clinical system evaluating the visual acuity through the cataract is developed [41], without the limitations of past technologies that have not demonstrated a clinically useful prediction of postoperative best-corrected visual acuity, such as the potential acuity meter and the visometer [42].

The gold standard for measuring the visual performance in clinical practice is the high contrast visual acuity (VA). Internal HOAs increase with age is related with a decrease of VA [38]. However, an increase of aberrations generating visual complains is not always related to a high contrast photopic VA deterioration [21]. Similarly, the increase in scattering has shown poor although statistically significant correlation with VA [30]. Therefore, VA provides an incomplete assessment of visual performance and other clinical tests, such as contrast sensitivity or straylight, should be added in the clinical evaluation of cataract [43]. In fact, despite the VA still remain as the gold standard for driving license (0.3 logMAR in Europe) [44], some researchers have claimed to include other metrics which have demonstrated a higher risk to be involved in car accidents, such as contrast sensitivity with Pelli Robson test (1.25 log cut-off value) [45, 46] and straylight (1.4 log cut-off value) [45], or motion sensitivity and mesopic high-contrast VA for driving at night [47].

The crystalline lens aging has a different impact factor on contrast sensitivity function (CSF) depending on the level of scattering or HOAs. Although both affect to CSF, Zhao et al. [48] reported that the loss in CSF when both scattering and HOAs are present cannot be explained as a summation of the single impact factor of scattering or HOAs. Indeed, less reduction can be obtained when combining scattering and HOAs than the impact factor of each one separately [48]. This suggests that there is a compensatory neural processing, with different impact for different spatial frequencies. While single analysis of HOAs has a higher impact on higher spatial frequencies, scattering has a more significant impact on middle spatial frequencies.

3. Objective Technologies for Lens Evaluation

Objective technologies for grading the development of cataract are based on the measure of these previous variables, internal aberrations and scattering. These technologies include densitometry measured with Scheimpflug camera devices or anterior segment optical coherence tomography (AS-OCT), internal wavefront aberrations obtained from the subtraction of the corneal from the total wavefront aberrations, and the direct measure of the point spread function with a double-pass system.

3.1. Densitometry. The objective lens densitometry (OLD) is measured by Scheimpflug camera-based devices. The Pentacam HR (Oculus Optikgeräte GmbH, Wetzlar, Germany) includes the pentacam nucleus staging (PNS) classification which evaluates the mean densitometry in a continuous scale from 0 to 100 [49] or in an ordinal classification from 0 to 5 [50]. The software automatically detects the nucleus location and measures the densitometry in a cylindrical three-dimensional template. A limitation of the software is that cortical cataracts can produce shadowing artefacts or misplacement of the reference template that may affect to the PNS [49]. Studies have found that the analysis of the nuclear region, as the PNS performs, has a higher correlation with visual performance than the average of the whole lens [51]. The average lens density at the nucleus location is correlated with VA ($r = 0.44$ [52], $r = 0.63$ [53], $r = 0.76$ [51]) as well as with contrast sensitivity for four spatial frequencies ($r = -0.30$ at 3 cpd, $r = -0.55$ at 6 cpd, $r = -0.60$ at 12 cpd, and $r = -0.48$ at 18 cpd) [51]. AS-OCT has been also proposed recently for grading the density of the lens with the purpose of predicting phacoemulsification energy; however, subjective grading through Lens Opacification System III (LOCS III) has resulted in higher correlations with the phacoemulsification energy than AS-OCT or Scheimpflug [54]. The latter is in controversy with the report by Faria-Correia et al. [49]. In any case, the grading of presbyopia and cataracts through AS-OCT seems to be a promising

technology, not only because of the OLD measure, but also due to the possibility to measure the dynamic changes of the crystalline lens during accommodation [55].

3.2. Wavefront Aberrometers. Nowadays, several devices subtract the corneal wavefront derived from corneal topography to the total wavefront directly obtained from raytracing or Hartman–Shack aberrometry. These devices include Irx3 (Hartmann–Shack; Imagine Eyes, Orsay, France), KR-1W (Hartmann–Shack, Topcon, Japan), Keratron (Hartmann–Shack; Optikon, Rome Italy) iTrace (ray-tracing; Tracey Technologies, Houston, TX), and OPD-Scan (Automated Retinoscopy; Nidek, Gamagori, Japan). In the early development of the measurement of internal aberrations, some caution was pointed out because of the lack of reliability of obtaining these from aberrometry and corneal topography (CT) [56]. The main problem of these devices was the two-step measurement that required a perfect realignment during topography and later measure of the wavefront [57]. In fact, internal aberration comparison between devices has led to significant differences [58], in some cases in a considerable degree [59]. However, it is also important to note that devices based on different technologies such as KR-1W or iTrace have reported similar results to describe an increase of negative internal spherical aberration in nuclear cataract [24–26, 28]. Based on the measurement of internal aberrations provided, some aberrometers such as the iTrace have developed an index that ranks overall lens performance from 0 (very poor) to 10 (excellent) points. This index has shown correlations with VA, ($r = -0.67$ [49], $r = -0.70$ [53]) but as far as we know, there are no studies showing the correlations of this index with other metrics such as contrast sensitivity.

3.3. Double-Pass System. The objective scatter index (OSI) comes from the double-pass technique that examines the forward-scattered light, which causes degradation of retinal images in eyes with cataract [60]. Unlike wavefront technologies, the double-pass technique also considers the scattered light; therefore, modulation transfer function in early stage cataract can be better related with visual function than the optical quality characterized using data from wavefront devices [61, 62]. OSI has been used to classify cataracts in normal (<1.0), early (from 1.0 to 2.9), mature (from 3.0 to 6.9), and severe (≥7.0) [60]. Control groups without cataract rarely shows an OSI value higher than 1.0, although some cases in control groups [63] or young subjects [64] can result in slight values over 1.0. A recent study has demonstrated that OSI has sensitivity and specificity values to discriminate healthy and cataractous eyes of 89% and 100%, respectively, when a cut-off value of 1.18 is used [4]. The mean cut-off value for early cataract differs among authors. While Artal et al. [60] reported a value around 2.0 for early cataract, Galliot et al. [65] classify early cataract with a mean OSI value of 3.7. The criteria for cataract classification should not be confused with the criteria for surgery. The cut-off value for which a cataract is recommended to be operated in a sample of subjects with decimal

VA > 0.5 was set by Paz et al. [66] at 2.1 considering two groups of subjects for which surgery was previously recommended or not according to conventional ophthalmological criteria (area under the receiver operating characteristic curve of 0.83). Zhang and Wang [67] also suggested conducting capsulotomy in patients operated on with cataract surgery when an OSI value of 3 was measured. Interestingly, they reported 5 cases of patients with subjective symptoms and VAs better than 0.15 logMAR but with OSI values above 3. In these cases, VAs remained constant after capsulotomy but with a decrease of OSI below 1.3 and with the resolution of symptoms.

The OSI has been also compared with LOCS III classification scale in nuclear (NC), cortical (CC), and posterior subcapsular (PSC) cataracts. Although there exists consensus about a clear correlation between OSI and LOCS III in NC, this is not as clear in PSC or CC [68, 69]. LOCS III is not always correlated with OSI because the central pupil area (4 mm) is not always covered by some types of cataracts [63]. An opacification can be detected on slit-lamp examination, but without induction of visual impairment in some cases. Indeed, Paz Filgueira et al. [68] reported that LOCS III in PSC was not correlated with psychophysical parameters, such as visual acuity, contrast sensitivity, and the straylight parameter ($\log(s)$). Likewise, Vilaseca et al. [63] found a greater dispersion of OSI and VA in eyes with PSC and CC.

The correlations of OSI and VA have been widely studied. Paz Filgueira et al. [68] reported nonsignificant linear correlations between OSI and VA, but these authors found a significant correlation between OSI and straylight parameter ($\log(s)$). Cochener et al. [70] reported a correlation of OSI and VA ($\rho = 0.48$, $P < 0.001$) similar to that reported by Crnej et al. [71] ($r = 0.45$). In contrast, Pan et al. [52] reported a correlation between OSI and VA of $r = 0.78$. Cabot et al. [69] reported that this correlation varied among nuclear ($\rho = 0.7$), cortical ($\rho = 0.5$), and posterior subcapsular ($\rho = 0.6$) cataracts. Similarly, Martínez-Roda et al. [4] also reported an OSI-VA correlation dependency on the type of cataract ($r = -0.40$ nuclear, $r = -0.38$ cortical, and $r = -0.48$ posterior subcapsular). Besides VA, correlations of OSI with contrast sensitivity have been also reported for nuclear cataract ($r = -0.56$ at 3 cpd, $r = -0.45$ at 6 cpd, $r = -0.39$ at 12 cpd, and $r = -0.40$ at 18 cpd), but these have been shown to increase for posterior subcapsular cataract, as happened with VA [51]. It is especially interesting the study of Vilaseca et al. [63] who reported an exponential decay model with correlations of $r = 0.88$, $r = 0.84$, and $r = 0.84$ for nuclear, cortical, and posterior subcapsular cataracts, respectively. The authors also remarked that in some cases, a dense cataract can drastically increase the OSI and therefore the intraocular scattering, whereas its impact on VA is not as strong.

The evaluation of the OSI has been also reported two months after cataract surgery with monofocal IOL implantation in eyes with a preoperative mean OSI around 11.5, showing significant differences between spherical (3.2 ± 0.8) and aspheric lenses (2.5 ± 0.8) that were not detected by means of visual acuity [72]. Park et al. [73] reported that only subjects above 70s resulted in a significant lower OSI after implantation of a monofocal IOL in comparison to nonimplanted subjects. However, Park et al. [73] reported a mean OSI in pseudophakic eyes of 2.21, and other authors have reported lower values, such as Jiménez et al. [74] who found a decrease in the mean OSI from 7.44 preoperatively to 1.48 at three months, or Lee et al. [75] who reported a mean OSI of 1.38 in pseudophakic eyes and Chen et al. [76] who found a mean OSI of 1.45 and 2.50 in eyes implanted with monofocal and multifocal IOLs, respectively. Lee et al. [77] also reported a mean OSI of 1.82 with multifocal IOLs. However, the validity of all these studies with MIOLs is questionable because of the known limitations of the near-infrared optical performance of diffractive multifocal intraocular lenses [78], or the first-pass in the double-pass technique that can be affected by the size of the first ring [79]. Finally, OSI has found to be correlated with straylight parameters and even related to driving safety [43]. Martínez-Roda et al. [44] estimated that an OSI of approximately 3 may be considered as a safe margin for driving.

3.4. Decision Criteria with Objective Systems. Decisions about crystalline lens surgery are based on a benefit/risk balance. Risks can be related to intraoperative or postoperative complications. Major complications are potentially sight-threatening and include infectious endophthalmitis (0.02%–0.05%) [80, 81], anterior segment syndrome [7], intraoperative suprachoroidal haemorrhage (0.46%) [82], cystoid macular edema (1.17%) [83], retinal detachment (0.03%) [64], persistent corneal edema, IOL dislocation, ptosis, corneal decompensation, diplopia, and blindness [7]. Other adverse events can be presented during the surgery, such as anterior capsular tears (0.55%–0.79%) [84, 85], posterior capsule tears or rupture with or without vitreous loss (1.8%–3.5%) [86, 87], or during the postoperative period, such as iritis (1.53%) [84], corneal edema (0.53%) [84], and posterior capsule opacification (4.2%) [87]. Considering that these complications have decreased with years [81, 82, 88], it is important to note that decisions should be taken considering the most recent evidence and also considering factors associated with the increase of incidence of complications, such as ocular comorbidities [87], age [89], sex [81], and combined surgery [81, 88].

Although new metrics have demonstrated superiority in the diagnosis of cataract [90], the common primary indicator for cataract surgery is still preoperative VA [91]. Kessel et al. [92] reported that there is a lack of scientific evidence supporting the use of preoperative VA to guide the clinician in the decision of recommending surgery or not. However, VA is effective for regulating the number of required surgeries in order to prevent an unmet population [93]. In Spain, VA of 0.4 decimal is considered the cut-off value for surgery indication in most of public hospitals, but this criterion is the result of the need for attending population within the possibilities of the health resources and therefore, the criteria can change depending on the possibilities of each country and the aging population with the potential of developing cataract [93]. Kessel et al. [94] also pointed out that evidence-based guidelines can change practice patterns unless they are counteracted by the reimbursement system. Therefore, the cut-off value of 0.4

TABLE 1: Monocular visual performance and optical quality in cataract and eyes implanted with multifocal intraocular lenses.

	CDVA	3 cpd	6 cpd	12 cpd	18 cpd	OSI
Control (52 to 65 years) [4]	−0.10	1.69	1.92	1.51	0.93	0.67
LOCS III (grade 1)	0.03	1.56	1.81	1.41	0.99	1.56
LOCS III (grade 2)	0.18	1.52	1.70	1.29	0.81	3.47
LOCS III (grade 3)	0.31	1.43	1.57	1.12	0.80	5.88
LOCS III (grade 4)	0.59	1.31	1.30	0.90	0.46	10.23
Multifocal						
Restor + 2.5 [109]	0.01	1.49	1.64	1.31	0.90	—
Restor + 3.0 [109]	0.01	1.51	1.65	1.22	1.07	—
Fine vision [109]	0.01	1.6	1.70	1.26	0.94	—
Tecnis symfony [110]	−0.04	1.6	1.69	1.31	0.89	—
Restor + 3.0 [111]	−0.13	1.73	1.93	1.56	1.12	—
Restor + 4.0 [111]	−0.13	1.70	1.92	1.54	1.09	—
Tecnis + 4.0 [112]	−0.03	1.86	1.99	1.68	1.21	—
Mean	−0.04	1.63	1.77	1.39	1.02	—

decimal used in public hospitals in Spain is more an economic point to prioritize surgeries in an ageing population than a risk-benefit balance based on health parameters. In fact, a cut-off value of VA is not recommended by the American Academy of Ophthalmology guidelines that recommends instead surgery when the visual function no longer meets the patients' needs [7].

If the preoperative VA is not a good indicator to guide the clinician in the recommendation of cataract surgery with monofocal IOLs, the recommendation of implantation of multifocal IOLs is even a more complicated process. The contraindication criteria for MIOLs have been well established [90], but the stage of DLS at which the patient will achieve a highest satisfaction after a MIOL implantation still remains unclear. Satisfaction after cataract surgery with MIOL implantation might be associated with nonvisual variables such as expectations considering the previous use of spectacles [95, 96] and quality of care given during the hospital stay [97]. The desire for achieving spectacle independence in a wide range of distances remains the most important issue for MIOLs indication, but since satisfaction with multifocal IOLs will vary due to nonrelated vision factors [90, 98, 99], other variables such as personality should be also considered [90, 100].

The DLS criteria suggest that refractive lens exchange (RLE) should be considered as a treatment alternative in Stage 2 when ocular scatter increases [1, 2] and some authors have suggested also in Stage 1 in subjects who have presbyopia and reduced visual quality under low light conditions, high hyperopia [101], or high myopia [6]. However, it is also important to note the risk factor associated to high hyperopia, such as choroidal effusion and macular edema [102], or in high myopia, such as the percentage of retinal detachment which is around 2–8% of eyes [6], and the risk factors associated to this detachment [102].

Besides risks of surgery, there are other vision-related adverse events due to MIOL implantation that can influence on patients' satisfaction. Adverse events of MIOLs include reduced contrast sensitivity, halos around point sources of light, multiple or ghosting images, and glare [7]. Halos and glare, also known as dysphotopsias, are intrinsically associated to the monofocal [103] or multifocal IOL technologies

[98, 99, 104], resulting in one of the most important complains [99, 103]. However, despite being intrinsically associated to the technology, not all the patients refer disturbances associated to dysphotopsias, probably because these phenomena are only perceived under certain conditions, such as driving at night looking at a bright light source against a dark background [104] due to neural adaptation [105] or due to patients' personality [100]. On the contrast, it is also important to note that some adverse effects produced by MIOLs, such as glare or contrast sensitivity reduction, also appear during cataract development. Thus, it is reasonable to expect that a patient with levels of contrast sensitivity, visual acuity, or dysphotopsia at far distance equal or better than those presented preoperatively will be more satisfied with a MIOL because a loss in visual quality at far would be not perceived as disturbing while an improvement at intermediate and near vision without spectacle would be perceived. Furthermore, it is important to note that a loss in contrast sensitivity is expected after MIOL implantation due to the lens split light in more than a focus, but this loss of energy at far distance will not be linearly correlated with the reduction in contrast sensitivity mainly due to optical quality in the normal eye is 10 times better than the capability of the neural system to process contrast [106]. Then, a reduction of energy of 50% will not correspond to a decrease of contrast sensitivity of 50%.

A wide knowledge of the visual quality at the preoperative stage and the achievable at the postoperative stage will lead to a benefit/risk based on vision-related adverse effects of MIOLs in addition to the benefit/risk based on surgery adverse events. In terms of dysphotopsia, Puell et al. [107] reported that halo radius started to increase exponentially from the age of 50 during cataract development. In this study, authors excluded cataracts below level 2 of LOCS III with independence of the age and they reported a maximum mean radius of 160 arcmin from 70 to 79 years. In another study, Palomo-Álvarez et al. [91] included subjects with cataract above level 2 of LOCS III obtaining a mean radius of 2.40 log arcmin (251 arcmin). The mean halo radii with monofocal IOL was 190 arcmin and with $a + 3.00$ D multifocal IOL was 225 arcmin [108]. Considering the values reported by these previous studies, we can consider that a cataract grade 2 is necessary to avoid exceeding the halo radii of the preoperative stage after cataract surgery with implantation either of monofocal or multifocal IOLs.

Our research group also conducted the same analysis for contrast sensitivity and visual acuity after MIOLs implantation (Table 1). The mean monocular contrast sensitivity and VA achieved with different MIOLs was close to those reported for grade 1 cataract by Martínez-Roda et al. [4] and the OSI was around 1.5. Therefore, considering the published literature, a cataract grade 1 would result in similar far contrast sensitivity than that achieved with a MIOL. However, the dysphotopsia associated to $a + 3.0$ D add bifocal IOL would be greater, being necessary a grade 2 cataract for obtaining a similar halo size. This conclusion should be interpreted with caution because it was obtained with different studies including different samples, and future paired design studies should be conducted including preoperative and postoperative halo ring size or contrast sensitivity in the same subjects.

4. Conclusions

The term dysfunctional lens syndrome (DLS) is commonly used in congresses instead of referring to presbyopia or cataracts [1, 2, 5, 101]. However, few research papers [49, 53, 113] use this term in studies linked with new objective technologies for grading the cataract development. The term DLS can be criticized by professionals and researchers arguing that this term was born with technology and not from evidence [114], even though some authors claimed that the term has been used for over 15 years [1]. In this review, we evaluated the current evidence around these new technologies in order to help the modern surgeon to take decisions about cataract and refractive lens exchange procedures based on these devices. However, there is still few studies addressing cut-off values recommended for implanting a monofocal or a multifocal IOL. Likewise, studies including benefits from surgery in patients measured preoperatively and postoperatively are required. Considering the limitations of these devices to measure optical quality after the implantation of a multifocal lens, the only mode to conduct this task is relating the preoperative objective with subjective measures of the visual performance, such as contrast sensitivity, and estimating the cut-off value based on their association with objective measures in the preoperative visit. In this sense, we can conclude according to literature that a preoperative OSI of 1.5 may be considered as a value equivalent to the visual performance achieved by the patient after the implantation of a MIOL as for this OSI value preoperative and postoperative contrast sensitivity are similar. However, this conclusion should be interpreted with caution because it is achieved by means of evaluating the results obtained from different studies, and future paired studies including information of the same eye during the preoperative and postoperative visit are required. Considering the current state of limited evidence on the potential usefulness of new technologies to characterize clinically age-related optical changes and the lack of a gold standard or clinical guidelines, the use of the term DLS should be used with caution in the scientific literature, being preferable the use of the terms presbyopia and cataract. A new terminology only should replace the previous one when this offer new evidence-based information not covered by the previous one.

Conflicts of Interest

The authors declare that they have no conflicts of interest.

Acknowledgments

The author David P. Piñero has been supported by the Ministry of Economy, Industry and Competitiveness of Spain within the program Ramón y Cajal, RYC-2016-20471.

References

[1] D. S. Durrie and M. Moshifar, "Dysfunctional lens syndrome," in *Proceedings of the Annual Meeting of ISRS. Pursuit of Perfection. Section II: Intraocular Refractive Surgery Topics*, Chicago, IL, USA, 2016.

[2] G. O. Waring, K. M. Rocha, D. S. Durrie, and V. M. Thompson, "Use of dysfunctional lens syndrome grading to guide decision making in the surgical correction of presbyopia," in *Proceedings of the ASCRS Meeting*, Los Ángeles, CA, USA, 2017.

[3] W. N. Charman, "Developments in the correction of presbyopia I: spectacle and contact lenses," *Ophthalmic and Physiological Optics*, vol. 34, no. 1, pp. 8–29, 2014.

[4] J. A. Martínez-Roda, M. Vilaseca, J. C. Ondategui et al., "Double-pass technique and compensation-comparison method in eyes with cataract," *Journal of Cataract and Refractive Surgery*, vol. 42, no. 10, pp. 1461–1469, 2016.

[5] V. M. Thompson, G. O. Waring, D. S. Durrie et al., "Adaptation of the diagnosis of presbyopia to the modern refractive cataract patient: dysfunctional lens syndrome," in *Proceedings of the ASCRS Meeting*, Los Ángeles, CA, USA, 2017.

[6] R. S. Chuck, D. S. Jacobs, J. K. Lee et al., "Refractive errors & refractive surgery preferred practice pattern®," *Ophthalmology*, vol. 125, no. 1, pp. P1–P104, 2018.

[7] R. J. Olson, R. Braga-Mele, S. H. Chen et al., "Cataract in the adult eye preferred practice pattern®," *Ophthalmology*, vol. 124, no. 1, pp. P1–P119, 2017.

[8] A. L. Petrou and A. Terzidaki, "A meta-analysis and review examining a possible role for oxidative stress and singlet oxygen in diverse diseases," *Biochemical Journal*, vol. 474, no. 16, pp. 2713–2731, 2017.

[9] M. G. Nye-Wood, J. M. Spraggins, R. M. Caprioli, K. L. Schey, P. J. Donaldson, and A. C. Grey, "Spatial distributions of glutathione and its endogenous conjugates in normal bovine lens and a model of lens aging," *Experimental Eye Research*, vol. 154, pp. 70–78, 2017.

[10] A. C. Grey, N. J. Demarais, B. J. West, and P. J. Donaldson, "A quantitative map of glutathione in the aging human lens," *International Journal of Mass Spectrometry*, 2017, In press.

[11] P. J. Donaldson, A. C. Grey, B. Maceo Heilman, J. C. Lim, and E. Vaghefi, "The physiological optics of the lens," *Progress in Retinal and Eye Research*, vol. 56, pp. e1–e24, 2017.

[12] G. Smith, M. J. Cox, R. Calver, and L. F. Garner, "The spherical aberration of the crystalline lens of the human eye," *Vision Research*, vol. 41, no. 2, pp. 235–243, 2001.

[13] P. Artal, E. Berrio, A. Guirao, and P. Piers, "Contribution of the cornea and internal surfaces to the change of ocular

aberrations with age," *Journal of the Optical Society of America A*, vol. 19, no. 1, pp. 137–143, 2002.

[14] J. L. Alió, P. Schimchak, H. P. Negri, and R. Montés-Micó, "Crystalline lens optical dysfunction through aging," *Ophthalmology*, vol. 112, no. 11, pp. 2022–2029, 2005.

[15] S. Amano, Y. Amano, S. Yamagami et al., "Age-related changes in corneal and ocular higher-order wavefront aberrations," *American Journal of Ophthalmology*, vol. 137, no. 6, pp. 988–992, 2004.

[16] R. Navarro, "The optical design of the human eye: a critical review," *Journal of Optometry*, vol. 2, no. 1, pp. 3–18, 2009.

[17] C. Qiu, B. Maceo Heilman, J. Kaipio, P. Donaldson, and E. Vaghefi, "Fully automated laser ray tracing system to measure changes in the crystalline lens GRIN profile," *Biomedical Optics Express*, vol. 8, no. 11, p. 4947, 2017.

[18] D. Siedlecki, A. de Castro, E. Gambra et al., "Distortion correction of OCT images of the crystalline lens," *Optometry and Vision Science*, vol. 89, no. 5, pp. E709–E718, 2012.

[19] B. Moffat, D. A. Atchison, and J. M. Pope, "Age-related changes in refractive index distribution and power of the human lens as measured by magnetic resonance micro-imaging in vitro," *Vision Research*, vol. 42, no. 13, pp. 1683–1693, 2002.

[20] R. C. Augusteyn, C. E. Jones, and J. M. Pope, "Age-related development of a refractive index plateau in the human lens: evidence for a distinct nucleus," *Clinical and Experimental Optometry*, vol. 91, no. 3, pp. 296–301, 2008.

[21] N. Sachdev, S. E. Ormonde, T. Sherwin, and C. N. J. McGhee, "Higher-order aberrations of lenticular opacities," *Journal of Cataract and Refractive Surgery*, vol. 30, no. 8, pp. 1642–1648, 2004.

[22] K. M. Rocha, W. Nosé, K. Bottós, J. Bottós, L. Morimoto, and E. Soriano, "Higher-order aberrations of age-related cataract," *Journal of Cataract and Refractive Surgery*, vol. 33, no. 8, pp. 1442–1446, 2007.

[23] J. Lee, M. J. Kim, and H. Tchah, "Higher-order aberrations induced by nuclear cataract," *Journal of Cataract and Refractive Surgery*, vol. 34, no. 12, pp. 2104–2109, 2008.

[24] J. H. Lee, H. G. Choo, and S. W. Kim, "Spherical aberration reduction in nuclear cataracts," *Graefe's Archive for Clinical and Experimental Ophthalmology*, vol. 254, no. 6, pp. 1127–1133, 2016.

[25] C.-Z. Wu, H. Jin, Z.-N. Shen, Y.-J. Li, and X. Cui, "Wavefront aberrations and retinal image quality in different lenticular opacity types and densities," *Scientific Reports*, vol. 7, no. 1, p. 15247, 2017.

[26] F. Faria-Correia, B. Lopes, T. Monteiro, N. Franqueira, and R. Ambrósio, "Scheimpflug lens densitometry and ocular wavefront aberrations in patients with mild nuclear cataract," *Journal of Cataract and Refractive Surgery*, vol. 42, no. 3, pp. 405–411, 2016.

[27] T. Kuroda, T. Fujikado, N. Maeda, T. Oshika, Y. Hirohara, and T. Mihashi, Wavefront analysis in eyes with nuclear or cortical cataract," *American Journal of Ophthalmology*, vol. 134, no. 1, pp. 1–9, 2002.

[28] X. Zhu, H. Ye, W. He, J. Yang, J. Dai, and Y. Lu, "Objective functional visual outcomes of cataract surgery in patients with good preoperative visual acuity," *Eye*, vol. 31, no. 3, pp. 452–459, 2017.

[29] T. Ritschel, M. Ihrke, J. R. Frisvad, J. Coppens, K. Myszkowski, and H.-P. Seidel, "Temporal glare: real-time dynamic simulation of the scattering in the human eye," *Computer Graphics Forum*, vol. 28, no. 2, pp. 183–192, 2009.

[30] T. J. T. P. van den Berg, "Intraocular light scatter, reflections, fluorescence and absorption: what we see in the slit lamp," *Ophthalmic and Physiological Optics*, vol. 38, no. 1, pp. 6–25, 2018.

[31] P. W. T. De Waard, J. K. Ijspeert, T. J. Van den Berg, and P. T. de Jong, "Intraocular light scattering in age-related cataracts," *Investigative Ophthalmology and Visual Science*, vol. 33, no. 3, pp. 618–625, 1992.

[32] T. Tanaka and G. B. Benedek, "Observation of protein diffusivity in intact human and bovine lenses with application to cataract," *Investigative Ophthalmology and Visual Science*, vol. 14, no. 6, pp. 449–456, 1975.

[33] G. B. Benedek, L. T. Chylack, T. Libondi, P. Magnante, and M. Pennett, "Quantitative detection of the molecular changes associated with early cataractogenesis in the living human lens using quasielastic light scattering," *Current Eye Research*, vol. 6, no. 12, pp. 1421–1432, 1987.

[34] R. Xu, "Light scattering: a review of particle characterization applications," *Particuology*, vol. 18, pp. 11–21, 2015.

[35] M. B. Datiles, R. R. Ansari, K. I. Suh et al., "Clinical detection of precataractous lens protein changes using dynamic light scattering," *Archives of Ophthalmology*, vol. 126, no. 12, pp. 1687–1693, 2008.

[36] M. B. Datiles, R. R. Ansari, J. Yoshida et al., "Longitudinal study of age-related cataract using dynamic light scattering," *Ophthalmology*, vol. 123, no. 2, pp. 248–254, 2016.

[37] A. B. Watson and J. I. Yellott, "A unified formula for light-adapted pupil size," *Journal of Vision*, vol. 12, no. 10, pp. 1–16, 2012.

[38] H. Namba, R. Kawasaki, A. Sugano et al., "Age-related changes in ocular aberrations and the Yamagata study (Funagata)," *Cornea*, vol. 36, pp. 34–40, 2017.

[39] E. Bellot, V. Coizet, J. Warnking, K. Knoblauch, E. Moro, and M. Dojat, "Effects of aging on low luminance contrast processing in humans," *NeuroImage*, vol. 139, pp. 415–426, 2016.

[40] C. Owsley, "Vision and aging," *Annual Review of Vision Science*, vol. 2, no. 1, pp. 255–271, 2016.

[41] P. Artal, S. Manzanera, K. Komar, A. Gambín-Regadera, and M. Wojtkowski, "Visual acuity in two-photon infrared vision," *Optica*, vol. 4, no. 12, p. 1488, 2017.

[42] O. Reid, D. A. L. Maberley, and H. Hollands, "Comparison of the potential acuity meter and the visometer in cataract patients," *Eye*, vol. 21, no. 2, pp. 195–199, 2007.

[43] T. Bal, T. Coeckelbergh, J. Van Looveren, J. J. Rozema, and M.-J. Tassignon, "Influence of cataract morphology on straylight and contrast sensitivity and its relevance to fitness to drive," *Ophthalmologica*, vol. 225, no. 2, pp. 105–111, 2011.

[44] European Coalition of Optometry and Optics (ECOO), *Visual Standards for Driving in Europe. A Consensus Paper*, 2017, http://www.ecoo.info/wp-content/uploads/2017/01/Visual-Standards-for-Driving-in-Europe-Consensus-Paper-January-2017....pdf.

[45] L. J. van Rijn, C. Nischler, R. Michael et al., "Prevalence of impairment of visual function in European drivers," *Acta Ophthalmologica*, vol. 89, no. 2, pp. 124–131, 2011.

[46] C. Owsley, B. T. Stalvey, J. Wells, M. E. Sloane, and G. McGwin, "Visual risk factors for crash involvement in older drivers with cataract," *Archives of Ophthalmology*, vol. 119, no. 6, pp. 881–887, 2001.

[47] J. A. Kimlin, A. A. Black, and J. M. Wood, "Nighttime driving in older adults: effects of glare and association with mesopic visual function," *Investigative Opthalmology and Visual Science*, vol. 58, no. 5, pp. 2796–2803, 2017.

[48] J. Zhao, F. Xiao, H. Zhao, Y. Dai, and Y. Zhang, "Effect of higher-order aberrations and intraocular scatter on contrast

sensitivity measured with a single instrument," *Biomedical Optics Express*, vol. 8, no. 4, p. 2138, 2017.

[49] F. Faria-Correia, I. Ramos, B. Lopes, T. Monteiro, N. Franqueira, and R. Ambrósio, "Correlations of objective metrics for quantifying dysfunctional lens syndrome with visual acuity and phacodynamics," *Journal of Refractive Surgery*, vol. 33, no. 2, pp. 79–83, 2017.

[50] D. R. Nixon, "Preoperative cataract grading by Scheimpflug imaging and effect on operative fluidics and phacoemulsification energy," *Journal of Cataract and Refractive Surgery*, vol. 36, no. 2, pp. 242–246, 2010.

[51] D. S. Grewal, G. S. Brar, and S. P. S. Grewal, "Correlation of nuclear cataract lens density using Scheimpflug images with lens opacities classification system III and visual function," *Ophthalmology*, vol. 116, no. 8, pp. 1436–1443, 2009.

[52] A. Pan, Q. Wang, F. Huang, J.-H. Huang, F.-J. Bao, and A.-Y. Yu, "Correlation among lens opacities classification system III grading, visual function index-14, pentacam nucleus staging, and objective scatter index for cataract assessment," *American Journal of Ophthalmology*, vol. 159, no. 2, pp. 241.e2–247.e2, 2015.

[53] F. Faria-Correia, I. Ramos, B. Lopes, T. Monteiro, N. Franqueira, and R. Ambrósio, "Comparison of dysfunctional lens index and Scheimpflug lens densitometry in the evaluation of age-related nuclear cataracts," *Journal of Refractive Surgery*, vol. 32, no. 4, pp. 244–248, 2016.

[54] N. Y. Makhotkina, T. T. J. M. Berendschot, F. J. H. M. van den Biggelaar, A. R. H. Weik, and R. M. M. A. Nuijts, "Comparability of subjective and objective measurements of nuclear density in cataract patients," *Acta Ophthalmologica*, 2018, In press.

[55] Y.-C. Chang, K. Liu, C. de Freitas et al., "Assessment of eye length changes in accommodation using dynamic extended-depth OCT," *Biomedical Optics Express*, vol. 8, no. 5, pp. 2709–2719, 2017.

[56] P. Gifford and H. A. Swarbrick, "Repeatability of internal aberrometry with a aberrometer/corneal topographer," *Optometry and Vision Science*, vol. 89, no. 6, pp. 929–938, 2012.

[57] N. Visser, T. T. J. M. Berendschot, F. Verbakel, A. N. Tan, J. de Brabander, and R. M. M. A. Nuijts, "Evaluation of the comparability and repeatability of four wavefront aberrometers," *Investigative Opthalmology and Visual Science*, vol. 52, no. 3, pp. 1302–1311, 2011.

[58] J. Hao, L. Li, F. Tian, and H. Zhang, "Comparison of two types of visual quality analyzer for the measurement of high order aberrations," *International Journal of Ophthalmology*, vol. 9, no. 2, pp. 292–297, 2016.

[59] J. B. Won, S. W. Kim, E. K. Kim, B. J. Ha, and T.-I. Kim, "Comparison of internal and total optical aberrations for 2 aberrometers: iTrace and OPD scan," *Korean Journal of Ophthalmology*, vol. 22, no. 4, pp. 210–213, 2008.

[60] P. Artal, A. Benito, G. M. Pérez et al., "An objective scatter index based on double-pass retinal images of a point source to classify cataracts," *PLoS One*, vol. 6, no. 2, Article ID e16823, 2011.

[61] L. Qiao, X. Wan, X. Cai et al., "Comparison of ocular modulation transfer function determined by a ray-tracing aberrometer and a double-pass system in early cataract patients," *Chinese Medical Journal*, vol. 127, no. 19, pp. 3454–3458, 2014.

[62] F. Díaz-Doutón, A. Benito, J. Pujol, M. Arjona, J. L. Guell, and P. Artal, "Comparison of the retinal image quality with a Hartmann–Shack wavefront sensor and a double-pass

instrument," *Investigative Opthalmology and Visual Science*, vol. 47, no. 4, pp. 1710–1716, 2006.

[63] M. Vilaseca, M. J. Romero, M. Arjona et al., "Grading nuclear, cortical and posterior subcapsular cataracts using an objective scatter index measured with a double-pass system," *British Journal of Ophthalmology*, vol. 96, no. 9, pp. 1204–1210, 2012.

[64] J. A. Martínez-Roda, M. Vilaseca, J. C. Ondategui et al., "Optical quality and intraocular scattering in a healthy young population," *Clinical and Experimental Optometry*, vol. 94, no. 2, pp. 223–229, 2011.

[65] F. Galliot, S. R. Patel, and B. Cochener, "Objective scatter index: working toward a new quantification of cataract?," *Journal of Refractive Surgery*, vol. 32, no. 2, pp. 96–102, 2016.

[66] C. Paz, R. F. Sánchez, E. Colombo, M. Vilaseca, J. Pujol, and L. A. Issolio, "Discrimination between surgical and non-surgical nuclear cataracts based on ROC analysis," *Current Eye Research*, vol. 39, no. 12, pp. 1187–1193, 2014.

[67] H. Zhang and J. Wang, "Visual quality assessment of posterior capsule opacification using optical quality analysis system (OQAS)," *Journal of Ophthalmology*, vol. 2017, Article ID 9852195, 4 pages, 2017.

[68] C. Paz Filgueira, R. F. Sánchez, L. A. Issolio, and E. M. Colombo, "Straylight and visual quality on early nuclear and posterior subcapsular cataracts," *Current Eye Research*, vol. 41, no. 9, pp. 1209–1215, 2016.

[69] F. Cabot, A. Saad, C. McAlinden, N. M. Haddad, A. Grise-Dulac, and D. Gatinel, "Objective assessment of crystalline lens opacity level by measuring ocular light scattering with a double-pass system," *American Journal of Ophthalmology*, vol. 155, no. 4, pp. 629.e2–635.e2, 2013.

[70] B. Cochener, S. R. Patel, and F. Galliot, "Correlational analysis of objective and subjective measures of cataract quantification," *Journal of Refractive Surgery*, vol. 32, no. 2, pp. 104–109, 2016.

[71] A. Crnej, N. Hirnschall, C. Petsoglou, and O. Findl, "Methods for assessing forward and backward light scatter in patients with cataract," *Journal of Cataract and Refractive Surgery*, vol. 43, no. 8, pp. 1072–1076, 2017.

[72] Y. Chen, X. Wang, C. D. Zhou, and Q. Wu, "Evaluation of visual quality of spherical and aspherical intraocular lenses by optical quality analysis system," *International Journal of Ophthalmology*, vol. 10, no. 6, pp. 914–918, 2017.

[73] C. W. Park, H. Kim, and C. K. Joo, "Assessment of optical quality at different contrast levels in pseudophakic eyes," *Journal of Ophthalmology*, vol. 2016, Article ID 4247973, 8 pages, 2016.

[74] R. Jiménez, A. Valero, J. Fernández, R. G. Anera, and J. R. Jiménez, "Optical quality and visual performance after cataract surgery with biaxial microincision intraocular lens implantation," *Journal of Cataract and Refractive Surgery*, vol. 42, no. 7, pp. 1022–1028, 2016.

[75] H. Lee, K. Lee, J. M. Ahn, E. K. Kim, B. Sgrignoli, and T.-I. Kim, "Double-pass system assessing the optical quality of pseudophakic eyes," *Optometry and Vision Science*, vol. 91, no. 4, pp. 437–443, 2014.

[76] T. Chen, F. Yu, H. Lin et al., "Objective and subjective visual quality after implantation of all optic zone diffractive multifocal intraocular lenses: a prospective, case-control observational study," *British Journal of Ophthalmology*, vol. 100, no. 11, pp. 1530–1535, 2016.

[77] H. Lee, K. Lee, J. M. Ahn, E. K. Kim, B. Sgrignoli, and T.-I. Kim, "Evaluation of optical quality parameters and ocular aberrations in multifocal intraocular lens implanted

eyes," *Yonsei Medical Journal*, vol. 55, no. 5, pp. 1413–1420, 2014.

[78] F. Vega, M. S. Millán, N. Vila-Terricabras, and F. Alba-Bueno, "Visible versus near-infrared optical performance of diffractive multifocal intraocular lenses," *Investigative Opthalmology and Visual Science*, vol. 56, no. 12, p. 7345, 2015.

[79] D. Gatinel, "Double pass-technique limitations for evaluation of optical performance after diffractive IOL implantation," *Journal of Cataract and Refractive Surgery*, vol. 37, no. 3, pp. 621-622, 2011.

[80] M. Jabbarvand, H. Hashemian, M. Khodaparast, M. Jouhari, A. Tabatabaei, and S. Rezaei, "Endophthalmitis occurring after cataract surgery: outcomes of more than 480,000 cataract surgeries, epidemiologic features, and risk factors," *Ophthalmology*, vol. 123, no. 2, pp. 295-301, 2016.

[81] C. Creuzot-Garcher, E. Benzenine, A. S. Mariet et al., "Incidence of acute postoperative endophthalmitis after cataract surgery a nationwide study in France from 2005 to 2014," *Ophthalmology*, vol. 123, no. 7, pp. 1414-1420, 2016.

[82] H. Hashemi, M. Khabazkhoob, F. Rezvan et al., "Complications of cataract surgery in Iran: trend from 2006 to 2010," *Ophthalmic Epidemiology*, vol. 23, no. 1, pp. 46–52, 2016.

[83] C. J. Chu, R. L. Johnston, C. Buscombe, A. B. Sallam, Q. Mohamed, and Y. C. Yang, "Risk factors and incidence of macular edema after cataract surgery a database study of 81984 eyes," *Ophthalmology*, vol. 123, no. 2, pp. 316-323, 2016.

[84] J. D. Stein, D. S. Grossman, K. M. Mundy, A. Sugar, and F. A. Sloan, "Severe adverse events after cataract surgery among medicare beneficiaries," *Ophthalmology*, vol. 118, no. 9, pp. 1716-1723, 2011.

[85] T. Ianchulev, D. Litoff, D. Ellinger, K. Stiverson, and M. Packer, "Office-based cataract surgery," *Ophthalmology*, vol. 123, no. 4, pp. 723-728, 2016.

[86] F. F. Marques, D. M. V. Marques, R. H. Osher, and J. M. Osher, "Fate of anterior capsule tears during cataract surgery," *Journal of Cataract and Refractive Surgery*, vol. 32, no. 10, pp. 1638-1642, 2006.

[87] A. C. Day, P. H. J. Donachie, J. M. Sparrow, and R. L. Johnston, "The Royal College of Ophthalmologists' national ophthalmology database study of cataract surgery: report 1, visual outcomes and complications," *Eye*, vol. 29, no. 4, pp. 552–560, 2015.

[88] S. E. Ti, Y. N. Yang, S. S. Lang, and S. P. Chee, "A 5-year audit of cataract surgery outcomes after posterior capsule rupture and risk factors affecting visual acuity," *American Journal of Ophthalmology*, vol. 157, no. 1, pp. 180.e1–185.e1, 2014.

[89] P. B. Greenberg, V. L. Tseng, W.-C. Wu et al., "Prevalence and predictors of ocular complications associated with cataract surgery in United States veterans," *Ophthalmology*, vol. 118, no. 3, pp. 507–514, 2011.

[90] R. Braga-Mele, D. Chang, S. Dewey et al., "Multifocal intraocular lenses: relative indications and contraindications for implantation," *Journal of Cataract and Refractive Surgery*, vol. 40, no. 2, pp. 313–322, 2014.

[91] C. Palomo-Álvarez and M. C. Puell, "Capacity of straylight and disk halo size to diagnose cataract," *Journal of Cataract and Refractive Surgery*, vol. 41, no. 10, pp. 2069-2074, 2015.

[92] L. Kessel, J. Andresen, D. Erngaard, P. Flesner, B. Tendal, and J. Hjortdal, "Indication for cataract surgery. Do we have evidence of who will benefit from surgery? A systematic review and meta-analysis," *Acta Ophthalmologica*, vol. 94, no. 1, pp. 10–20, 2016.

[93] M. Comas, R. Román, F. Cots et al., "Unmet needs for cataract surgery in Spain according to indication criteria. Evaluation through a simulation model," *British Journal of Ophthalmology*, vol. 92, no. 7, pp. 888–892, 2008.

[94] L. Kessel, D. Erngaard, P. Flesner, J. Andresen, and J. Hjortdal, "Do evidence-based guidelines change clinical practice patterns?," *Acta Ophthalmologica*, vol. 95, no. 4, pp. 337–343, 2017.

[95] C. K. Pager, "Expectations and outcomes in cataract surgery. a prospective test of 2 models of satisfaction," *Archives of Ophthalmology*, vol. 122, no. 12, pp. 1788–1792, 2004.

[96] M. J. Hawker, S. N. Madge, P. A. Baddeley, and S. R. Perry, "Refractive expectations of patients having cataract surgery," *Journal of Cataract and Refractive Surgery*, vol. 31, no. 10, pp. 1970–1975, 2005.

[97] M. D. Nijkamp, R. M. M. A. Nuijts, B. van den Borne, C. A. B. Webers, F. van der Horst, and F. Hendrikse, "Determinants of patient satisfaction after cataract surgery in 3 settings," *Journal of Cataract and Refractive Surgery*, vol. 26, no. 9, pp. 1379–1388, 2000.

[98] M. A. Woodward, J. B. Randleman, and R. D. Stulting, "Dissatisfaction after multifocal intraocular lens implantation," *Journal of Cataract and Refractive Surgery*, vol. 35, no. 6, pp. 992–997, 2009.

[99] N. E. De Vries, C. A. B. Webers, W. R. H. Touwslager et al., "Dissatisfaction after implantation of multifocal intraocular lenses," *Journal of Cataract and Refractive Surgery*, vol. 37, no. 5, pp. 859–865, 2011.

[100] U. Mester, T. Vaterrodt, F. Goes et al., "Impact of personality characteristics on patient satisfaction after multifocal intraocular lens implantation: results from the "happy patient study"," *Journal of Refractive Surgery*, vol. 30, no. 10, pp. 674–678, 2014.

[101] D. S. Durrie, "Developing a treatment algorithm for stage 1 dysfunctional lens syndrome," in *Proceedings of the ASCRS Meeting*, Los Angeles, CA, USA, May 2017.

[102] J. L. Alió, A. Grzybowski, and D. Romaniuk, "Refractive lens exchange in modern practice: when and when not to do it?," *Eye and Vision*, vol. 1, no. 1, p. 10, 2014.

[103] C. Kirwan, J. M. Nolan, J. Stack, T. C. B. Moore, and S. Beatty, "Determinants of patient satisfaction and function related to vision following cataract surgery in eyes with no visually consequential ocular co-morbidity," *Graefe's Archive for Clinical and Experimental Ophthalmology*, vol. 253, no. 10, pp. 1735–1744, 2015.

[104] F. Alba-Bueno, N. Garzón, F. Vega, F. Poyales, and M. S. Millán, "Patient-perceived and laboratory-measured halos associated with diffractive bifocal and trifocal intraocular lenses," *Current Eye Research*, vol. 42, no. 1, pp. 35–42, 2017.

[105] A. M. Rosa, Â. C. Miranda, M. Patrício et al., "Functional magnetic resonance imaging to assess the neurobehavioral impact of dysphotopsia with multifocal intraocular lenses," *Ophthalmology*, vol. 124, no. 9, pp. 1–10, 2017.

[106] F. W. Campbell and D. G. Green, "Optical and retinal factors affecting visual resolution," *Journal of Physiology*, vol. 181, no. 3, pp. 576–593, 1965.

[107] M. C. Puell, M. J. Pérez-Carrasco, A. Barrio, B. Antona, and C. Palomo-Alvarez, "Normal values for the size of a halo produced by a glare source," *Journal of Refractive Surgery*, vol. 29, no. 9, pp. 618–622, 2013.

[108] M. C. Puell, M. J. Pérez-Carrasco, F. J. Hurtado-Ceña, and L. Álvarez-Rementería, "Disk halo size measured in individuals with monofocal versus diffractive multifocal

intraocular lenses," *Journal of Cataract and Refractive Surgery*, vol. 41, no. 11, pp. 2417–2423, 2015.

[109] M. R. Sedaghat, H. Momeni-Moghaddam, S. S. Naroo, H. Ghavamsaeedi, and A. Vahedi, "Dysfunctional lens syndrome," *International Ophthalmology*, pp. 1–5, 2017, In press.

[110] M. Mark Packer, *Dysfunctional Lens Syndrome Paradox*, Ophthalmology Times, New York, NY, USA, 2015, http://ophthalmologytimes.modernmedicine.com/ophthalmologytimes/news/dysfunctional-lens-syndrome-paradox?page=full.

[111] R. Bilbao-Calabuig, F. González-López, F. Amparo, G. Alvarez, S. R. Patel, and F. Llovet-Osuna, "Comparison between mix-and-match implantation of bifocal intraocular lenses and bilateral implantation of trifocal intraocular lenses," *Journal of Refractive Surgery*, vol. 32, no. 10, pp. 659–663, 2016.

[112] E. Pedrotti, E. Bruni, E. Bonacci, R. Badalamenti, R. Mastropasqua, and G. Marchini, "Comparative analysis of the clinical outcomes with a monofocal and an extended range of vision intraocular lens," *Journal of Refractive Surgery*, vol. 32, no. 7, pp. 436–442, 2016.

[113] K. Nakamura, H. Bissen-Miyajima, M. Yoshino, and S. Oki, "Visual performance after contralateral implantation of multifocal intraocular lenses with +3.0 and +4.0 diopter additions," *Asia-Pacific Journal of Ophthalmology*, vol. 4, no. 6, pp. 329–333, 2015.

[114] J. S. M. Chang, J. C. M. Ng, V. K. C. Chan, and A. K. P. Law, "Visual outcomes, quality of vision, and quality of life of diffractive multifocal intraocular lens implantation after myopic laser in situ keratomileusis: a prospective, observational case series," *Journal of Ophthalmology*, vol. 2017, Article ID 6459504, 12 pages, 2017.

14

The Influence of Lunar Phases on Complications in Cataract Surgery: An Analysis of 16,965 Patients

Eva-Maria Faschinger,[1,2] Pia Veronika Vécsei-Marlovits,[1,2] Dieter Franz Rabensteiner,[3] and Birgit Weingessel[1,2]

[1]Department of Ophthalmology, KH Hietzing, Wolkersbergenstrasse 1, 1130 Vienna, Austria
[2]Karl Landsteiner Institute of Process Optimization and Quality Management in Cataract-Surgery, Wolkersbergenstrasse 1, 1130 Vienna, Austria
[3]Department of Ophthalmology, Medical University of Graz, Auenbruggerplatz 4, 8036 Graz, Austria

Correspondence should be addressed to Birgit Weingessel; birgit.weingessel@gmail.com

Academic Editor: Lisa Toto

Purpose. Popular beliefs exert an impact of lunar phases on elective surgery. The aim of our study was to evaluate potential correlations between complications in cataract surgery and the phases of the moon during its passage through the zodiac and Fridays that fall on the 13th. *Methods.* Patients with complications during cataract surgery were extracted retrospectively from the clinical database from 2010 to 2014. The dates of surgeries were viewed in relation to the phase and the position of the moon (sign of the zodiac). *Results.* Of 16,965 cataract surgeries, 132 eyes developed complications. 0.70% developed complications with a waxing moon, and 0.87% with a waning moon ($p = 0.745$). After Bonferroni correction, there were no statistically significant differences between the numbers of complications under the different signs of the zodiac and no complications on Fridays that fell on the 13th. *Conclusions.* The analysis of "non-moon-fitting days" for surgery showed quantitative differences, without statistically significant findings. Our results revealed more complications when the moon was waning, which is in contrast to esoteric belief. Patients may be informed that phases of the moon, signs of the zodiac, or a particular date will have no impact on their surgeries.

1. Introduction

Lunar effects on health and human behavior have been postulated for centuries [1]. Superstition, moon calendars, and popular beliefs exert a considerable impact on evidence-based medicine, especially on elective surgery [2]. Public interest in the impact of the moon is persistently high. Many individuals believe in correlations or even causality between the course of the moon and their personal lives [3].

In the course of its 29.5-day cycle, the moon passes through its phases. It waxes after new moon and wanes after full moon. In the course of this cycle, the moon also changes roughly every second day from one of the twelve signs of the zodiac to the next. According to esoteric belief, there is a relationship between the phases of the moon and the factors of everyday life such as the quality of sleep and hair growth, as

well as the frequency of accidents and surgical complications, seizures, mood disorders, and even a more frequent occurrence of myocardial infarction [4–7]. This may cause patients to request a change in the date of their elective surgery because of the moon being in an unfavorable constellation [7, 8]. Many patients are afraid of the wrong timing of surgery with respect to moon phases and thus influence surgeons as well as other medical staff [9]. According to the moon calendar, surgeries should only be performed on days when the moon is waning because complications are more common and recovery is prolonged when the moon is waxing [8]. For eye surgery, the days when the moon is waxing and in Aries are considered especially unfavorable [8].

In some rural areas, nearly one fifth of the population believes in the impact of moon phases on the outcome of medicine [1]. More than 40% of medical staffs believe that lunar phases affect human behavior [2]. Ten percent of the German population believes in the effects of lunar phases on disease [3, 4]. In a survey conducted in a German hospital, 21.3% of the in-hospital patients had a moon calendar and scheduled their operations according to lunar cycles [10].

Since cataract surgery is one of the most commonly performed procedures and can be timed by the patient, we viewed the frequency of complications following cataract surgery with reference to the phases of the moon and the ruling house (signs of zodiac) on the day of surgery. We also looked for any correlation with Fridays that fall on the 13th of a month.

2. Material and Methods

A retrospective, single-center study was performed: Intraoperative complications were retrieved from the records of all cataract surgeries performed at the Department of Ophthalmology, Hietzing Hospital, Vienna, Austria, in the 5-year period from 2010 to 2014. All phacoemulsification were performed by 11 experienced surgeons who had a record of more than 500 operations. However, some members of the surgical team had not been active during the entire 5-year period. Our statistical evaluation of all surgeries showed no difference in the complication rates of the different surgeons.

The analyzed complications included ruptures of the posterior capsule and surgically induced zonulysis with vitreous prolapse requiring vitrectomy. Congenital cataracts in children and combined operations were excluded from the analysis.

The lunar phases for the days in question were taken from moon calendars for Middle Europe. The waxing or waning phase of the moon, the zodiac house it was in, and the time points of complications were correlated to each other. Surgical complications on Fridays that fell on the 13th of a given month were also noted. Every year has at least one and as many as three Fridays that fall on the 13th.

All procedures performed were in accordance with the ethical standards of the institutional and national research committee (EK-17-073-VK), the 1964 Helsinki Declaration, and its subsequent amendments.

Statistics were analyzed with the SPSS Statistics 23 program (IBM, USA). Pearson's chi-square test was used to determine whether the distribution of a dichotomous characteristic (waxing or waning moon; complications yes or no) was identical in both groups. The level of statistical significance was set to $p < .05$. A Bonferroni correction was carried out to neutralize cumulative alpha error due to multiple comparisons.

3. Results

The evaluation included 16,965 cataract operations and 132 eyes with complications (0.78%) (see Figure 1 for the individual years).

Complications were somewhat more frequent during a waning moon ($n = 68$) than a waxing moon ($n = 64$). However, 7842 operations were performed during a waning moon and 9123 operations during a waxing moon. In percentages,

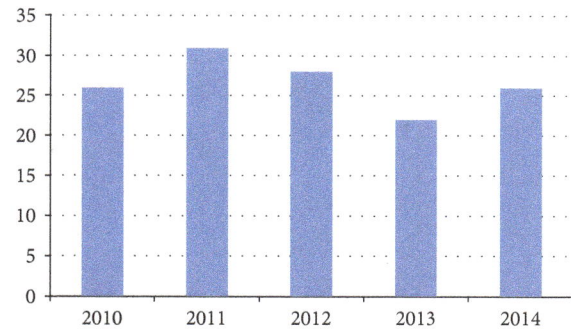

FIGURE 1: Number of complications during phacoemulsification per year (2010–2014).

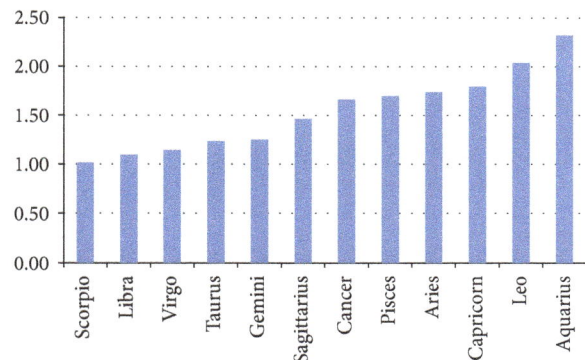

FIGURE 2: Percent frequency of complications during phacoemulsification per sign (sum of waxing and waning moon, by frequency): least complications in Scorpio, most common in Aquarius.

this amounted to 0.87% complications in a waning moon and 0.70% in a waxing moon ($p = .745$, not significant).

With regard to the twelve zodiac signs (sum of the waxing and waning moon), complications were most rare in Scorpio (1.01%) and most common in Aquarius (2.32%) (Figure 2). The difference was just slightly nonsignificant ($p = .051$). Listed in chronological sequence, the signs showed the following percentages of complications: Capricorn 1.79, Aquarius 2.32, Pisces 1.69, Aries 1.74, Taurus 1.23, Gemini 1.25, Cancer 1.66, Leo 2.03, Virgo 1.14, Libra 1.09, Scorpio 1.10, and Sagittarius 1.46%.

Viewing the waxing and waning phases of the moon separately, complications were most frequent with a waxing moon in Leo (1.4%) and Aries (1.25%) and with a waning moon in Aquarius (1.24%). The fewest complications were noted with a waxing moon in Taurus (0.31%), Libra (0.32%), and Sagittarius (0.45%) (Figure 3).

Statistically, there were no significant differences between a waxing and a waning moon for the respective zodiac signs (Capricorn $p = .199$, Aquarius $p = .770$, Pisces $p = .576$, Aries $p = .130$, Taurus $p = .149$, Gemini $p = .737$, Cancer $p = .803$, Leo $p = .162$, Virgo $p = .990$, Libra $p = .269$, Scorpio $p = .993$, and Sagittarius $p = .226$).

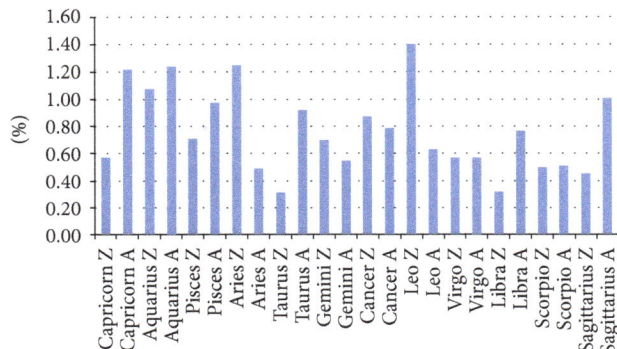

FIGURE 3: Percent frequency of complications with waxing (Z) and waning (A) moon per zodiac sign: least complications in Taurus (Z, waxing), most common in Leo (Z, waxing).

TABLE 1: Comparison of the three maximum values for complications under the zodiac signs and phase of the moon (Z = waxing, A = waning) to the three minimum values for complications, with reference to the zodiac sign and the phase of the moon. *Statistically significant in Pearson's chi-square test.

Maximum values	Minimum values	Significance
1st max. Leo Z	1st min. Taurus Z	0.029*
1st max. Leo Z	2nd min. Libra Z	0.035*
1st max. Leo Z	3rd min. Sagittarius A	0.065
2nd max. Aries Z	1st min. Taurus Z	0.047*
2nd max. Aries Z	2nd min. Libra Z	0.056
3rd max. Aquarius A	1st min. Taurus Z	0.051
3rd max. Aquarius A	2nd min. Libra Z	0.061

3.1. Subgroup Analyses. A significant difference ($p = .029$) was noted when comparing the first maximal value (Leo, waxing moon) with the first minimum value (Taurus, waxing) as well as with the second minimal value (Libra, waxing, $p = .035$), but no longer with the third minimum value (Sagittarius, waxing $p = .065$). The comparison of the second maximum value (Aries, waxing) with the first minimum value (Taurus, waxing) again yielded a significant difference ($p = .047$), but not with the second minimum value (Libra, waxing, $p = .056$). Comparing the third maximal value (Aquarius, waning) with the first minimum value (Taurus, waxing) yielded no significant result ($p = .051$), nor did a comparison with the second minimum value (Libra, waxing, $p = .061$) (Table 1).

3.2. Bonferroni Correction. Twelve zodiac signs and two moon states (waxing and waning) produced 24 groups that, when compared, would lead to 276 possible analogies. Dividing the assumed alpha error of 0.05 by 276, statistical significance was only achieved with $p < .00018$. In these circumstances, none of the results were statistically significant.

During the five-year period of the study, twelve Fridays fell on the 13th of a month (August 2010; January, May, and October 2011; January, April, and July 2012; September

and December 2013; and March, June, and November 2014). No complications occurred on Friday the 13th.

4. Discussion

Based on the Internet and other publications, many patients request to be operated on days when the moon is "favorable" because they believe that the phases of the moon and the respective signs of the zodiac influence the results of surgery [1–3, 8]. There are many more relevant esoteric Internet sites than there are academic, medical, or natural science-oriented publications, and critical opinions on the subject are few and far between [3, 11].

Our retrospective study on cataract surgeries scheduled in relation to the phases of the moon showed a percentage difference in complications with a waxing moon (0.70%) and a waning moon (0.87%), but the difference was not significant. As the moon passed through the twelve signs of the zodiac, complications were most frequent in Leo, Aries, and Aquarius and least frequent in Taurus, Libra, and Sagittarius. There were no significant differences with the zodiacs and no significant difference depending on whether the moon in the respective house was waxing or waning. Complications within the various zodiac signs were considered in the subgroup analyses. The zodiac sign with the highest number of complications and with the least complications and the phase of the moon (such as a waxing moon in Leo or Aries) revealed a few statistically significant results. However, the results were no longer significant after Bonferroni correction.

Our data showed more complications with a waning moon and do not agree with esoteric beliefs which recommend operations when the moon is waning [8]. The sign of Aries with a waxing moon was associated with the second highest number of complications and was not the most frequent period, as reported in the esoteric literature. We noted the most frequent complications with a waxing moon in Leo. One publication has partly confirmed our data. Gerstmeyer and Lehri checked 8212 surgical reports of phacoemulsification and found no correlations with the lunar phases (waxing and waning). However, they did not take the moon's passage through the zodiac into account, which seems to be important from the patients' point of view [11].

Studies investigating the influence of the moon and its passage through the zodiac are controversial. The majority of them have reported no influence of the lunar phase on survival or complications: Kühnl et al. concluded, from their study in patients with lung cancer, that the moon had no significant effect on intra- and postoperative complications or morbidity and mortality [12]. Wolbank et al. performed a 6-year retrospective investigation of frequency distribution in 11,134 patients presenting for emergency treatment. Clusters were seen (especially for lung diseases), but no relationship was observed between moon phases, the moon's passage through the zodiac, and the number of emergency patients [13]. Another study by Schuld et al. comprising 27,914 emergency cases including blood loss, aortic aneurysm, and gastrointestinal perforations mentions the same conclusion. Besides the moon and zodiac signs, Fridays that fell on the 13th of the month in the nine-year period also showed no accumulation of emergency cases [2]. A retrospective study by Peters-Engl et al. reported no significant difference in survival in breast cancer patients during a waxing (1904 operations) and waning (1853 operations) moon [14]. No significant difference in progression-free survival was noted in 452 patients after radical cystectomy [9]. The very scant literature on the subject also showed no association between surgical complications or medical emergencies and phases of the moon and zodiac signs [13]. A meta-analysis of 37 publications mentioned no connection between lunar phases and "lunatic" behavior (psychiatric disorders and crises, murder, or other criminal behavior) [15]. Lunar phases were not associated with psychiatric admissions or emergency presentation in 8473 psychiatric patients and 1909 emergency psychiatric evaluations [16]. Komann et al. investigated the effect of lunar phases on acute postsurgical pain and treatment-related side effects and assessed datasets of 12,224 patients from 10 international hospitals [3]. The authors disputed the claimed differences in surgical outcomes between lunar phases and concluded that none of the results would justify delaying or skipping surgeries because of moon phases [3].

Some authors report a possible impact: Joswig et al. performed a retrospective analysis of 924 elective spine surgeries and found no influence of unfavorable lunar or zodiac constellations that would justify a moon-calendar-based selection of elective surgery dates, but they also noted that patients undergoing surgery during a waxing moon experienced more intraoperative complications [7]. In a retrospective investigation of 15,985 patients with acute myocardial infarction, Wende et al. observed a possible cardioprotective time of three days after a new moon [17]. The odds of death were reduced at full moon in 210 patients who had undergone repair for dissection in the ascending aorta [18]. A significantly higher number of admissions were noted at full moon in 7219 patients with medically unexplained acute stroke symptoms [1]. A significant clustering of seizures around the full moon period was noted in a review of 859 patients admitted to an emergency unit for seizure [19].

All in all, after cataract operations, we observed nonsignificant differences in intraoperative complications with reference to the phases of the moon (waxing or waning) and its passage through the zodiac. In the subgroup analysis (comparison of the signs with the most numerous complications to those with the least), no significant differences were noted even after Bonferroni correction.

The strength of the present study is the large number of operations. Its weakness is the possible inhomogeneity in the skills of the operating surgeons. No individual quality analyses were performed for the 11 surgeons in respect of the frequency of complications. However, all of the surgeons were experienced. A study with fewer surgeons would possibly provide more conclusive data. We also had no data on the number of risk factors, such as pseudoexfoliation, narrow pupils, or a hard nucleus [20]. Since a surgeon's physical and mental states in terms of his/her concentration abilities, stress, and time constraints vary from day to day, it would be difficult to evaluate these factors. Prospective studies involving one or very few surgeons, with a homogeneous risk profile for the respective eye, would produce more solid results.

Patients who have concerns about a cataract operation planned for an "unfavorable" day with reference to the moon may be informed that there are no conclusive data at the present time to substantiate their concerns. A patient who insists on a more favorable day for the operation can, however, be accommodated when possible.

Conflicts of Interest

The authors declare that they have no conflicts of interest.

References

[1] F. Ahmad, T. J. Quinn, J. Dawson, and M. Walters, "A link between lunar phase and medically unexplained stroke symptoms: an unearthly influence?" *Journal of Psychosomatic Research*, vol. 65, no. 2, pp. 131–133, 2008.

[2] J. Schuld, J. E. Slotta, S. Schuld, O. Kollmar, M. K. Schilling, and S. Richter, "Popular belief meets surgical reality: impact of lunar phases, Friday the 13th and zodiac signs on emergency operations and intraoperative blood loss," *World Journal of Surgery*, vol. 35, pp. 1945–1949, 2011.

[3] M. Komann, C. Weinmann, and W. Meissner, "Howling at the moon? The effect of lunar phases on post-surgical pain outcome," *British Journal of Pain*, vol. 8, no. 2, pp. 72–77, 2014.

[4] R. G. Holzheimer, C. Nitz, and U. Gresser, "Lunar phase does not influence surgical quality," *European Journal of Medical Research*, vol. 8, pp. 414–418, 2003.

[5] M. Zimecki, "The lunar cycle: effects on human and animal behavior and physiology," *Postepy higieny i medycyny doswiadczalnej*, vol. 60, pp. 1–7, 2006.

[6] A. W. Yang, J. D. Johnson, C. M. Fronczak, and C. A. LaGrange, "Lunar phases and emergency department visits for renal colic due to ureteral calculus," *PLoS One*, vol. 11, no. 6, article e0157589, 2016.

[7] H. Joswig, M. N. Stienen, C. Hock, G. Hildebrandt, and W. Surbeck, "The influence of lunar phases and zodiac sign "Leo" on perioperative complications and outcome in elective spine surgery," *Acta Neurochirurgica*, vol. 158, no. 6, pp. 1095–1101, 2016.

[8] J. Paungger and T. Poppe, *Vom richtigen Zeitpunkt: Die Anwendung des Mondkalenders im täglichen Leben*, Hugendubel Verlag, München, 1996.

[9] M. May, K. P. Braun, C. Helke et al., "Lunar phases and zodiac signs do not influence quality of radical cystectomy—a statistical analysis of 452 patients with invasive bladder cancer," *International Urology and Nephrology*, vol. 39, no. 4, pp. 1023–1030, 2007.

[10] A. Ficklscherer, A. Angermann, P. Weber, B. Wegener, M. Pietschmann, and P. Müller, "Lunar phase does not influence perioperative complications in total hip arthroplasty," *Archives of Medical Science*, vol. 8, no. 1, pp. 111–114, 2011.

[11] K. Gerstmeyer and S. Lehri, "Der entzauberte Mythos: Lunarphase und operative Komplikationen bei Kataraktoperationen," *Klinische Monatsblätter für Augenheilkunde*, vol. 227, article V24, 2010.

[12] A. Kühnl, M. Herzog, M. Schmidt et al., "The dark side of the moon: impact of moon phases and long-term survival,

mortality and morbidity of surgery for lung cancer," *European Journal of Medical Research*, vol. 14, pp. 178–181, 2009.

[13] S. Wolbank, G. Prause, F. Smolle-Jüttner et al., "The influence of lunar phenomena on the incidence of emergency cases," *Resuscitation*, vol. 58, pp. 97–102, 2003.

[14] C. Peters-Engl, W. Frank, F. Kerschbaum, U. Denison, M. Medl, and P. Sevelda, "Lunar phases and survival of breast cancer patients—a statistical analysis of 3,757 cases," *Breast Cancer Research and Treatment*, vol. 70, pp. 131–135, 2001.

[15] J. Rotton and I. W. Kelly, "Much ado about the full moon: a meta-analysis of lunar-lunacy research," *Psychological Bulletin*, vol. 97, pp. 286–306, 1985.

[16] R. N. McLay, A. A. Daylo, and P. S. Hammer, "No effect of lunar cycle on psychiatric admissions or emergency evaluations," *Military Medicine*, vol. 171, no. 12, pp. 1239–1242, 2006.

[17] R. Wende, S. Klotvon, I. Kirchberger et al., "The influence of lunar phases on the occurrence of myocardial infarction: fact or myth? The MONICA/KORA Myocardial Infarction Registry," *European Journal of Preventive Cardiology*, vol. 20, no. 2, pp. 268–274, 2013.

[18] J. H. Shuhaiber, J. L. Fava, T. Shin et al., "The influence of seasons and lunar cycle on hospital outcomes following ascending aortic dissection repair," *Interactive Cardiovascular and Thoracic Surgery*, vol. 17, no. 5, pp. 818–822, 2013.

[19] P. Polychronopoulos, A. A. Argyriou, V. Sirrou et al., "Lunar phases and seizure occurrence: just an ancient legend?" *Neurology*, vol. 66, no. 9, pp. 1442-1443, 2006.

[20] B. J. Shingleton, M. C. Marvin, J. S. Heier et al., "Pseudoexfoliation: high risk factors for zonule weakness and concurrent vitrectomy during phacoemulsification," *Journal of Cataract and Refractive Surgery*, vol. 36, pp. 1261–1269, 2010.

15

Modified Vitrectomy Technique for Phakic Rhegmatogenous Retinal Detachment with Intermediate Break

Vincenza Bonfiglio,[1] Mario D. Toro [ID],[1,2] Antonio Longo [ID],[1] Teresio Avitabile,[1] Robert Rejdak [ID],[2] Katarzyna Nowomiejska [ID],[2,3] Tomasz Choragiewicz [ID],[2] Andrea Russo,[1] Matteo Fallico,[1] Agnieszka Kaminska,[4] Elina Ortisi,[1] Stefano Zenoni,[5] and Michele Reibaldi [1]

[1]Eye Clinic, University of Catania, Catania, Italy
[2]Department of General Ophthalmology, Medical University of Lublin, Lublin, Poland
[3]Institute for Ophthalmic Research, University Eye Hospital, Tuebingen, Germany
[4]Faculty of Family Studies, Cardinal Stefan Wyszynski University, Warsaw, Poland
[5]Life Clinic, Milano, Italy

Correspondence should be addressed to Mario D. Toro; toro.mario@email.it

Academic Editor: Elad Moisseiev

Purpose. To evaluate the effects of a modification of the traditional 25-gauge pars plana vitrectomy technique in the treatment of uncomplicated macula-on rhegmatogenous retinal detachment (RRD) with intermediate retinal break(s) and marked vitreous traction in the phakic eye. *Methods.* Prospective, noncomparative, and interventional case series. All consecutive phakic eyes with primary uncomplicated macula-on RRD with intermediate retinal break(s) and marked vitreous traction, with at least 1 year of postoperative follow-up, were enrolled. In all eyes, "localized 25-gauge vitrectomy" under air infusion with localized removal of the vitreous surrounding the retinal break(s), in association with laser photocoagulation and air tamponade, was performed. The primary end point was the rate of primary retinal attachment. Secondary end points were cataract progression and assessed by digital Scheimpflug lens photography (mean change of nuclear density units) and the rate of complications. *Results.* Thirty-two phakic eyes were included in the final analysis. At 12 months, the primary outcome of anatomical success was achieved in 94% of eyes. The mean nuclear density units did not change significantly at any time point during the follow-up. After localized vitrectomy, one eye developed an epiretinal membrane, and one eye developed cystoid macular edema; no other significant complications were reported. *Conclusions.* "Localized vitrectomy" has a high anatomical success rate in phakic eyes with primary uncomplicated macula-on RRD with intermediate retinal break(s) and marked vitreous traction, without causing progression of cataract.

1. Introduction

Scleral buckling (SB), primary pars plana vitrectomy (PPV), and pneumoretinopexy (PR) are the surgical procedures to treat primary rhegmatogenous retinal detachment (RRD). In the last few decades, primary PPV is the method of choice to manage RRD for several reasons including technical advances, lower postoperative inflammation, less patient discomfort, and greater familiarity of surgeons with this technique compared to the SB procedure [1–3]. The major disadvantages of primary PPV are cataract progression and iatrogenic retinal breaks [1].

The location and size of the retinal break(s) is one of the clinical features that influence the choice of treatment [1].

The scleral buckling versus primary vitrectomy in rhegmatogenous retinal detachment (SPR) study [4] included primary medium-severe RRD with intermediate breaks, described as "breaks between the equator and major vessel arcades."

In the management of RRD, the SPR study [5] suggested that the SB procedure in the phakic eyes shows a better postoperative visual acuity while the vitrectomy technique in the pseudophakic eyes shows better anatomical outcomes. However, no correlation about choice of treatment between

SB and PPV, and between visual and anatomic outcomes, according to the location of breaks was made in this study specifically.

SB is difficult to perform in cases involving an intermediate location of the break(s), and it is associated with many possible complications [6–10].

However, SB has the advantage of less risk of cataract development and substantially lower cost over PPV [1, 11].

In this study, the authors describe a new technique called "localized vitrectomy," used to treat uncomplicated macula-on primary RRD with intermediate break(s) and marked vitreous traction, in the phakic eyes. This procedure is a modification of the traditional 25-gauge PPV, consisting of a mini-invasive vitrectomy with a limited vitreous removal surrounding the retinal break(s), without core vitrectomy or shaving the vitreous base over 360°. Furthermore, the authors have evaluated the efficacy of this procedure, including visual and anatomic results, complication rate, and postoperative cataract progression.

2. Methods

In this prospective study, all consecutive phakic eyes that underwent 25-gauge PPV for primary macula-on primary RRD with intermediate break(s) and marked vitreous traction at the Ophthalmological Clinic of Catania between January 2014 and September 2016 were included. The risks and benefits of the treatment were explained to the patients, and a written consent was obtained in accordance with the Helsinki Declaration before the procedures. The Institutional Review Board/Ethics Committee approved the design of the study.

The inclusion criteria were as follows:

(1) Phakic eye

(2) Primary uncomplicated macula-on RRD including PVR grade A or B with one or more contiguous intermediate retinal break(s), defined as breaks between the equator and major vessel arcades [2], and with marked vitreous traction

(3) Presence of posterior vitreous detachment (PVD)

(4) Absent-to-moderate cataract (grade 0.0 to 2.0 in the Thompson classification) in the RRD eye and in the controlateral eye [12]

(5) Minimum follow-up of 12 months

Patients were excluded if they had secondary retinal detachment, previous ocular surgery, amblyopia, other rhegmatogenous retinal lesions, posterior retinal breaks (macular hole or between the major vessel arcades), giant breaks, or vitreous hemorrhage that required complete PPV.

Primary end point was the rate of primary retinal attachment; secondary end points were cataract progression and the rate of complications.

Two experienced vitreoretinal surgeons evaluated all primary RRD at the Ophthalmological Clinic of Catania between January 2014 and September 2016 and independently assessed and identified macula-on primary RRD with intermediate break(s) and marked vitreous traction.

All cases in which surgeons differed in their clinical assessment of degree of the RRD, with inconsistence decisions, were excluded.

We divided fundus drawings into 4 quadrants centered at the fovea, superotemporal (ST), superonasal (SN), inferotemporal (IT), and inferonasal (IN), respectively, and recorded the location of each break in the 4 quadrants.

As superior break, we defined a retinal break located between 9 and 3 o'clock meridian, and as inferior break, a retinal break between 4 and 8 o'clock meridian.

Before vitrectomy, an independent, experienced retinal specialist (M. F.) assessed the presence of PVD using a slit-lamp biomicroscopy with an external lens of 78 diopters to identify the presence of the Weiss ring and the visible posterior vitreous cortex. A second retinal specialist (A. R.) performed 10 MHz B-scan ultrasonography (Cinescan S HF, Quantel Medical, Clermont-Ferrand, France) using transverse and longitudinal scans. Only eyes with PVD confirmed by both techniques were enrolled in the study.

All patients underwent a complete ophthalmic evaluation including measurement of best-corrected visual acuity (BCVA) and intraocular pressure (IOP) and examination of the anterior segment and dilated fundus preoperatively (at baseline) and at 1 day, 1 week, and 3, 6, 9, and 12 months after surgery.

BCVA was measured using early treatment diabetic retinopathy study charts by a single well-trained and experienced ophthalmologist (M. T.). Vision results were quantified as a logarithm of the minimum angle of resolution (logMAR).

IOP was measured by the Goldmann applanation tonometry. Hypotony was defined as an IOP of 5 mmHg or less.

In all patients, the lens status evaluation was performed with digital Scheimpflug lens photography at the baseline and at 3, 6, and 12 months after surgery. The nuclear density was assessed in the vitrectomized eye (study group) and in the fellow eye (control group). Lens images were obtained and analyzed by using a Nidek EAS-1000 anterior segment analysis system (Nidek, Gamagori, Japan). All lens images were taken by the same observer (A. L.) after pupillary dilation and at the same settings, as previously described by Sawa et al. [13] and Vivino et al. [14]. The opacification value of the nuclear region was expressed in nuclear density units (NDUs).

All preoperative, intraoperative, and postoperative data including patient demographics (age and sex) and postoperative complications were recorded in a database. The incidence, timing, and causes of retinal redetachment were also registered.

2.1. Surgical Technique. All patients underwent 3-port 25-gauge vitrectomy with a valved trocar system performed by the same surgeon (T. A.) under local sub-Tenon's anesthesia (using 10 ml of a 50 : 50 mixture of 2% lidocaine and 0.5% bupivacaine with 150 IU hyaluronidase). Surgical procedures were performed using the Stellaris PC under a Resight 700 noncontact panoramic viewing system

(Carl Zeiss Meditec). The sclerotomy was placed 4 mm posterior to the limbus. With closed infusion, the retinal break(s) were localized, the eye was rotated in order to position the region of the retinal break as high as possible, and air infusion was started with a pressure of 30–35 mmHg. Localized removal of the vitreous surrounding the retinal break(s) was performed, and a complete release of the vitreoretinal adhesion surrounding the retinal break(s) was obtained. Finally, the subretinal fluid was drained with a needle through the retinal break. Neither core vitrectomy nor shaving of the vitreous base was performed.

After complete retinal attachment was achieved, endolaser photocoagulation was applied around the retinal break(s). Tamponade was performed with filtered air. Transconjunctival sutures were placed only in two eyes, in which leakage at the sclerotomy sites was observed. All patients were asked to maintain a specific head position, according to the location of the retinal break, for 3 days after surgery. In particular, patients with inferior break(s) were instructed to maintain a face-down and lateral position, while patients with superior break to maintain upright and lateral position depending on the quadrant o'clock meridian.

2.2. Statistical Analysis.

2.2. Statistical Analysis. Measured Snellen visual acuity values were converted to the logMAR values for subsequent analysis. The analysis of variance (ANOVA) was used to compare the mean values of pre- and postoperative BCVA and IOP in the vitrectomized eyes (study group) and to compare the mean NDUs of the study group eyes with that of the control group eyes (fellow eyes) at baseline and at 3, 6, and 12 months after treatment. Multiple comparisons were performed using the Tukey HSD test, if the differences were significant. Student's *t*-test was used to compare the mean NDUs detected in the two groups. *P* values <0.05 were considered significant. The data were analyzed using the Statistical Packages for the Social Sciences for Windows (v.17.0; SPSS, Chicago, IL, USA).

3. Results

Of the 46 phakic consecutive eyes with uncomplicated macula-on RRD and intermediate retinal break(s) with marked vitreous traction, 11 eyes were excluded (5 eyes did not have PVD, 4 eyes had cataract more than grade 0.0–2.0, and 2 patients declined to participate), and 35 eyes addressed the inclusion criteria and were enrolled in the study. Of the these 35 eyes recruited for surgery, only 32 eyes were included in the analysis because 2 patients were lost during the follow-up period, and one patient had intraoperative vitreous hemorrhage during surgery and required conversion to standard PPV (Figure 1). Of the 32 eyes with RRD, 22 (68.7%) had superior retinal breaks and 10 (31.3%) had inferior retinal breaks. In particular, 19 eyes (59.3%) had retinal break(s) located in the ST quadrant, 7 eyes (21.8%) had break(s) in the IT quadrant, 3 eyes (9.3%) in the SN, and 3 eyes (9.3%) in the IN quadrant.

The mean (SD) age of patients was 61.5 ± 13.3 years; 18 patients (56%) were men, and 14 (44%) were women.

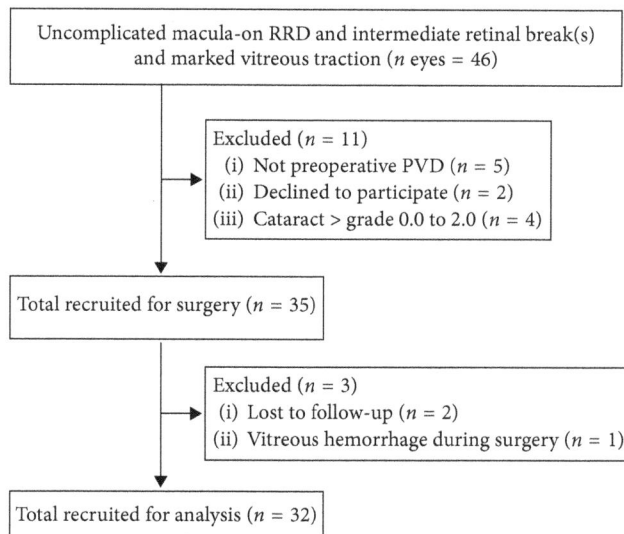

```
┌─────────────────────────────────────────────────┐
│ Uncomplicated macula-on RRD and intermediate    │
│ retinal break(s) and marked vitreous traction   │
│ (n eyes = 46)                                   │
└─────────────────────────────────────────────────┘
                     │
                     │    ┌──────────────────────────────────┐
                     ├───▶│ Excluded (n = 11)                │
                     │    │  (i) Not preoperative PVD (n = 5)│
                     │    │  (ii) Declined to participate    │
                     │    │       (n = 2)                    │
                     │    │  (iii) Cataract > grade 0.0 to   │
                     │    │        2.0 (n = 4)               │
                     │    └──────────────────────────────────┘
                     ▼
┌─────────────────────────────────────────────────┐
│ Total recruited for surgery (n = 35)            │
└─────────────────────────────────────────────────┘
                     │
                     │    ┌──────────────────────────────────┐
                     ├───▶│ Excluded (n = 3)                 │
                     │    │  (i) Lost to follow-up (n = 2)   │
                     │    │  (ii) Vitreous hemorrhage during │
                     │    │       surgery (n = 1)            │
                     │    └──────────────────────────────────┘
                     ▼
┌─────────────────────────────────────────────────┐
│ Total recruited for analysis (n = 32)           │
└─────────────────────────────────────────────────┘
```

FIGURE 1: Flow diagram of the study (enrollment).

3.1. Primary Anatomical Success Rate.

3.1. Primary Anatomical Success Rate. The primary anatomical success rate, defined as retinal reattachment at the final follow-up of 12 months after a single operation, was 94% (30 of 32 eyes): 95 4% of eyes with superior retinal breaks (21 of 22 eyes) and 90% of eyes with inferior retinal breaks (9 eyes of 10), respectively (*P* = 0.534). Recurrence of RRD occurred in 2 eyes (6%) during the follow-up period: one eyes with preoperative ST retinal break and one eye with preoperative IT retina break. Both occurred within 1 month after the first operation. The redetachment was attributed to development of grade C PVR in one eye and to a new peripheral retinal break in the inferior quadrant in the other eye. Both of these eyes were reoperated by 25-gauge vitrectomy and SF6 tamponade; the retinal reattachment was obtained in both eyes. Thus, the final anatomical success rate, defined as retinal attachment at the final follow-up without regard to additional procedures, was 100% (32 of 32 eyes).

3.2. Visual Acuity.

3.2. Visual Acuity. ANOVA showed no change in the mean BCVA from the baseline to 12 months after surgery. The mean ± SD logMAR BCVA was 0.17 ± 0.13 logMAR, 0.17 ± 0.12 logMAR, 0.16 ± 0.12 logMAR, and 0.16 ± 0.1 logMAR, respectively, at the baseline and 3, 6, and 12 months, without significant difference (ANOVA, *P* = 0.973).

3.3. Progression of Lens Opacity.

3.3. Progression of Lens Opacity. At the baseline, the mean ± SD NDU was 68 ± 12 in the study group and 69 ± 14 in the control group (*t*-test *P* = 0.933) (Table 1). ANOVA showed that the mean NDUs did not change significantly in either group during the follow-up (study group *P* = 0.523; control group *P* = 0.725). No difference in NDUs was found between two groups at 3, 6, and 12 months.

No intraoperative complications were observed.

No significant IOP changes were detected during the follow-up period (ANOVA, *P* = 0.781). The mean ± SD preoperative and postoperative IOP at 1 day, 1 week, and 1, 3, 6, and 12 months, were 13.6 ± 3.1 mmHg, 13.1 ± 4.5 mmHg,

TABLE 1: NDUs at the baseline and at 3, 6, and 12 months after surgery.

NDUs (range, 0 to 255 steps) (mean ± SD)	Vitrectomy group	Control group	P^*
Baseline	68 ± 12	69 ± 14	0.933
3 months	70 ± 12	69 ± 16	0.779
6 months	72 ± 18	71 ± 11	0.875
12 months	73 ± 15	72 ± 9	0.724

* t-test.

13.7 ± 3.2 mmHg, 14.2 ± 5.2 mmHg, 14.7 ± 4.7 mmHg, 14.4 ± 3.9 mmHg, and 14.2 ± 4.5 mmHg, respectively. No hypotony was detected in any eyes, and none of the patients had endophthalmitis after surgery.

One eye developed an epiretinal membrane (ERM) 3 months after surgery and one eye showed cystoid macular edema at 1 month-follow up examination, resolved after topical therapy. No other postoperative complications were registered.

4. Discussion

Our study showed that a "localized vitrectomy" was effective in the treatment of primary macula-on RRDs, with superior and inferior, intermediate break(s) and marked vitreous traction in the phakic eyes and did not cause significant progression of cataract.

To date, no study has evaluated the efficacy of different surgical techniques in presence of uncomplicated RRD and intermediate retinal break(s).

PR is a well-accepted alternative surgical technique to scleral buckling and vitrectomy for RRDs with one or more retinal breaks within one clock hour; however, it is contraindicated in the eyes with inferior retinal break(s) and in which breaks are held open by vitreous traction [15].

The SPR study evaluated the phakic eyes with medium-severe primary RRD and intermediate break(s) [3] and shows better functional outcomes with the SB procedure than PPV. However, SPR study analysis included primary RRD with many different preoperative variables, such as macula-on only in 42.9% of eyes, RD with multiple breaks in different quadrants, bullous RD, intermediate breaks with marked vitreous traction, and RD with unclear hole situations. Furthermore, in the SPR study, no subanalysis of postoperative outcomes was conducted to identify any relation between choice of treatment and location of break(s), in particular intermediate break(s) [3].

The surgical SB procedure to treat primary RRD is very challenging in the eyes with intermediate break(s). Despite the advantages of not increasing the risk of cataract and being less expensive than PPV, SB can cause several possible complications, such as myopic shift in refraction (68%) [6], diplopia with extraocular muscle dysfunction (3%–50%) [6–8], choroidal detachment (23%–44%) [7], subretinal hemorrhage (3%–5.1%) [8, 9], iatrogenic scleral break (2%) [10], accidental subretinal fluid drainage (5%–8%) [8, 10], retinal breaks (0.54%–4%) [8], choroidal hemorrhage (2%)

[10], retinal incarceration (2.2%–3%) [8], explant exposure (6%) [10], macular pucker (2%) [6, 9], and PVR (5%–21%) [6, 9].

Moreover, breaks between the equator and major vessel arcades are commonly supported by one or more large radial sponges that need a surgical familiarity for the correct sponge placement with a potential risk of compression of the vortex veins [1].

In a previous study, Uemura and Nakao showed that, in the eyes with uncomplicated RRD caused by a posterior retinal break, both procedures SB and PPV had a similar visual recovery but the vitrectomized eyes had less severe intraoperative complications compared with SB [16].

Vitrectomy offers some advantages such as easy access to intermediate retinal breaks and greater familiarity with this technique compared with SB [1, 4]. However, PPV is known to cause cataract progression and may cause several other complications such as glaucoma (8.9%) [17], choroidal hemorrhage (0.8%) [18], diplopia/EOM dysfunction (0.5%–7%) [6, 9], cataract (70%) [9], macular pucker (9%) [7], postoperative PVR (6%–18%) [6, 7], and iatrogenic retinal breaks (6%–15.7%) [7, 19].

Our small gauge-modified vitrectomy showed a single-operation anatomical success rate of 94%, which is consistent with the rates of 74–93.9% for repair of primary RRD in other reports of conventional small-gauge vitrectomy [20–22] and did not cause significant progression of cataract.

We observed only one case with intraoperative hemorrhage requiring conversion to standard PPV and that was excluded by the analysis.

Moreover, no statistically significant difference between eyes with superior retinal break(s) and eyes with inferior retinal break(s) in terms of primary anatomical success rate ($P = 0.534$) was noted in our study. However, this topic is still controversial; in fact, despite Goto et al. [23] reported that inferior retinal breaks were significantly associated with a lower success anatomic comparing with superior retinal breaks (80% versus 98%, $P = 0.012$), the other authors [24] showed inferior breaks do not represent a risk factor for worse anatomical and functional results (96.5% versus 93.3%, respectively, in superior and inferior retinal breaks).

It is well established that vitrectomy increases lens opacity in most eyes when assessed at 6 months regardless of the caliber of the instrument [25].

In our study, no progression of nuclear sclerosis was observed through the 12 months of follow-up, and the NDUs at 12 months did not differ between the vitrectomized and fellow eyes. Our result is consistent with previous studies that found no progression of cataract in the eyes that had undergone removal of the ERM without vitrectomy [26, 27].

The mechanism underlying cataract progression after vitrectomy is not completely understood. One hypothesis is that, in the absence of vitreous gel, molecular oxygen from the retinal vasculature reaches the lens and promotes oxidative damage of the lens nucleus and nuclear sclerotic cataract [28]. According to this hypothesis, the very limited amount of vitreous removal in our modified vitrectomy, with core and vitreous base preservation, could explain the absence of progression of cataract.

Our choice to use air as tamponade was supported by findings of previous studies reporting favorable results with air tamponade in the management of RRD, with a single-operative success rate from 84.38% to 94.4% [29]. Air used as gas tamponade showed no inferior results to long-acting gas because of the adhesion between retina and retinal pigment epithelium (RPE) occurring within 24 hours. Moreover, long-acting and expansive gas could cause vitreous disturbance and increase the risks of elevated IOP, PVR, and new or missed tears [30].

Despite the recent evolution of vitreoretinal surgical techniques, the incidence of "new" retinal breaks has been reported for small-gauge PPV in up to 15.7% of eyes [19]. Although the sample number was small in our study, we found new retinal breaks in only 1 eye (3%) during the 12-month follow-up and suggests that the residual vitreous does not cause secondary vitreous traction in these eyes. Similarly, previous reports of no vitrectomizing vitreous surgery for ERM have also reported no new retinal breaks during the long follow-up [31].

In our series, ERM developed in 3% of eyes. This is a lower percentage than the 3.6–12.8% reported by others [32, 33]. The most likely explanation for the development of ERM is that the retinal pigment epithelial cells migrate to the surface of the posterior pole of the retina by diffusing into the vitreous cavity through the break or through fibrosis [33]. In our modified technique, the remaining vitreous probably prevented such diffusion into the vitreous cavity.

Furthermore, a potential advantage of our new technique of "localized vitrectomy," without core and vitreous base removing, is that it still allows intravitreal injections in the eyes experiencing the onset of neovascular age-related macular degeneration, which can be difficult to treat after previous conventional PPV. Experimental studies have shown a reduction in the intravitreal half-life of drugs in the vitrectomized eyes due to significantly faster clearance rates of the drugs after vitrectomy, which could make them less effective [34, 35], and it may require more frequent treatment regimen of anti-VEGF therapy [34, 35].

The main limitations of this study are the small number of patients enrolled and the lack of an interventional control group. Large studies should also evaluate the efficacy and rate of postoperative complications.

5. Conclusion

"Localized vitrectomy" seems to be an effective surgical procedure to treat uncomplicated macula-on primary RRD with intermediate break(s), marked vitreous traction, and PVD in the phakic eyes, achieving a high anatomical success rates without progression of cataract.

Conflicts of Interest

The authors declare that they have no conflicts of interest with this submission.

Authors' Contributions

All authors listed on the title page have read the manuscript and agreed to its submission. VB, MDT, AL, TA, and MR did conception, design, statistical analysis drafting, and critical revision. RR, KN, AR, MF, TC, AK, EO, and SZ performed drafting, data acquisition, and critical revision. All authors approved the final version of the manuscript.

References

[1] I. Kreissig, "View 1: minimal segmental buckling without drainage," British Journal of Ophthalmology, vol. 87, no. 6, pp. 782–784, 2003.

[2] D. McLeod, "Is it time to call time on the scleral buckle?," British Journal of Ophthalmology, vol. 88, no. 11, pp. 1357–1359, 2004.

[3] L. Kellner, B. Wimpissinger, U. Stolba, W. Brannath, and S. Binder, "25-gauge vs 20-gauge system for pars plana vitrectomy: a prospective randomised clinical trial," British Journal of Ophthalmology, vol. 91, no. 7, pp. 945–948, 2007.

[4] N. Feltgen, C. Weiss, S. Wolf, D. Ottenberg, H. Heimann, and SPR Study Group, "Scleral buckling versus primary vitrectomy in rhegmatogenous retinal detachment study (SPR Study): recruitment list evaluation. Study report no. 2," Graefe's Archive for Clinical and Experimental Ophthalmology, vol. 245, no. 6, pp. 803–809, 2007.

[5] H. Heimann, K. U. Baertz-Schmidt, N. Bronfeld, C. Weiss, R. D. Hilgers, and M. H. Foerster, "Scleral buckling versus primary vitrectomy in rhegmatogenous retinal detachment: a prospective randomized multicenter clinical study," Ophthalmology, vol. 114, no. 12, pp. 2142.e4–2154.e4, 2007.

[6] D. Steel, "Retinal detachment," BMJ Clinical Evidence, vol. 3, 2014.

[7] The SPR Study Study Group, "View 2: the case for primary vitrectomy," British Journal of Ophthalmology, vol. 87, no. 6, pp. 784–787, 2003.

[8] E. R. Holz and W. F. Mieler, "View 3: the case for pneumatic retinopexy," British Journal of Ophthalmology, vol. 87, no. 6, pp. 787–789, 2003.

[9] Z. Lv, Y. Li, Y. Wu, and Y. Qu, "Surgical complications of primary rhegmatogenous retinal detachment: a meta-analysis," PLoS One, vol. 10, no. 3, Article ID e0116493, 2015.

[10] A. S. Abdullah, S. Jan, M. S. Qureshi, M. T. Khan, and M. D. Khan, "Complications of conventional scleral buckling occurring during and after treatment of rhegmatogenous retinal detachment," Journal of the College of Physicians and Surgeons Pakistan, vol. 20, no. 5, pp. 321–326, 2010.

[11] M. I. Seider, A. Naseri, and J. M. Stewart, "Cost comparison of scleral buckle versus vitrectomy for rhegmatogenous retinal detachment repair," American Journal of Ophthalmology, vol. 156, no. 4, pp. 661–666, 2013.

[12] J. T. Thompson, B. M. Glaser, R. N. Sjaarda, and R. P. Murphy, "Progression of nuclear sclerosis and long-term visual results of vitrectomy with transforming growth factor beta-2 for macular holes," American Journal of Ophthalmology, vol. 119, no. 1, pp. 48–54, 1995.

[13] M. Sawa, Y. Saito, A. Hayashi, S. Kusaka, M. Ohji, and Y. Tano, "Assessment of nuclear sclerosis after non-vitrectomizing vitreous surgery," *American Journal of Ophthalmology*, vol. 132, no. 3, pp. 356–362, 2001.

[14] M. A. Vivino, S. Chintalagiri, B. Trus, and M. Datiles, "Development of a Scheimpflug slit lamp camera system for quantitative densitometric analysis," *Eye*, vol. 7, no. 6, pp. 791–798, 1993.

[15] C. K. Chan, S. G. Lin, A. S. Nuthi, and D. M. Salib, "Pneumatic retinopexy for the repair of retinal detachments: a comprehensive review (1986–2007)," *Survey of Ophthalmology*, vol. 53, no. 5, pp. 443–478, 2008.

[16] A. Uemura and K. Nakao, "A comparison between scleral buckling procedure and vitrectomy for the management of uncomplicated retinal detachment caused by posterior retinal break," *Nippon Ganka Gakkai Zasshi*, vol. 99, no. 10, pp. 1170–1174, 1995.

[17] S. A. Mansukhani, A. J. Barkmeier, S. J. Bakri et al., "The risk of primary open angle glaucoma following vitreoretinal surgery: a population-based study," *American Journal of Ophthalmology*, vol. 193, pp. 143–155, 2018.

[18] M. Reibaldi, A. Longo, M. R. Romano et al., "Delayed suprachoroidal hemorrhage after pars plana vitrectomy: five-year results of a retrospective multicenter cohort study," *American Journal of Ophthalmology*, vol. 160, no. 6, pp. 1235.e1–1242.e1, 2015.

[19] R. Ehrlich, Y. W. Goh, N. Ahmad, and P. Polkinghorne, "Retinal breaks in small-gauge pars plana vitrectomy," *American Journal of Ophthalmology*, vol. 153, no. 5, pp. 868–872, 2012.

[20] S. A. Lewis, D. M. Miller, C. D. Riemann, R. E. Foster, and M. R. Petersen, "Comparison of 20-, 23-, and 25-gauge pars plana vitrectomy in pseudophakic rhegmatogenous retinal detachment repair," *Ophthalmic Surgery, Lasers, and Imaging*, vol. 42, no. 2, pp. 107–113, 2011.

[21] S. Rezar, S. Sacu, R. Blum, K. Eibenberger, U. Schmidt-Erfurth, and M. Georgopoulos, "Macula-on versus macula-off pseudophakicrhegmatogenous retinal detachment following primary 23-gaugevitrectomy plus endotamponade," *Current Eye Research*, vol. 41, no. 4, pp. 543–550, 2016.

[22] S. Mehta, K. J. Blinder, G. K. Shah, and M. G. Grand, "Pars plana vitrectomy versus combined pars plana vitrectomy and scleral buckle for primary repair of rhegmatogenous retinal detachment," *Canadian Journal of Ophthalmology*, vol. 46, no. 3, pp. 237–241, 2011.

[23] T. Goto, T. Nakagomi, and H. Iijima, "A comparison of the anatomic successes of primary vitrectomy for rhegmatogenous retinal detachment with superior and inferior breaks," *Acta Ophthalmologica*, vol. 91, no. 6, pp. 552–556, 2013.

[24] P. Stavrakas, P. Tranos, A. Androu et al., "Anatomical and functional results following 23-Gauge primary pars plana vitrectomy for rhegmatougenous retinal detachment: superior versus inferior breaks," *Journal of Ophthalmology*, vol. 2017, Article ID 2565249, 7 pages, 2017.

[25] H. Feng and R. A. Adelman, "Cataract formation following vitreoretinal procedures," *Clinical Ophthalmology*, vol. 8, pp. 1957–1965, 2014.

[26] M. Reibaldi, A. Longo, T. Avitabile et al., "Transconjunctival non vitrectomizing vitreous surgery versus 25-gauge vitrectomy in patients with epiretinal membrane: a prospective randomized study," *Retina*, vol. 35, no. 5, pp. 873–879, 2015.

[27] M. Sawa, M. Ohji, S. Kusaka et al., "Nonvitrectomizing vitreous surgery for epiretinal membrane long-term follow-up," *Ophthalmology*, vol. 112, no. 8, pp. 1402–1408, 2005.

[28] S. Milazzo, "Pathogenesis of cataract after vitrectomy," *French Journal of Ophthalmology*, vol. 37, no. 3, pp. 243-244, 2014.

[29] C. Zhou, Q. Qiu, and Z. Zheng, "Air versus gas tamponade in rhegmatogenous retinal detachment with inferior breaks after 23-gauge pars plana vitrectomy: a prospective, randomized comparative interventional study," *Retina*, vol. 35, no. 5, pp. 886–891, 2015.

[30] K. Y. Pak, S. J. Lee, H. J. Kwon, S. W. Park, I. S. Byon, and J. E. Lee, "Use of air as gas tamponade in rhegmatogenous retinal detachment," *Journal of Ophthalmology*, vol. 2017, Article ID 1341948, 5 pages, 2017.

[31] Y. Saito, J. M. Lewis, I. Park et al., "Nonvitrectomizing vitreous surgery: a strategy to prevent postoperative nuclear sclerosis," *Ophthalmology*, vol. 106, no. 8, pp. 1541–1545, 1999.

[32] R. C. Katira, M. Zamani, D. M. Berinstein, and R. A. Garfinkel, "Incidence and characteristics of macular pucker formation after primary retinal detachment repair by pars plana vitrectomy alone," *Retina*, vol. 28, no. 5, pp. 744–748, 2008.

[33] K. Y. Nam and J. Y. Kim, "Effect of internal limiting membrane peeling on the development of epiretinal membrane after pars plana vitrectomy for primary rhegmatogenous retinal detachment," *Retina*, vol. 35, no. 5, pp. 880–885, 2015.

[34] S. Gisladottir, T. Loftsson, and E. Stefansson, "Diffusion characteristics of vitreous humor and saline solution follow the Stokes Einstein equation," *Graefe's Archive for Clinical and Experimental Ophthalmology*, vol. 247, no. 12, pp. 1677–1684, 2009.

[35] J. B. Christoforidis, M. M. Williams, J. Wang et al., "Anatomic and pharmacokinetic properties of intravitreal bevacizumab after vitrectomy and lensectomy," *Retina*, vol. 33, no. 5, pp. 946–952, 2013.

16

Bimanual Microincision Cataract Surgery versus Coaxial Microincision Cataract Surgery

Chenxi Fu, Naipin Chu, Xiaoning Yu, and Ke Yao

Eye Center, Second Affiliated Hospital, School of Medicine, Zhejiang University, Hangzhou, China

Correspondence should be addressed to Ke Yao; xlren@zju.edu.cn

Academic Editor: Tamer A. Macky

Purpose. This meta-analysis was conducted to compare the intraoperative and postoperative outcomes of bimanual microincision cataract surgery (B-MICS) and coaxial microincision cataract surgery (C-MICS). *Methods.* Three databases were searched for papers that compared B-MICS and C-MICS from inception to June 2016. The following intraoperative and postoperative outcomes were included in the final meta-analysis: ultrasound time (UST), effective phacoemulsification time (EPT), balanced salt solution use (BSS use), mean surgery time, best-corrected visual acuity (BCVA), central corneal thickness (CCT), and increased CCT. *Results.* There were no statistically significant differences in mean surgery time, UST, BSS use, BCVA, CCT, or increased CCT (one subgroup at postoperative day 7-8 and another subgroup at postoperative day 30). However, there was less EPT needed during surgery ($p < 0.01$) and lower levels of increased CCT at postoperative day 1 ($p = 0.02$) in the B-MICS group compared with the C-MICS group. *Conclusions.* The EPT was shorter and increased CCT was less at postoperative day 1 in the B-MICS group. There were no statistically significant differences in other intraoperative and postoperative outcomes between the B-MICS group and the C-MICS group. B-MICS is an efficient and safe cataract surgery procedure.

1. Introduction

With the development of equipment for cataract surgery and increased requirements for visual outcome, the main recent change in cataract surgical procedure aims to decrease the size of the clean corneal incision. In coaxial microincision cataract surgery (C-MICS), irrigation, aspiration, and phacoemulsification are performed with the same instruments, which is similar to standard coaxial small incision cataract surgery (C-SICS) but provides a smaller incision [1, 2]. Less surgically induced astigmatism (SIA) and faster wound healing are expected from incision sizes below 2.2 mm, which makes C-MICS more popular among ophthalmologists around the world [3]. For B-MICS, the separate irrigating hand piece port can be supplementary during phacoemulsification, and the same size of two incisions and hand piece ports makes the interchange of the two ports possible during surgery [4, 5]. However, the extra step of enlarging the main

incision or making a third incision is a drawback of the pervasiveness of the B-MICS.

According to a recent study [6], there are new aspheric intraocular lenses that are small enough to fit through a 1.4 mm incision, which saves the trouble of having an extra step for the IOL implant. Since the trend in cataract surgery has been to minimize the corneal incision, the 1.4 mm incision of B-MICS may have advantages in refractive surgery [4, 5]. Two published meta-analysis studies have compared the outcomes of B-MICS versus C-SICS and C-MICS versus C-SICS. To our knowledge, there has not been a meta-analysis comparing the outcomes of B-MICS and C-MICS [7, 8]. Several clinical studies have compared the intraoperative and postoperative outcomes of B-MICS and C-MICS, but there has been no clear conclusion. This meta-analysis was performed to compare the outcomes of B-MICS with C-MICS to make recommendations for improvements in cataract surgery.

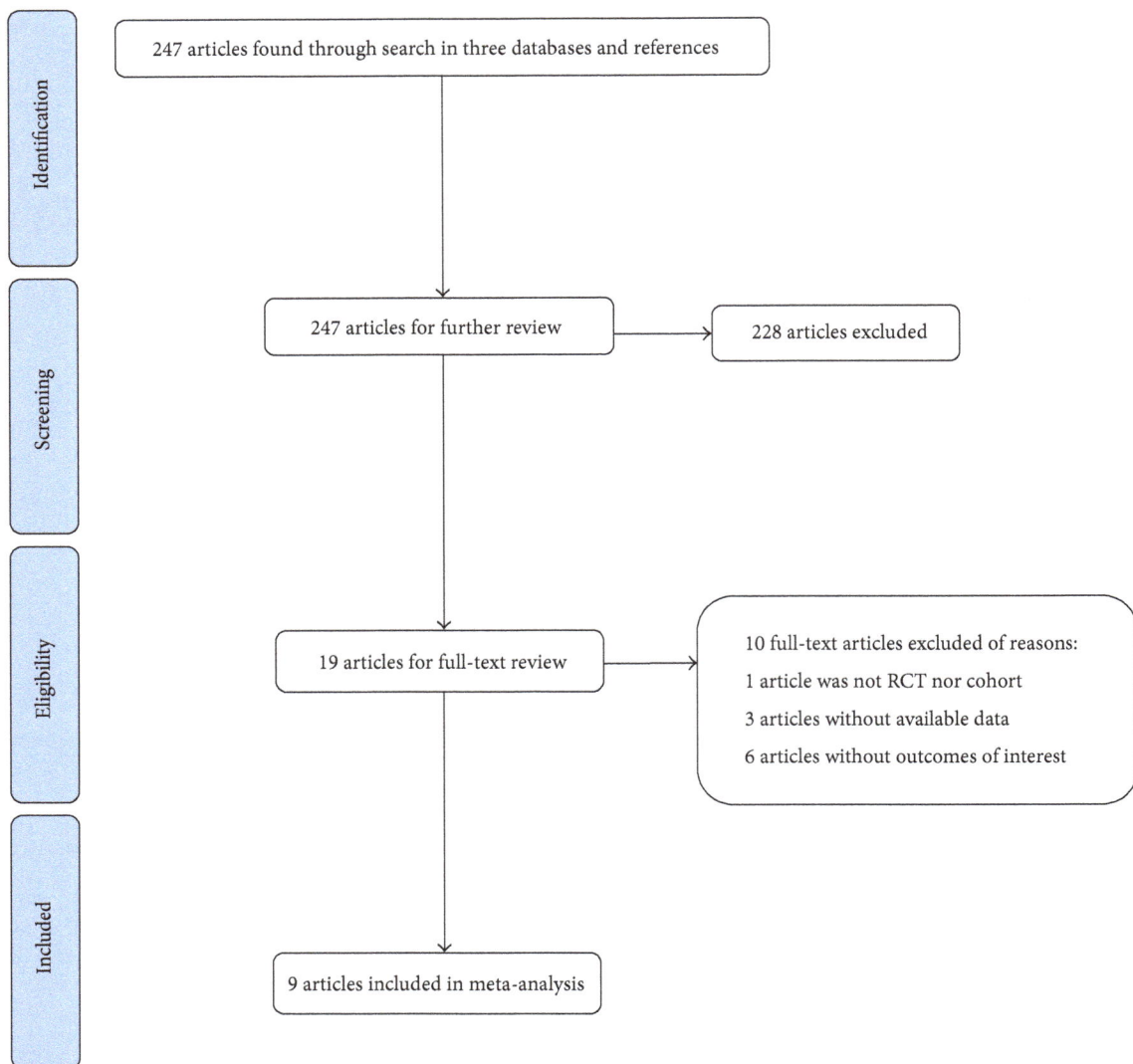

FIGURE 1: Flow diagram of study selection progress.

2. Materials and Methods

This meta-analysis was performed according to the Preferred Reporting Items for Systematic Reviews and Meta-Analyses (PRISMA) statement [9].

The following terms were searched in PubMed, Web of Science, and the Cochrane Library: "bimanual microincision," "biaxial microincision," "bimanual microincisional cataract surgery," "bimanual phacoemulsification," "biaxial phacoemulsification," "coaxial microincision," "coaxial microincisional cataract surgery," and "coaxial phacoemulsification." Papers published before July 2016 were included in the search. The references of the included papers were reviewed to seek papers that were missed in the primary search. The papers included in the meta-analysis met the following criteria: (1) the incision of the coaxial microincision cataract surgery (C-MICS) was less than 2.2 mm and (2) patients in the study had no other ocular diseases other than cataracts. Two

investigators (Fu and Chu) searched the three databases in all fields independently.

After scanning the titles and abstracts, Fu and Chu obtained access to the full text of the papers that compared outcomes of C-MICS and B-MICS. After reading the full text, papers were included in the meta-analysis based on the criteria listed above. The search and exclusion process was conducted as shown in Figure 1. The basic information and the data on intraoperative and postoperative outcomes, including EPT, mean surgery time, BBS use, UST, BCVA, CCT, and increased CCT, were extracted from the papers independently by two investigators. If there were any disagreements, Fu and Chu double-checked the related papers for data verification. For B-MICS, the sizes of the first-made incision and the extended or the third incision for the IOL implant were both recorded if they were reported in the papers. The BCVA data extracted from all papers were reported in the logMAR system. To avoid extracting repetitious data, two investigators double-checked the sources and characteristics of the patients in the studies with the same subject and author. Seven RCTs were evaluated according to the Jadad score system, and studies of three or more points were of good quality.

The data on all outcomes were analysed using Stata software (version 12.0, StataCorp, College Station, TX, USA). The means and SDs of outcomes were extracted from the papers to obtain the weighted mean difference (WMD) with a 95% confidence interval (CI). Except for heterogeneity and metaregression analyses of the data, the statistical significance level was set at $p < 0.01$. For heterogeneity among studies, the significance level was set at $p < 0.10$ for Cochran's Q statistic and $I^2 > 50\%$ for the I^2 index score [10]. A fixed-effects model based on the inverse variance method was used for continuous data unless the heterogeneity among the studies was high (I^2 score $> 50\%$), in which case, a random-effects model based on the DerSimonian and Laird method was used [11]. To assess the robustness of the results, a sensitivity analysis was performed on all results by excluding one study at a time. Egger's linear regression and Begg's rank correlation tests were performed to assess the potential publication bias [12, 13]. The statistical analysis procedures described above were repeated by two investigators independently.

3. Results

Among the included papers, there were seven randomized controlled trials (RCTs) [3, 14–19] and two cohort studies [20, 21]. Basic information on the nine articles is provided in Table 1. The included studies reported on a total of 711 eyes (356 eyes in the B-MICS group and 355 eyes in the C-MICS group).

3.1. Intraoperative Outcomes

3.1.1. Effective Phacoemulsification Time (EPT). In seven studies reporting on 589 eyes, the EPT was longer in the C-MICS group than in the B-MICS group in the fixed-effects model (Figure 2, WMD: −1.18, 95% CI: −1.66 to −0.70, $p \leq 0.001$, $I^2 = 49.3\%$, $P_{heterogeneity} = 0.066$).

3.1.2. Mean Surgery Time. In four studies that reported on 330 eyes, the mean surgery time was recorded. The forest plot showed that there was no statistically significant difference between the B-MICS group and the C-MICS group in the random-effects model (Figure 2, WMD: 0.55, 95% CI: −0.20 to 1.31, $p = 0.338$, $I^2 = 91.1\%$, $P_{heterogeneity} = 0.001$).

3.1.3. Use of Balanced Salt Solution (BSS). As shown in Figure 3, there was no statistically significant difference in BBS use in the random-effects model (Figure 3, WMD: 21.963, 95% CI: −6.150 to 50.076, $p = 0.126$, $I^2 = 95.4\%$, $P_{heterogeneity} = 0.001$).

3.1.4. Ultrasound Time (UST). Three studies reported UST, and significant heterogeneity in UST among these studies was found. As shown in Figure 3, there was no statistically significant difference between the two groups in the random-effects model (Figure 3, WMD: −12.79, 95% CI: −31.37 to 5.78, $p = 0.177$, $I^2 = 83.6\%$, $P_{heterogeneity} = 0.002$).

3.2. Postoperative Outcomes

3.2.1. Best-Corrected Visual Acuity (BCVA). In five studies, the BCVA was measured at postoperative day 1, day 7, day 30, day 60, and day 90. Subgroup meta-analysis was performed for two subgroups: BCVA within 7 postoperative days (222 eyes) and BCVA at day 30 (160 eyes). In both groups, no statistically significant difference was found between the B-MICS group and the C-MICS group in the fixed-effects model (Figure 4, within 7 days: WMD: −0.007, 95% CI: −0.045 to 0.032, $p = 0.735$, $I^2 = 0.0\%$, $P_{heterogeneity} = 0.570$; at day 30: WMD: −0.003, 95% CI: −0.021 to 0.014, $p = 0.697$, $I^2 = 8.9\%$, $P_{heterogeneity} = 0.334$).

3.2.2. Central Corneal Thickness. CCT was measured in three studies. We used data from two studies that recorded the precise CCT measuring time for 82 and 90 eyes, respectively, and analysed the postoperative CCT in the day 1 subgroup and the after day 30 subgroup. As shown in the forest plot, no statistically significant difference was found in either subgroup (Figure 5, at day 1: WMD: 1.991, 95% CI: −18.148 to 22.130, $p = 0.846$, $I^2 = 0.0\%$, $P_{heterogeneity} = 0.461$; after day 30: WMD: 4.409, 95% CI: −8.081 to 16.899, $p = 0.479$, $I^2 = 0.0\%$, $P_{heterogeneity} = 0.797$).

3.2.3. Increased Central Corneal Thickness. In two studies, one reporting on 60 eyes and one reporting on 90 eyes, increased CCT was measured and calculated. Three subgroups (day 1, day 7-8, and day 30) were assessed. There were no statistically significant differences in the day 7-8 subgroup or in the day 30 subgroup. And for the subgroup day 1, the forest plot showed that increased CCT was less common in the B-MICS group than in the C-MICS group in the fixed-effects model (Figure 6, day 1: WMD: −24.715, 95% CI: −45.569 to −3.861, $p = 0.020$, $I^2 = 0.0\%$, $P_{heterogeneity} = 0.355$; day 7-8: WMD: −2.495, 95% CI: −10.724 to 5.733, $p = 0.552$, $I^2 = 0.0\%$, $P_{heterogeneity} = 0.779$; day 30: WMD: 3.431, 95% CI: −2.223 to 9.085, $p = 0.903$, $I^2 = 0.0\%$, $P_{heterogeneity} = 0.903$).

3.3. Sensitivity Analysis and Publication Bias.
After excluding one study at a time, the results of different outcomes all fell in the 95% CI of all articles, except for the postoperative BCVA at day 30 (estimate −0.477, 95% CI: −0.2067 to 0.0138).

No publication biases were found for any of the results of the intraoperative and postoperative outcomes.

4. Discussion

For the pooled results of the B-MICS and C-MICS in this meta-analysis, no statistically significant differences were found in mean surgery time, UST, BSS use, postoperative BCVA (within 7 days and at day 30), postoperative CCT (at day 1 and after day 30), and postoperative increased CCT (at day 7-8 and day 30). Figure 2 demonstrates that less EPT was needed in the B-MICS group. Less increased CCT at postoperative day 1 was found in the B-MICS group, as shown in Figure 6.

The shorter EPT in B-MICS may be due to the "cold" phacoemulsification mode used in B-MICS, or it may be

TABLE 1: Characteristics of 9 studies included in the meta-analysis.

Source (publication year, country)	Number of eyes B-MICS/C-MICS	Age (year) B-MICS/C-MICS	Gender (M/F) B-MICS/C-MICS	First incision size B-MICS/C-MICS	Final incision size B-MICS/C-MICS	Follow-up (day)	Jadad score
Cavallini et al. (2007, Italy)	50/50	NA	Total: 15/35	1.4/2.2	$2.24 \pm 0.04/2.29 \pm 0.08$	90	$1+1-0+0+0-1+1$
Wilczynski et al. (2009, Poland)	50/58	$67.8 \pm 9.5/73.8 \pm 8.4$	(35/15)/(33/25)	1.7/1.8	NA	30	
Wilczynski et al. (2009, Poland)	50/51	$67 \pm 10/73 \pm 8$	(9/41)/(19/32)	1.7/1.8	NA	30	
Elkady et al. (2009, Spain)	25/15	$1.73 \pm 0.08/2.24$	(5/11)/(9/9)	1.4/2.2	$1.73 \pm 0.08/2.24$	30	$1+1-0+0+0-1+1$
Can et al. (2010, Turkey)	45/45	$61.5 \pm 8.1/65.8 \pm 13.2$	(17/14)/(14/18)	NA	$1.89 \pm 0.21/2.26 \pm 0.07$	90	$1+0-1+0+0-0+1$
Can et al. (2011, Turkey)	30/30	$63.6 \pm 15.5/69.1 \pm 9.1$	(13/12)/(13/13)	1.2–1.4/1.6–1.8	NA	30	$1+1-0+0+0-1+1$
Can et al. (2012, Turkey)	40/40	$65.29 \pm 8.24/63.59 \pm 11.77$	(16/12)/(17/15)	1.2–1.4/1.6–1.8	NA	30	$1+1-0+0+0-1+1$
Wang et al. (2012, China)	41/41	Total: 67 ± 10	NA	1.3/2.2	NA	30	$1+0-1+0+0-0+1$
Alió et al. (2014, Egypt)	25/25	$67.60 \pm 8.46/70.50 \pm 8.88$	NA	1.0/2.2	NA	30	$1+1-0+0+0-1+1$

Study ID	WMD (95% CI)	Weight%
EPT (S)		
Alio (2014)	-3.00 (-4.19, -1.81)	16.24
Can (2012)	-1.14 (-2.34, 0.06)	15.92
Can (2011)	-1.48 (-3.88, 0.92)	4.00
Can (2010)	-0.69 (-1.47, 0.09)	38.11
Wilczynski (2009)	-0.68 (-2.54, 1.18)	6.65
Wilczynski (2009)	-0.37 (-1.99, 1.25)	8.76
Cavallini (2007)	-1.08 (-2.57, 0.41)	10.32
Overall ($I^2 = 49.3\%$, $p = 0.066$)	-1.18 (-1.66, -0.70)	100.00
Surgery time (min)		
Can (2012)	1.30 (-0.11, 2.71)	25.60
Can (2011)	0.09 (-1.35, 1.53)	25.52
Can 2010)	5.78 (3.58, 7.98)	23.08
Cavallini (2007)	-1.65 (-2.99, -0.31)	25.80
Overall ($I^2 = 91.1\%$, $p = 0.001$)	0.55 (-0.20, 1.31)	100.00

-7.98　　　0　　　7.98

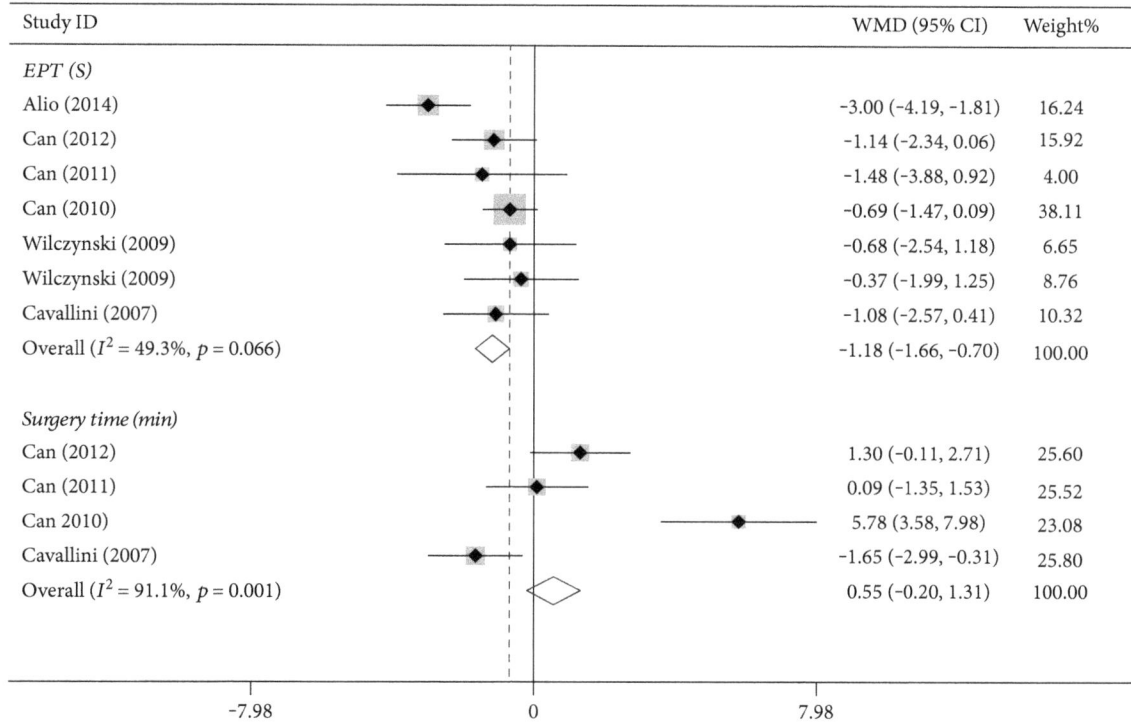

FIGURE 2: Effective phacoemulsification time and surgery time between bimanual microincision cataract surgery and coaxial microincision cataract surgery.

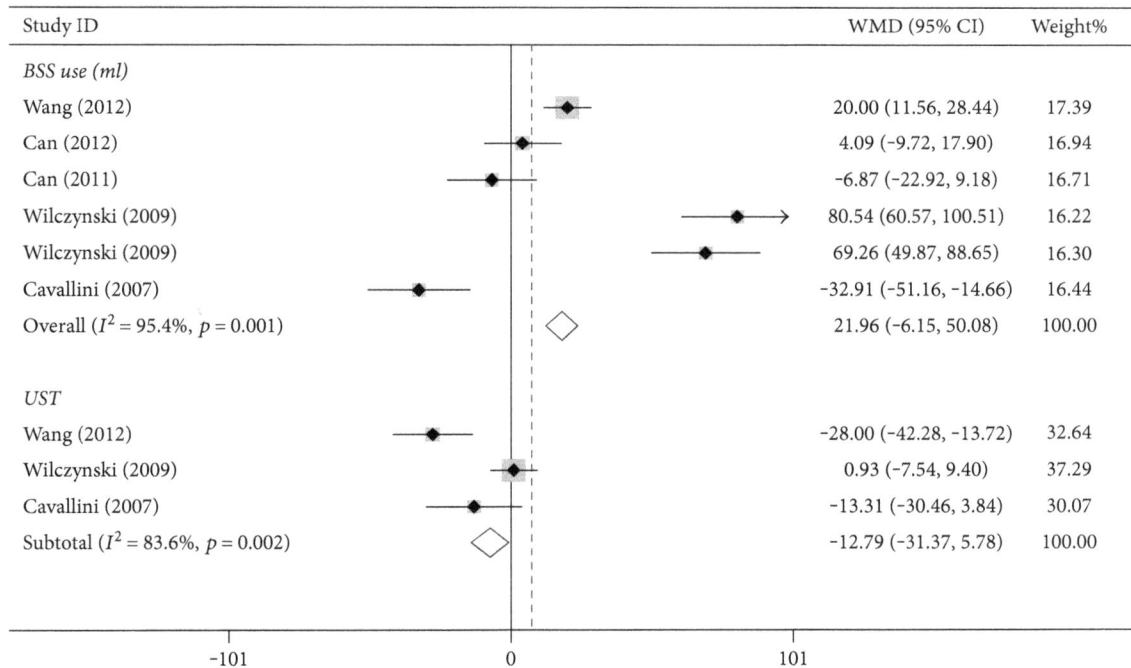

Study ID	WMD (95% CI)	Weight%
BSS use (ml)		
Wang (2012)	20.00 (11.56, 28.44)	17.39
Can (2012)	4.09 (-9.72, 17.90)	16.94
Can (2011)	-6.87 (-22.92, 9.18)	16.71
Wilczynski (2009)	80.54 (60.57, 100.51)	16.22
Wilczynski (2009)	69.26 (49.87, 88.65)	16.30
Cavallini (2007)	-32.91 (-51.16, -14.66)	16.44
Overall ($I^2 = 95.4\%$, $p = 0.001$)	21.96 (-6.15, 50.08)	100.00
UST		
Wang (2012)	-28.00 (-42.28, -13.72)	32.64
Wilczynski (2009)	0.93 (-7.54, 9.40)	37.29
Cavallini (2007)	-13.31 (-30.46, 3.84)	30.07
Subtotal ($I^2 = 83.6\%$, $p = 0.002$)	-12.79 (-31.37, 5.78)	100.00

-101　　　0　　　101

FIGURE 3: Balanced saline use and ultrasound time between bimanual microincision cataract surgery and coaxial microincision cataract surgery.

due to the separation of the irrigation port from the aspiration port in B-MICS, which can avoid a competing current from the phacoemulsification tip and assist in the emulsification and aspiration process. Moreover, the separation and exchangeable hand pieces can provide surgeons with more flexibility to clean the subincisional cortex and residual viscoelastic material [4, 5, 19, 22]. The decrease in EPT caused less damage to the cornea, which was reflected by lower levels of

Study ID		WMD (95% CI)	Weight
BCVA within 7 days			
Wang (2012)		0.01 (-0.04, 0.06)	54.59
Elkady (2009)		-0.06 (-0.20, 0.08)	7.56
Cavallini (2007)		-0.02 (-0.08, 0.04)	37.86
Overall ($I^2 = 0.0\%$, $p = 0.570$)		-0.01 (-0.05, 0.03)	100.00
BCVA day 30			
Can (2012)		-0.04 (-0.11, 0.03)	5.80
Elkady (2009)		-0.08 (-0.23, 0.07)	1.39
Cavallini (2007)		0.00 (-0.02, 0.02)	92.81
Overall ($I^2 = 8.9\%$, $p = 0.334$)		-0.00 (-0.02, 0.01)	100.00

-0.226　　　　　0　　　　　0.226

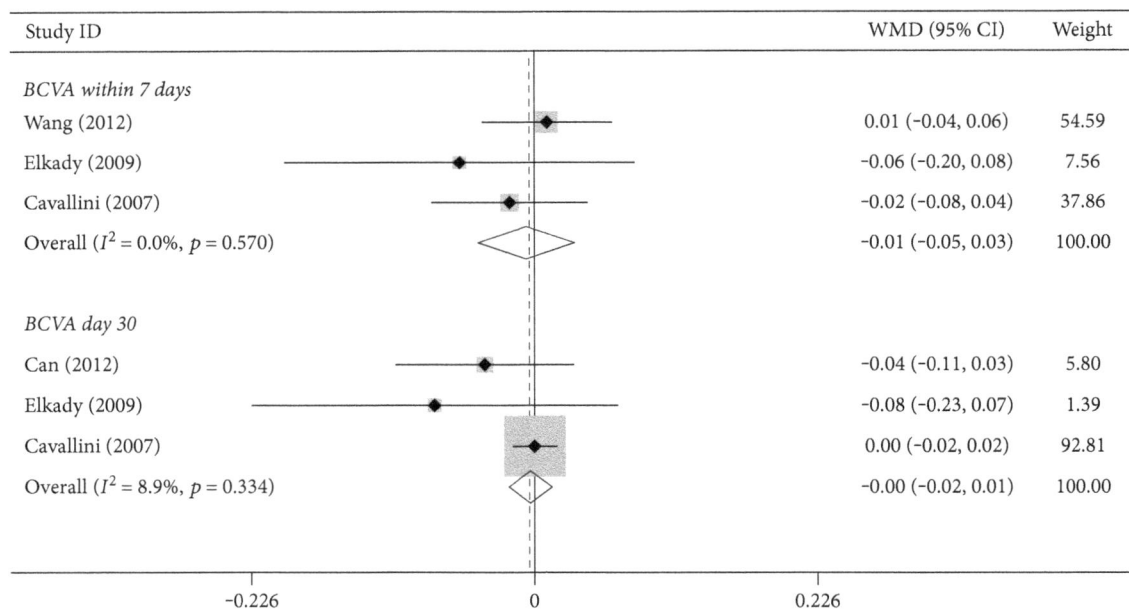

FIGURE 4: Best-corrected visual acuity between bimanual microincision cataract surgery and coaxial microincision cataract surgery.

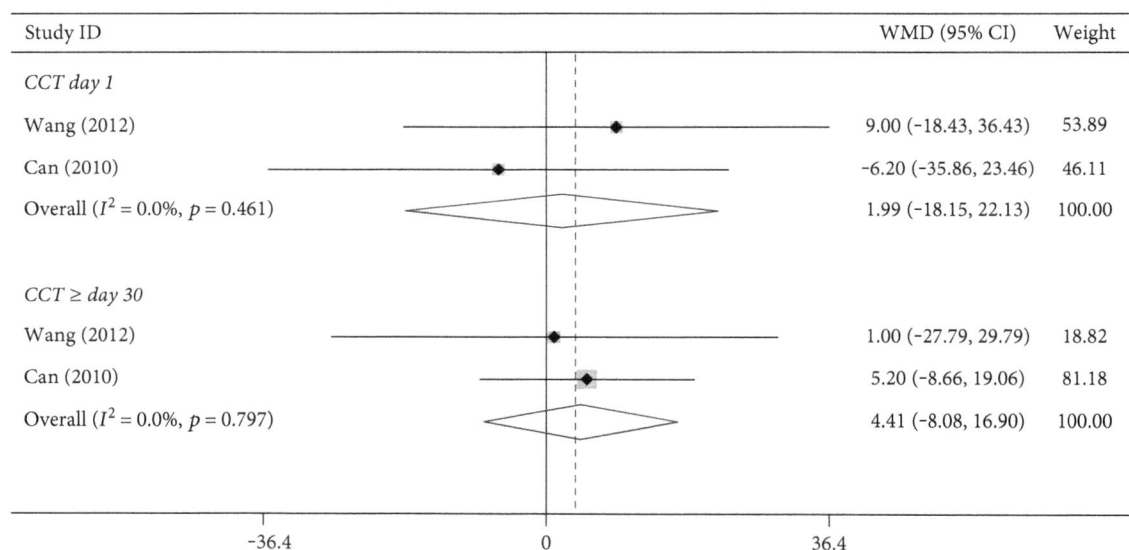

Study ID		WMD (95% CI)	Weight
CCT day 1			
Wang (2012)		9.00 (-18.43, 36.43)	53.89
Can (2010)		-6.20 (-35.86, 23.46)	46.11
Overall ($I^2 = 0.0\%$, $p = 0.461$)		1.99 (-18.15, 22.13)	100.00
CCT ≥ day 30			
Wang (2012)		1.00 (-27.79, 29.79)	18.82
Can (2010)		5.20 (-8.66, 19.06)	81.18
Overall ($I^2 = 0.0\%$, $p = 0.797$)		4.41 (-8.08, 16.90)	100.00

-36.4　　　　　0　　　　　36.4

FIGURE 5: Increased central corneal thickness between bimanual microincision cataract surgery and coaxial microincision cataract surgery.

postoperative increased CCT. The shorter EPT and the lower levels of postoperative increased CCT in the B-MICS group may accelerate the healing of the corneal wound and reduce the endothelial cell loss percentage (ECL %).

The intraoperative and postoperative complications were not analysed because the incidence of intraoperative complications was quite low, and long-term postoperative complications such as posterior capsule opacification (PCO) were rarely found during follow-up in the included studies. PCO develops several months to a few years after uneventful cataract surgeries, but the longest follow-up time in the included studies was three months. Among all cases reported in the studies, three cases in the B-MICS group (6.6%) and one

(2.2%) in the C-MICS group from the Can et al. study suffered from intraoperative complications [16]. In all four cases, IOL were implanted successfully during the surgery, and related postoperative complications were not reported. Can et al. also reported postoperative complications in three cases (anterior chamber inflammation in 2 eyes, posterior capsule opacification in 1 eye). No intraoperative or postoperative complications were reported in the other studies. It seems that there were more complications in the B-MICS group. However, in some studies [23–25], less posterior wound retraction, less intraoperative and postoperative inflammation, and lower risk of endophthalmitis were observed, which implied a faster and better recovery of the

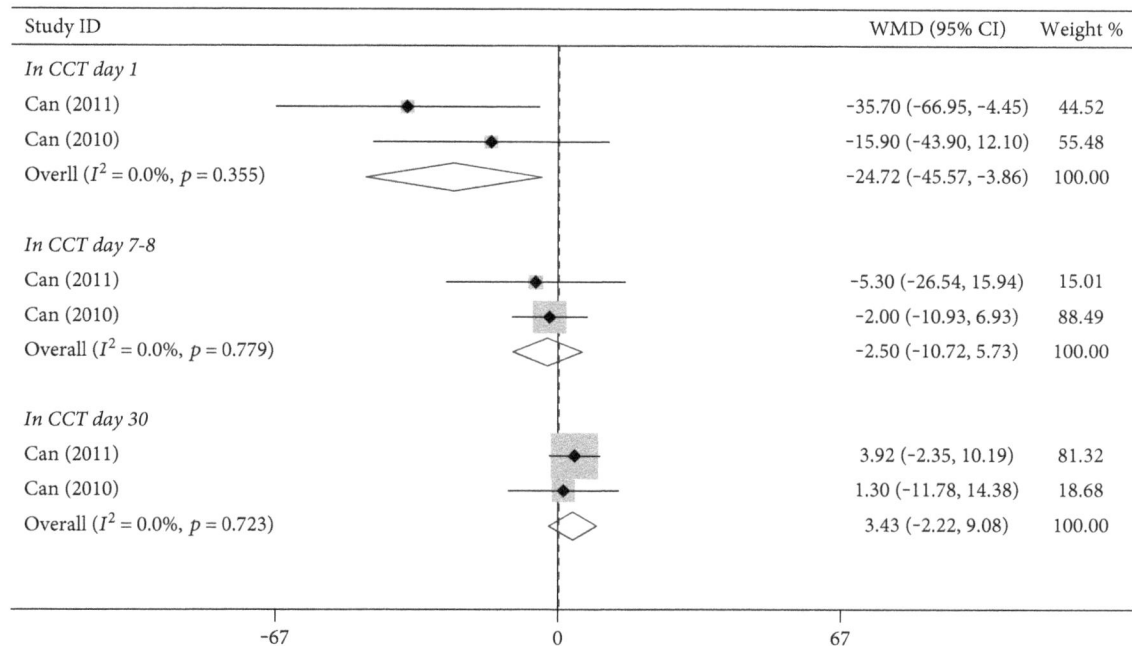

Study ID		WMD (95% CI)	Weight %
In CCT day 1			
Can (2011)		-35.70 (-66.95, -4.45)	44.52
Can (2010)		-15.90 (-43.90, 12.10)	55.48
Overll ($I^2 = 0.0\%$, $p = 0.355$)		-24.72 (-45.57, -3.86)	100.00
In CCT day 7-8			
Can (2011)		-5.30 (-26.54, 15.94)	15.01
Can (2010)		-2.00 (-10.93, 6.93)	88.49
Overall ($I^2 = 0.0\%$, $p = 0.779$)		-2.50 (-10.72, 5.73)	100.00
In CCT day 30			
Can (2011)		3.92 (-2.35, 10.19)	81.32
Can (2010)		1.30 (-11.78, 14.38)	18.68
Overall ($I^2 = 0.0\%$, $p = 0.723$)		3.43 (-2.22, 9.08)	100.00

FIGURE 6: Central corneal thickness between bimanual microincision cataract surgery and coaxial microincision cataract surgery.

corneal wound. Based on the sample size and number of studies included, studies with large sample sizes and with longer follow-up times are necessary for the comparison of the two surgery techniques.

Four papers included in this meta-analysis reported SIA [14, 16, 18], which could not be analysed statistically because the SIA measurement time points were different and the studies adopted two different methods for IOL implant. Lower levels of SIA were found in the B-MICS group in the Cavallini et al. study [14] (at postoperative day 7 and 1 month), the Can et al. study [16] (at postoperative 3 months), and the Can et al. study [18] (at postoperative 1 month), whereas higher levels of SIA were reported in the Cavallini et al. study [14] (at postoperative day 1 and 3 months) and the Wilczynski et al. study [21] (at postoperative day 1). However, no difference was observed in postoperative clinical visual quality. In some earlier studies [15, 26], there were no statistically significant differences found in corneal power and postoperative astigmatism changes between the B-MICS and C-MICS group; the authors also claimed that both techniques were able to provide an astigmatically neutral incision. The IOL implant procedure of B-MICS in the included studies all required the step of expansion of the initial incision or making a third incision. Because the smaller corneal wound is known to be associated with lower levels of SIA [27, 28], the use of the new IOL injectable directly through a 1.4 mm incision, which allows surgeons to skip the extra damage step to the cornea, may cause less SIA than C-MICS with a 1.8 mm corneal incision.

Because the incision sizes of B-MICS and C-MICS are both micro, SIA or BCVA may not be precise enough to detect differences between the two procedures. In three studies [15, 17, 18], corneal optical coherence tomography

and corneal topography were used to measure parameters such as the detachment rate of the Descemet's membrane, endothelial gaps, epithelial gaps, and surgery-induced corneal coma to compare the two microincision techniques. Lower levels of surgery-induced corneal coma were reported in the B-MICS group in one study [17], which was consistent with the results of the Eliwa and Hamza study [29].

Although the incision of cornea is 2.0 mm or less in the original definition of MICS [30, 31], a few papers extended the range to 2.2 mm due to difference in machine settings and the following phacoemulsification and implantation procedures enlarging the incision a little bit. So, we adopted less than 2.2 mm as the range of MICS in this paper. Among all results, high heterogeneity was detected in mean surgery time, UST, and BSS use. The high levels of heterogeneity may be due to the number of papers reporting data on individual outcomes, characteristics of patients, and locations of different studies. Our study was limited by the number of studies available and the data recorded in each study. Only a few studies included analysis of the outcomes of mean surgery time, EPT, UST, CCT, and increased CCT. Further studies are needed to confirm the conclusions of our meta-analysis. We were not able to conduct statistical analyses for some postoperative outcomes, such as SIA, average ultrasound power (AVE), and ECL%. Further studies comparing the two techniques are necessary.

There are some advantages to our study. All nine studies included in this meta-analysis were prospective, and seven of the studies were randomized trials. The operations in the B-MICS and C-MICS groups were performed by the same experienced surgeon in the majority of the included studies [3, 14–18], which avoided the bias of the proficiency level of different surgeons. For the data on postoperative outcomes such as BCVA, CCT, and increased CCT, subgroup analyses were performed on the basis of time slot of follow-up, which avoided the bias of different follow-up times.

The learning curve is also considered to be a drawback of the pervasiveness of B-MICS. Some related studies have been conducted. In one long-term follow-up study comparing the clinical results, such as PCO incidence and clear corneal incision (CCI) architecture of B-MICS, between surgeons in training and experienced surgeons [32], the PCO incidence was higher and corneal incisions were shorter and less angled for less experienced surgeons. The higher PCO incidence may be due to insufficient cleaning of the posterior capsule; the different CCI architectures may be induced by the difficulty in using the nondominant hand. However, in the long-term follow-up, there were no statistically significant differences in BCVA, SIA, and corneal pachymetry changes between surgeons in training and experienced surgeons. This study indicated that there was a process of experience accumulation for inexperienced surgeons. However, there was no such difference in skill acquisition between the two techniques. One recent study reported no significant difference in visual outcomes and complication rates between B-MICS performed by surgeons in training and C-MICS performed by surgeons in training that reported before [33]. Therefore, the results of both studies suggest that B-MICS can be considered as a safe and effective surgery performed by surgeons in training.

In this meta-analysis, there was a shorter EPT and lower levels of increased CCT at postoperative day 1 in the B-MICS group, but other main clinical outcomes of B-MICS and C-MICS were not significantly different. Thus, both cataract surgery techniques are efficient, safe, and appropriate for cataract surgery.

Conflicts of Interest

The authors declare that there is no conflict of interest regarding the publication of this paper.

References

[1] R. H. Osher and V. P. Injev, "Microcoaxial phacoemulsification part 1: laboratory studies," *Journal of Cataract and Refractive Surgery*, vol. 33, pp. 401–407, 2007.

[2] J. L. Alio, J. L. Rodriguez-Prats, A. Vianello, and A. Galal, "Visual outcome of microincision cataract surgery with implantation of an Acri. Smart lens," *Journal of Cataract and Refractive Surgery*, vol. 31, pp. 1549–1556, 2005.

[3] Y. Wang, Y. Xia, X. Liu, D. Zheng, L. Luo, and Y. Liu, "Comparison of bimanual and micro-coaxial phacoemulsification with torsional ultrasound," *Acta Ophthalmologica*, vol. 90, pp. 184–187, 2012.

[4] T. Paul and R. Braga-Mele, "Bimanual microincisional phacoemulsification: the future of cataract surgery?," *Current Opinion in Ophthalmology*, vol. 16, pp. 2–7, 2005.

[5] M. P. Weikert, "Update on bimanual microincisional cataract surgery," *Current Opinion in Ophthalmology*, vol. 17, pp. 62–67, 2006.

[6] C. von Sonnleithner, R. Bergholz, J. Gonnermann, M. K. Klamann, N. Torun, and E. Bertelmann, "Clinical results and higher-order aberrations after 1.4-mm biaxial cataract surgery and implantation of a new aspheric intraocular lens," *Ophthalmic Research*, vol. 53, pp. 8–14, 2015.

[7] C. Chen, M. Zhu, Y. Sun, X. Qu, and X. Xu, "Bimanual microincision versus standard coaxial small-incision cataract surgery: meta-analysis of randomized controlled trials," *European Journal of Ophthalmology*, vol. 25, pp. 119–127, 2015.

[8] X. Shentu, X. Zhang, X. Tang, and X. Yu, "Coaxial microincision cataract surgery versus standard coaxial small-incision cataract surgery: a meta-analysis of randomized controlled trials," *PLoS One*, vol. 11, article e0146676, 2016.

[9] D. Moher, A. Liberati, J. Tetzlaff, D. G. Altman, and PRISMA Group, "Preferred reporting items for systematic reviews and meta-analyses: the PRISMA statement," *International Journal of Surgery*, vol. 8, pp. 336–341, 2010.

[10] J. P. Higgins, S. G. Thompson, J. J. Deeks, and D. G. Altman, "Measuring inconsistency in meta-analyses," *British Medical Journal*, vol. 327, pp. 557–590, 2003.

[11] R. Der Simonian and R. Kacker, "Random-effects model for meta-analysis of clinical trials: an update," *Contemporary Clinical Trials*, vol. 28, pp. 105–114, 2007.

[12] M. Egger, G. Davey Smith, M. Schneider, and C. Minder, "Bias in meta-analysis detected by a simple, graphical test," *British Medical Journal*, vol. 315, pp. 629–634, 1997.

[13] C. B. Begg and M. Mazumdar, "Operating characteristics of a rank correlation test for publication bias," *Biometrics*, vol. 50, pp. 1088–1101, 1994.

[14] G. M. Cavallini, L. Campi, C. Masini, S. Pelloni, and A. Pupino, "Bimanual microphacoemulsification versus coaxial miniphacoemulsification: prospective study," *Journal of Cataract and Refractive Surgery*, vol. 33, pp. 387–392, 2007.

[15] B. Elkady, D. Pinero, and J. L. Alio, "Corneal incision quality: microincision cataract surgery versus microcoaxial phacoemulsification," *Journal of Cataract and Refractive Surgery*, vol. 35, pp. 466–474, 2009.

[16] I. Can, T. Takmaz, Y. Yildiz, H. A. Bayhan, G. Soyugelen, and B. Bostanci, "Coaxial, microcoaxial, and biaxial microincision cataract surgery: prospective comparative study," *Journal of Cataract and Refractive Surgery*, vol. 36, pp. 740–746, 2010.

[17] I. Can, H. A. Bayhan, H. Celik, and B. Bostanci Ceran, "Anterior segment optical coherence tomography evaluation and comparison of main clear corneal incisions in microcoaxial and biaxial cataract surgery," *Journal of Cataract and Refractive Surgery*, vol. 37, pp. 490–500, 2011.

[18] I. Can, H. A. Bayhan, H. Celik, and B. B. Ceran, "Comparison of corneal aberrations after biaxial microincision and microcoaxial cataract surgeries: a prospective study," *Current Eye Research*, vol. 37, pp. 18–24, 2012.

[19] J. L. Alió, F. Soria, A. A. Abdou, P. Peña-García, R. Fernández-Buenaga, and J. Javaloy, "Comparative outcomes of bimanual MICS and 2.2-mm coaxial phacoemulsification assisted by femtosecond technology," *Journal of Refractive Surgery*, vol. 30, pp. 34–40, 2014.

[20] M. Wilczynski, E. Supady, P. Loba, A. Synder, D. Palenga-Pydyn, and W. Omulecki, "Comparison of early corneal endothelial cell loss after coaxial phacoemulsification through 1.8 mm microincision and bimanual phacoemulsification through 1.7 mm microincision," *Journal of Cataract and Refractive Surgery*, vol. 35, pp. 1570–1574, 2009.

[21] M. Wilczynski, E. Supady, L. Piotr, A. Synder, D. Palenga-Pydyn, and W. Omulecki, "Comparison of surgically induced astigmatism after coaxial phacoemulsification through 1.8 mm microincision and bimanual phacoemulsification through 1.7 mm microincision," *Journal of Cataract and Refractive Surgery*, vol. 35, pp. 1563–1569, 2009.

[22] I. H. Fine, R. S. Hoffman, and M. Packer, "Optimizing refractive lens exchange with bimanual microincision phacoemulsification," *Journal of Cataract and Refractive Surgery*, vol. 30, pp. 550–554, 2004.

[23] G. M. C. L. Cavallini, G. Torlai, M. Forlini, and E. Fornasari, "Clear corneal incisions in bimanual microincision cataract surgery: long-term wound-healing architecture," *Journal of Cataract and Refractive Surgery*, vol. 38, pp. 1743–1748, 2012.

[24] A. Behrens, W. J. Stark, K. A. Pratzer, and P. J. McDonnell, "Dynamics of small-incision clear cornea wounds after phacoemulsification surgery using optical coherence tomography in the early postoperative period," *Journal of Refractive Surgery*, vol. 24, pp. 46–49, 2008.

[25] S.-P. Chee and K. Bacsal, "Endophthalmitis after microincision cataract surgery," *Journal of Cataract and Refractive Surgery*, vol. 31, pp. 1834-1835, 2005.

[26] J. L. Alio, B. Elkady, and D. Ortiz, "Corneal optical quality following sub 1.8 mm micro-incision cataract surgery vs. 2.2 mm mini-incision coaxial phacoemulsification," *Middle East African Journal of Ophthalmology*, vol. 17, pp. 94–99, 2010.

[27] Y. Jiang, Q. Le, J. Yang, and Y. Lu, "Changes in corneal astigmatism and high order aberrations after clear corneal tunnel phacoemulsification guided by corneal topography," *Journal of Refractive Surgery*, vol. 22, pp. S1083–S1088, 2006.

[28] K. Yao, X. Tang, and P. Ye, "Corneal astigmatism, high order aberrations, and optical quality after cataract surgery: microincision versus small incision," *Journal of Refractive Surgery*, vol. 22, pp. S1079–S1082, 2006.

[29] T. F. E. M. Eliwa and I. Hamza, "Effect of biaxial versus coaxial microincision cataract surgery on optical quality of the cornea," *Indian Journal of Ophthalmology*, vol. 63, pp. 487–490, 2015.

[30] J. L. R. P. J. Alio and A. Galal, Eds., *MICS: MicroIncision Cataract Surgery*, Highlights of Ophthalmology International, El Dorado, Panama, 2004.

[31] J. L. F. H. Alio, Ed., *Minimizing Incisions and Maximizing Outcomes in Cataract Surgery*, Springer-Verlag, Berlin, Germany, 2010.

[32] G. M. Cavallini, T. Verdina, M. Forlini et al., "Long-term follow-up for bimanual microincision cataract surgery: comparison of results obtained by surgeons in training and experienced surgeons," *Clinical Ophthalmology*, vol. 10, pp. 979–987, 2016.

[33] G. M. Cavallini, V. Volante, T. Verdina et al., "Results and complications of surgeons-in-training learning bimanual microincision cataract surgery," *Journal of Cataract and Refractive Surgery*, vol. 41, pp. 105–115, 2015.

17

Impact of B-Scan Averaging on Spectralis Optical Coherence Tomography Image Quality before and after Cataract Surgery

Dominika Podkowinski, Ehsan Sharian Varnousfaderani, Christian Simader, Hrvoje Bogunovic, Ana-Maria Philip, Bianca S. Gerendas, Ursula Schmidt-Erfurth, and Sebastian M. Waldstein

Christian Doppler Laboratory for Ophthalmic Image Analysis, Vienna Reading Center, Department of Ophthalmology, Medical University of Vienna, Spitalgasse 23, 1090 Vienna, Austria

Correspondence should be addressed to Sebastian M. Waldstein; sebastian.waldstein@meduniwien.ac.at

Academic Editor: Patrik Schatz

Background and Objective. To determine optimal image averaging settings for Spectralis optical coherence tomography (OCT) in patients with and without cataract. *Study Design/Material and Methods.* In a prospective study, the eyes were imaged before and after cataract surgery using seven different image averaging settings. Image quality was quantitatively evaluated using signal-to-noise ratio, distinction between retinal layer image intensity distributions, and retinal layer segmentation performance. Measures were compared pre- and postoperatively across different degrees of averaging. *Results.* 13 eyes of 13 patients were included and 1092 layer boundaries analyzed. Preoperatively, increasing image averaging led to a logarithmic growth in all image quality measures up to 96 frames. Postoperatively, increasing averaging beyond 16 images resulted in a plateau without further benefits to image quality. Averaging 16 frames postoperatively provided comparable image quality to 96 frames preoperatively. *Conclusion.* In patients with clear media, averaging 16 images provided optimal signal quality. A further increase in averaging was only beneficial in the eyes with senile cataract. However, prolonged acquisition time and possible loss of details have to be taken into account.

1. Introduction

Spectral-domain optical coherence tomography (SD-OCT) is the most important imaging modality for diagnosis and management of retinal diseases [1]. Recent technical advances have significantly improved the image resolution, contrast, scanning speed and angle, depth penetration, and automated analysis techniques in OCT imaging [2]. In order to allow precise identification of fine clinical details and robust automated segmentation, improvements in image quality are a main focus of research in OCT technology.

One important reason for low image quality in OCT is speckle noise, that is, random granular noise [3]. Based on the assumption that noise must be randomly distributed in an image, averaging of several images of the same object can be applied to enhance image quality [4]. Some current OCT devices include an image averaging function in their software and are able to provide averaged images based on the scanning protocol selection. If combined with the built-in eye tracking technology, images of the same retinal location can be acquired several times and image averaging of identical retinal regions is feasible. This concept, termed "automated real time averaging" (ART), is widely used in clinical practice and research studies. However, there are no solid data or guidelines available regarding the impact of averaging extent on image quality. Inadequately selected averaging settings may result in unnecessarily poor image quality, patient overexposure, or inefficient use of resources.

To allow a comprehensive evaluation of image quality characteristics, standardized parameters measuring the various aspects of image quality are required. Frequently used parameters for quantitative analysis are the signal-to-noise ratio (SNR) and, as a surrogate variable, the reproducibility of retinal thickness measurements. Moreover, some studies rely on subjective grading for the assessment of image quality [5,6]. However, using subjective scores can be variable even for trained experts.

Most retinal diseases occur with exceeding frequency in elderly patients, a patient group where media opacities, in particular cataract, are common [7]. Previous studies have demonstrated that cataract can affect the OCT image quality as well as the reproducibility of retinal thickness measurements [5,8-10]. However, these studies did not consider the role of image averaging.

The purpose of our study was to establish optimal image averaging settings in retinal OCT acquisition based on objective parameters for the assessment of image quality. Furthermore, we evaluated the optimal settings for image averaging in patients with and without cataract.

2. Patients/Materials and Methods

This study was a prospective, observational, noninterventional case series. The study protocol was prospectively approved by the Ethics Committee of the Medical University of Vienna. All study procedures complied with the tenets set forth in the Declaration of Helsinki. Prior to inclusion, all patients provided written informed consent to participate.

Patients with the diagnosis of senile cataract and planned cataract surgery at the Medical University of Vienna, Austria, were included into the study between March and October 2013. Exclusion criteria were retinal pathologies, which could influence central fixation, and optical media abnormalities apart from cataract that could influence imaging quality. Only one eye per patient was included.

2.1. Examination and Imaging Procedure. A complete ophthalmic examination, including slit lamp examination and fundus biomicroscopy, was performed in all patients one week before and one week after uncomplicated cataract surgery. All surgeries were performed by a single, experienced surgeon (CS) using clear corneal or scleral corneal incisions, phacoemulsification, and implantation of an acrylic intraocular lens into the capsular bag. Preoperatively, cataracts were classified according to the Lens Opacities Classification System III (LOCS III) as nuclear (N), cortical (C), or posterior (P) [11]. If the LOCS III score was >N3, <C3, and <P3, the cataract was categorized as nuclear; if C was equal to or higher than 3, it was categorized as cortical; and if P was equal to or higher than 3, the categorization was posterior [5].

After pupil dilatation, OCT scans were acquired at each visit following a standardized acquisition protocol by a single investigator (DP). The Spectralis™ HRA+OCT (Heidelberg Engineering, Dossenheim, Germany) was used to scan repeated patterns of 512 A-scans in a single horizontal line of 6 mm length corresponding to an angle of 20°. For each repetition, the automated real-time averaging (ART) feature was employed with systematically varying the number of averaged B-scans as follows: The degree of averaging was selected according to a logarithmically escalating scale with seven steps using 2, 4, 8, 16, 32, 48,

and 96 frames. Thus, seven scans were acquired at each visit for each patient. The order of scans was randomized to counteract potential systematic bias. The first scan acquired was set as a reference, and the built-in device follow-up function was used to align all following scans (before and after surgery) to the identical retinal position. All scans were exported as TIFF files for further processing as shown in Figure 1.

To be able to assess the contrast and distinction between the individual retinal layers, the following layer boundaries were manually annotated by a single investigator (DP) in Adobe Photoshop version CS6 (Figure 2): boundaries between vitreous and nerve fiber layer (NFL), border between nerve fiber layer and ganglion cell layer (GCL), border between inner plexiform layer and inner nuclear layer (INL), border between inner nuclear layer and outer plexiform layer (OPL), border between outer plexiform layer and outer nuclear layer (ONL), and border between outer nuclear layer and external limiting membrane (ELM). Reproducibility data on the annotation procedure has been reported previously [12].

2.2. Image Quality Quantification. Three different measures were employed for quantitative image quality analysis: [1] signal-to-noise ratio (SNR), [2] Cohen's *d* value, and [3] automated layer segmentation performance. All computations were performed with the MATLAB software (version R2013a, The MathWorks Inc., Natick, Massachusetts, USA). The measures are defined as follows.

2.2.1. Signal-to-Noise Ratio (SNR). The SNR compares the level of a desired signal in the image to the level of noise. It is computed individually for each manually annotated intraretinal layer as

$$\text{SNR} = \frac{\mu_l}{\sigma_l}, \tag{1}$$

where μ_l and σ_l are the mean and the standard deviation of the grey values within a single layer. Under the assumption of signal and noise being uncorrelated, the SNR is expected to increase with the square root of the number of averaging frames, resulting in a favorable appearance of the image. The SNR of an image was computed by averaging the SNR values of all the layers.

2.2.2. Cohen's d Value. The dissimilarity of individual retinal layers based on their grey values was assessed by measuring the overlap of the image intensity distributions between neighboring manually annotated layers. It is measured using Cohen's *d* value, which is inversely proportional to the overlap of distributions, and it is computed for two neighboring layers L_1 and L_2 as

$$d(L_1, L_2) = \frac{\mu_{l1} - \mu_{l2}}{\sqrt{\left((N_{l1} - 1)\sigma_{l1}^2 + (N_{l2} - 1)\sigma_{l2}^2\right)/(N_{l1} + N_{l2} - 2)}}, \tag{2}$$

where μ_{l1}, σ_{l1}^2, and N_{l1} are the mean, the variance, and the sample size of an intensity distribution that are generated

B-scans	Before surgery	After surgery
2		
4		
8		
16		
32		
48		
96		

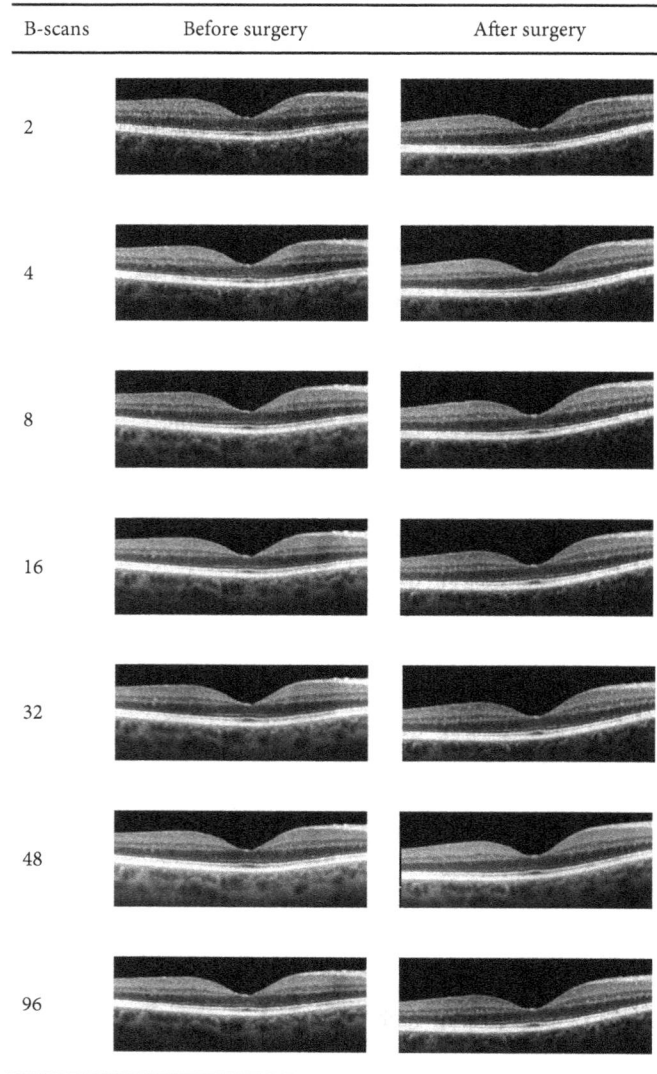

FIGURE 1: Exemplar OCT scans of a study patient acquired with different averaging settings. Left: number of B-scans averaged. Middle: images acquired before cataract surgery with turbid media. Right: images acquired after cataract extraction.

from pixels forming layer L_1 (resp., for L_2). A high value of Cohen's d indicates that the neighboring layer intensity distributions are well separated and thus their distinction is high. For each manually annotated layer, the d value was computed as the average of the two d values with its two neighboring layers above and below. The Cohen's d value of an image was computed by averaging the values of all the layers.

2.2.3. Automated Layer Segmentation Performance.
The ability to differentiate between the individual retinal layers based on their appearance was further assessed by measuring the performance of an automated segmentation method in correctly segmenting each layer. The automated segmentation method is based on pixel classification. Segmentation of a layer was computed by first learning Gaussian mixture model representation of its intensity distribution as well as those of the two neighboring layers. Each intensity distribution was modeled using three Gaussian components. Then, the pixels

were classified to a particular layer by maximum likelihood criteria. Accuracy of automated segmentation method is evaluated with the Dice index, which computes the similarity between two sets of pixels corresponding to automatically segmented layer S_{auto} and the manually denoted one S_{manual} (taken as the ground truth) as

$$\text{Dice}(S_{auto}, S_{manual}) = 2\frac{|S_{auto} \cap S_{manual}|}{|S_{auto}| + |S_{manual}|}. \qquad (3)$$

The Dice index is in the range [0,1] with higher values denoting better segmentations. It was computed separately for each layer. The Dice index of an image was computed as the average of all the layers.

2.3. Statistical Analysis.
Statistical analysis was performed using the SPSS V.22 statistical package (IBM CROP, Armonk, NY, USA). The impact of the varying degrees of averaging on the three different image quality measures was

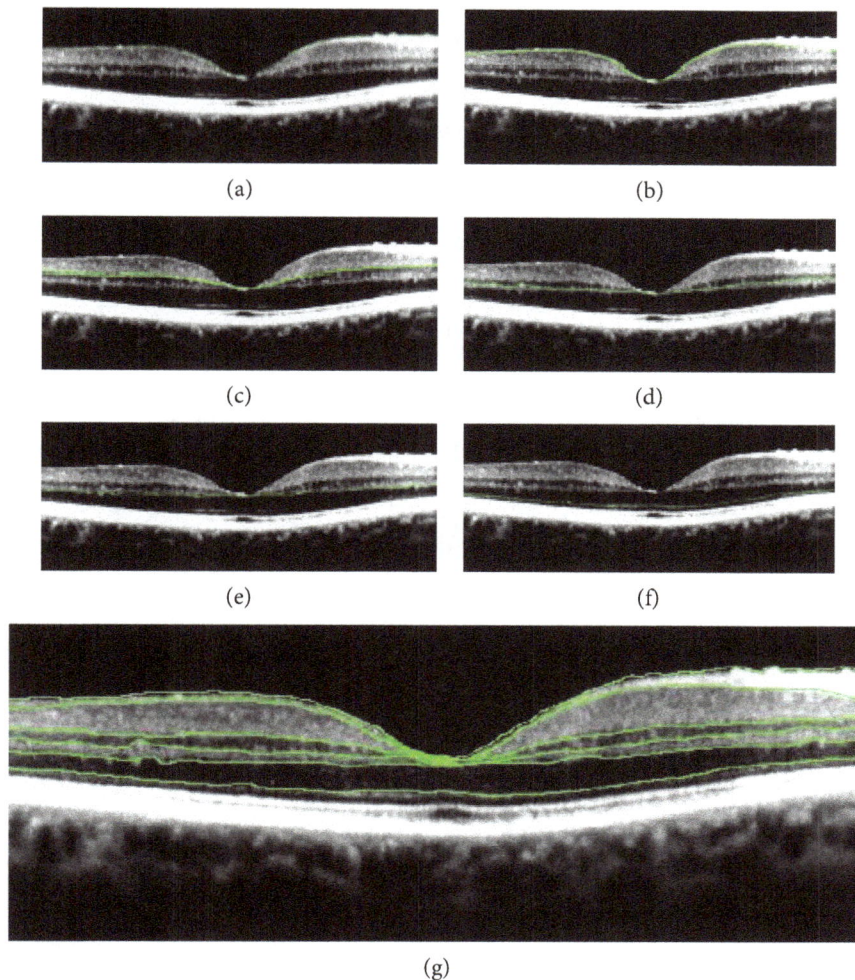

FIGURE 2: Example of manually annotated borders of the individual retinal layers on an optical coherence tomography scan. (a) Border between vitreous and NFL, (b) border between NFL and GCL, (c) border between IPL and INL, (d) border between INL and OPL, (e) border between OPL and ONL, (f) border between ONL and ELM, and (g) all annotated borders. Annotations were performed on each scan with different averaging settings; thus, on 7 scans preoperatively and 7 scans postoperatively for each patient.

assessed by descriptive statistics and performed separately for preoperative and postoperative acquisitions shown in the histograms and graphs using different matrices described in the results section. In addition, we computed for each eye which degree of preoperative averaging reached the quality of the postoperative setting.

3. Results

Thirteen eyes of 13 patients were included. Nine participants were female and five were male. The mean ± standard deviation patient age was 68.3 ± 8.7 years. Eight of the cataracts were classified as nuclear, four as cortical, and one as posterior. The classification is based on the highest score in one of the three categories according to the LOCS III grading. All included cataracts were of mixed type. For each eye, 5 individual layers with 6 boundaries were annotated on each baseline and follow-up scan using 7 different averaging settings. This resulted in a total of 14 B-scans,

70 individual layers, and 84 layer boundaries that were analyzed for each patient. In total, 1092 layer annotations were performed.

3.1. Signal-to-Noise Ratio. Preoperatively, a seemingly linear increase in SNR was seen with escalating averaging settings, with an increase in SNR at each averaging increment.

Postoperatively, an increase was detected until 16 averaged frames. Thereafter, a further increase in averaging did not result in SNR changes, resembling a logarithmic growth pattern with saturation at 16 averaged frames (Figure 3). Preoperatively, all the eyes required equal or more averaged frames to achieve the same levels of SNR as 16 averaged frames postoperatively (Figure 4).

3.2. Cohen's d Value. The differentiation of the individual retinal layers based on the overlap of image intensity distribution as measured by Cohen's *d* value increased logarithmically pre- and postoperatively, with progressive

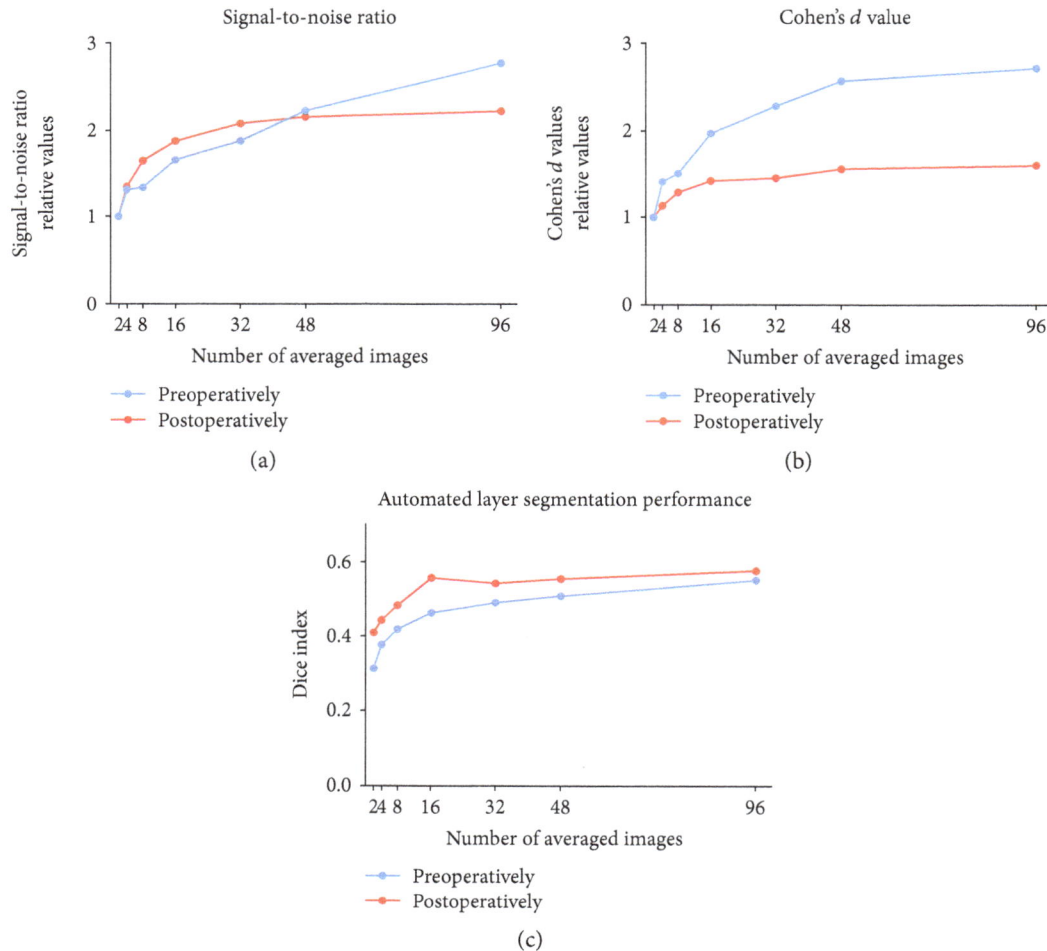

FIGURE 3: Quantitative measures of image quality. The graphs show signal-to-noise ratio (SNR; (a)), the Cohen's *d* value (b), and intraretinal layer segmentation performance (c). SNR and Cohen's *d* are computed relative to the baseline at two averaged frames. The SNR compares the level of a desired signal in the image to the level of noise. Cohen's *d* value describes the dissimilarity of individual retinal layers based on their grey values and is inversely proportional to the overlap of distributions. It is computed for two neighboring layers. The ability to differentiate between the individual retinal layers based on their appearance was further assessed by measuring the performance of an automated computer algorithm on correctly segmenting each layer based on pixel classification. Cohen's *d* value and the automated layer segmentation performance are demonstrated as relative values. Results are shown as mean for each averaging frame increment, separately for pre- and postoperative results overall patients and all layers.

saturation achieved at 48 averaged frames (Figure 3). Pre-operatively, all but one eye required more averaged frames to achieve the same Cohen's *d* value as 16 averaged frames postoperatively, shown in Figure 4.

3.3. Layer Segmentation Performance. The ability to segment the individual retinal layers as measured by the Dice index showed a strongly logarithmic growth pattern both preoperatively and postoperatively (Figure 3). Preoperatively, the Dice index saturated at 48 averaged frames. Postoperatively, the increase in the Dice index was substantial from two to 16 averaged frames, with only minimal improvement with further increasing image averaging. Preoperatively, all but one eye required more averaged frames to achieve the same segmentation performance as 16 averaged frames postoperatively (Figure 4).

4. Discussion

This study provides evidence for the selection of optimal image averaging settings in retinal OCT acquisition based on objective parameters for the assessment of image quality in patients with and without cataract. In the eyes with clear optical media, image averaging using 16 frames resulted in high levels of SNR and good distinction between the individual retinal layers. A further increase in the degree of image averaging did not provide additional benefit in image quality. On the other hand, in the eyes with senile cataract, higher degrees of image averaging allowed a further increase in image quality and may therefore be clinically useful. Our findings may be of relevance for the selection of OCT scanning protocols in clinical research and practice. If the image quality achieved with higher averaging settings

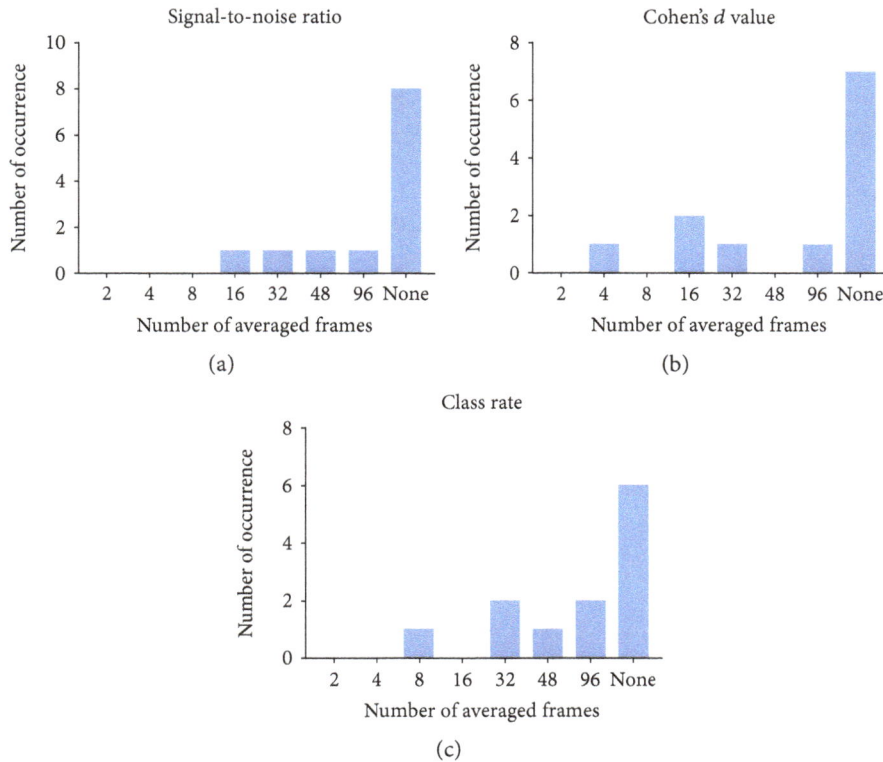

FIGURE 4: Intraindividual evaluation of quantitative measures of image quality for all 13 patients. On the *x*-axis, the number of averaged frames preoperatively is shown, which is needed to achieve the same result as an average of 16 frames postoperatively. A 16-frame scan provides the most beneficial setting after cataract surgery. Comparison is computed individually for each patient. On the *y*-axis, the number of cases is shown. "None" indicates that there was no averaging setting preoperatively, which achieved the same result as postoperatively.

is similar to the image quality at lower averaging settings, it is beneficial to use the settings which are quicker to acquire based on time and compliance; therefore, a lower number of averaging is to favor.

Few studies have addressed the impact of B-scan averaging on image quality in retinal OCT previously. A retrospective study by Pappuru et al. demonstrated significantly improved distinction between the retinal layers using image averaging in healthy eyes [13]. While scan averaging at four frames resulted in a significant improvement of image quality, an increase to 20 frames showed no significant change. Similar results were reported in a study by Sakamoto et al. [14]. These previous findings are corroborated by our study for the eyes with clear optical media; however, in the eyes with cataract, our study demonstrated that further averaging may be of value for image quality. B-scan averaging had no significant influence on RNFL thickness measurements in one study, although another study demonstrated superior reproducibility of RNFL measurements by averaging 100 frames [15,16]. In both studies, only patients with clear media were included.

Several studies investigated the influence of senile cataract on the image quality of retinal OCT. van Velthofen et al. used a subjective grading of the scans prior to surgery as well as the objective parameter signal strength and SNR to determine the image quality changes before

and after cataract surgery [5]. The objective image quality parameters improved postoperatively, similarly to our study. The largest influence on the image quality was demonstrated for nuclear cataract; although due to the small study size, the statistical subgroup analysis was inconclusive. An analysis of the different subtypes of cataracts was not within the scope of our study, also due to limitations in the sample size.

The other available studies focused mainly on the reproducibility of retinal thickness measurements as a surrogate variable for image quality relating to cataract surgery. A study by Bambo et al. demonstrated improved reproducibility of thickness measurements with clear optical media. Preoperatively, reproducibility was superior using Spectralis OCT compared to Cirrus OCT, presumably due to the eye tracking function in Spectralis OCT [17]. Similar results were shown by other published studies, where patients with different diseases, such as diabetes, retinitis pigmentosa, and multiple sclerosis, were included [18-20].

In our study, we employed three different measures for the assessment of image quality in retinal OCT: the SNR and two different measures to assess the ability to distinguish between the individual retinal layers, that is, Cohen's *d* value and layer segmentation Dice index. All three measures are well-established in image analysis. In clinical practice, particularly the ability to discern fine anatomical detail is critically important for the evaluation of imaging biomarkers for disease management [21]. In clear optical media, optimal levels of these two parameters were achieved by averaging 16 image frames. Furthermore, high image averaging settings result in prolonged acquisition times, which may lead to unnecessarily lengthy visits, reduced patient compliance, and compromised image quality. Higher degrees of image averaging may lead to excessive smoothing of the image. Such smoothing of the Spectralis OCT image may be caused by the repeated scanning not capturing the identical anatomical position and may result in unwanted loss of morphologic detail [22].

Based on the data provided by our study, a setting of 16 averaged frames seems to provide a solid balance between the advantages and disadvantages of image averaging in patients with clear optical media. Concerning eyes with optical media opacities with an increase in image averaging may result in a good balance regarding the investigated image quality parameters.

Even more for clinical practice, an evidence-based selection of OCT scanner settings is particularly relevant in large scale multicenter clinical trials. The advent of automated large-scale three-dimensional computerized analysis of OCT data highlights the critical need for standardized scanning protocols. In the future, population-level research may become increasingly relevant with the establishment of large publicly available image data bases consisting of highly standardized data repositories.

This study is mainly limited by its sample size. However, it should be noted that an extensive scanning protocol was used and laborious manual annotations of several individual retinal layers were undertaken. This resulted in 1092 annotations and data points for analysis, allowing solid conclusions. Furthermore, our results show a slight decrease in Cohen's d value at 32 averaged frames postoperatively. This unexpected decrease may be associated with ocular surface changes as a consequence of cataract surgery. This diagnosis is to be expected after surgery [23]. The order of scan acquisition with the different image averaging settings was randomized in our study to avoid confounding effects of dry eye disease. A further potential limitation of this study is the lack of annotations for the photoreceptor and retinal pigment epithelium (RPE) layers. However, we expect OCT signal properties to be stable across the retinal structures at least in healthy cases.

In conclusion, our study suggests that 16 averaged frames may provide optimal image quality in the examination of patients with clear optical media by Spectralis OCT. Excessive image averaging did not deliver corresponding image quality benefits, led to disadvantageous smoothing effects, and should be avoided in clinical practice. However, in patients with media opacities, such as senile cataract, a higher degree of image averaging may result in a further increase in image quality. Our results may be of value in designing standardized OCT scanning protocols in clinical practice and future clinical trials.

Disclosure

This study was presented at the annual meeting of the Association for Research in Vision and Ophthalmology, May 2014, Orlando, FL [24]. The funding organization had no role in the design or conduct of this research.

Conflicts of Interest

The authors declare that there is no conflict of interest regarding the publication of this paper.

Acknowledgments

The authors received funding from Austrian Federal Ministry of Economy, Family and Youth, National Foundation for Research, Technology and Development.

References

[1] W. Geitzenauer, C. K. Hitzenberger, and U. M. Schmidt-Erfurth, "Retinal optical coherence tomography: past, present and future perspectives," The British Journal of Ophthalmology, vol. 95, no. 2, pp. 171–177, 2011.

[2] P. A. Keane and S. R. Sadda, "Retinal imaging in the twenty-first century: state of the art and future directions," Ophthalmology, vol. 121, no. 12, pp. 2489–2500, 2014.

[3] J. M. Schmitt, S. H. Xiang, and K. M. Yung, "Speckle in optical coherence tomography," Journal of Biomedical Optics, vol. 4, no. 1, pp. 95–105, 1999.

[4] B. Sander, M. Larsen, L. Thrane, J. L. Hougaard, and T. M. Jorgensen, "Enhanced optical coherence tomography imaging by multiple scan averaging," The British Journal of Ophthalmology, vol. 89, no. 2, pp. 207–212, 2005.

[5] M. E. van Velthoven, M. H. van der Linden, M. D. de Smet, D. J. Faber, and F. D. Verbraak, "Influence of cataract on optical coherence tomography image quality and retinal thickness," The British Journal of Ophthalmology, vol. 90, no. 10, pp. 1259–1262, 2006.

[6] S. Liu, A. S. Paranjape, B. Elmaanaoui et al., "Quality assessment for spectral domain optical coherence tomography (OCT) images," Proceedings of SPIE, vol. 7171, p. 71710x, 2009.

[7] B. E. Klein, R. Klein, and K. L. Linton, "Prevalence of age-related lens opacities in a population. The beaver dam eye study," Ophthalmology, vol. 99, no. 4, pp. 546–552, 1992.

[8] C. Cagini, T. Fiore, B. Iaccheri, F. Piccinelli, M. A. Ricci, and D. Fruttini, "Macular thickness measured by optical coherence tomography in a healthy population before and after uncomplicated cataract phacoemulsification surgery," Current eye Research, vol. 34, no. 12, pp. 1036–1041, 2009.

[9] P. H. Kok, H. W. van Dijk, T. J. van den Berg, and F. D. Verbraak, "A model for the effect of disturbances in the optical media on the OCT image quality," Investigative Ophthalmology & Visual Science, vol. 50, no. 2, pp. 787–792, 2009.

[10] M. Esmaeelpour, B. Povazay, B. Hermann et al., "Three-dimensional 1060-nm OCT: choroidal thickness maps in normal subjects and improved posterior segment visualization in cataract patients," Investigative Ophthalmology & Visual Science, vol. 51, no. 10, pp. 5260–5266, 2010.

[11] L. T. Chylack Jr., J. K. Wolfe, D. M. Singer et al., "The lens opacities classification system III. The longitudinal study of

cataract study group," *Archives of Ophthalmology*, vol. 111, no. 6, pp. 831–836, 1993.

[12] E. S. Varnousfaderani, J. Wu, W.-D. Vogl et al., "A novel benchmark model for intelligent annotation of spectral-domain optical coherence tomography scans using the example of cyst annotation," *Computer Methods and Programs in Biomedicine*, vol. 130, pp. 93–105, 2016.

[13] R. R. Pappuru, C. Briceno, Y. Ouyang, A. C. Walsh, and S. R. Sadda, "Clinical significance of B-scan averaging with SD-OCT," *Ophthalmic Surgery, Lasers & Imaging*, vol. 43, no. 1, pp. 63–68, 2012.

[14] A. Sakamoto, M. Hangai, and N. Yoshimura, "Spectral-domain optical coherence tomography with multiple B-scan averaging for enhanced imaging of retinal diseases," *Ophthalmology*, vol. 115, no. 6, pp. 1071–1078, 2008.

[15] C. Ye, D. S. Lam, and C. K. Leung, "Retinal nerve fiber layer imaging with spectral-domain optical coherence tomography: effect of multiple B-scan averaging on RNFL measurement," *Journal of Glaucoma*, vol. 21, no. 3, pp. 164–168, 2012.

[16] B. Pemp, R. H. Kardon, K. Kircher, E. Pernicka, U. Schmidt-Erfurth, and A. Reitner, "Effectiveness of averaging strategies to reduce variance in retinal nerve fibre layer thickness measurements using spectral-domain optical coherence tomography," *Graefe's Archive for Clinical and Experimental Ophthalmology*, vol. 251, no. 7, pp. 1841–1848, 2013.

[17] M. P. Bambo, E. Garcia-Martin, S. Otin et al., "Influence of cataract surgery on repeatability and measurements of spectral domain optical coherence tomography," *The British Journal of Ophthalmology*, vol. 98, no. 1, pp. 52–58, 2014.

[18] E. Garcia-Martin, J. Fernandez, L. Gil-Arribas et al., "Effect of cataract surgery on optical coherence tomography measurements and repeatability in patients with non-insulin-dependent diabetes mellitus," *Investigative Ophthalmology & Visual Science*, vol. 54, no. 8, pp. 5303–5312, 2013.

[19] E. Garcia-Martin, D. Rodriguez-Mena, I. Dolz et al., "Influence of cataract surgery on optical coherence tomography and neurophysiology measurements in patients with retinitis pigmentosa," *American Journal of Ophthalmology*, vol. 156, no. 2, pp. 293–303, 2013, e292.

[20] J. H. Na, K. R. Sung, and Y. Lee, "Factors associated with the signal strengths obtained by spectral domain optical coherence tomography," *Korean Journal of Ophthalmology*, vol. 26, no. 3, pp. 169–173, 2012.

[21] U. Schmidt-Erfurth and S. M. Waldstein, "A paradigm shift in imaging biomarkers in neovascular age-related macular degeneration," *Progress in Retinal and eye Research*, vol. 50, pp. 1–24, 2016.

[22] S. Vongkulsiri, M. Suzuki, and R. F. Spaide, "Colocalization error between the scanning laser ophthalmoscope infrared reflectance and optical coherence tomography images of the Heidelberg Spectralis," *Retina*, vol. 35, no. 6, pp. 1211–1215, 2015.

[23] A. Movahedan and A. R. Djalilian, "Cataract surgery in the face of ocular surface disease," *Current Opinion in Ophthalmology*, vol. 23, no. 1, pp. 68–72, 2012.

[24] D. Podkowinski, S. M. Waldstein, E. S. Varnousfaderani et al., "Quantitative evaluation of Spectralis optical coherence tomography image quality with systematic variation of B-scan averaging before and after cataract surgery," *Investigative Ophthalmology & Visual Science*, vol. 55, no. 13, p. 4804, 2014 http://iovs.arvojournals.org/article.aspx?articleid=2270354.

18

The Effect of Anterior Capsule Polishing on Capsular Contraction and Lens Stability in Cataract Patients with High Myopia

Dandan Wang,[1,2] Xiaoyu Yu [ID],[1,2] Zhangliang Li [ID],[1,2] Xixia Ding,[1,2] Hengli Lian,[1,2] Jianyang Mao,[1,2] Yinying Zhao,[1,2] and Yun-E. Zhao [ID][1,2]

[1]School of Optometry and Ophthalmology and Eye Hospital, Wenzhou Medical University, Wenzhou, Zhejiang, China
[2]Key Laboratory of Vision Science, Ministry of Health P.R. China, Wenzhou, Zhejiang, China

Correspondence should be addressed to Yun-E. Zhao; zyehzeye@126.com

Academic Editor: Florence Cabot

Purpose. To evaluate the effect of anterior capsule polishing in patients with high myopia after cataract surgery. *Setting.* The Eye Hospital of Wenzhou Medical University, Zhejiang, China. *Design.* Prospective study. *Methods.* High myopic patients with a bilateral cataract who underwent phacoemulsification with 360° anterior capsular polishing in one eye and without polishing in the contralateral eye were recruited. The following parameters were recorded at 1, 3, and 6 months postoperatively, including the area and diameter of the anterior capsule opening (area and D), IOL tilt and decentration, refraction, and postoperative aqueous depth (PAD). *Results.* Paired samples of 38 eyes of 19 patients were enrolled. The area decreased significantly in both the polished group and unpolished group, whereas the diameter reduced more in the unpolished group. The IOL tilt and decentration at 3-month and 6-month follow-up showed significant differences between two groups. In the unpolished group, the IOL decentration firstly appeared between one-month to three-month visit, while the refraction error, PAD, and IOL tilt were significantly different between the three-month and six-month visits. *Conclusion.* 360° anterior capsule polishing can effectively reduce the extent of the anterior capsule contraction and increase the stability of IOL. The study was registered at http://www.clinicaltrials.gov, and the clinical trial accession number is NCT 03142269.

1. Introduction

Phacoemulsification has been referred to as a refractive surgery due to the development of surgical techniques and refraction-correcting IOLs. An accurate prediction of postoperative refraction is important in refractive cataract surgery. The anterior capsule contraction syndrome (ACCS) is a well-recognized postoperative complication. The outcomes of ACCS are opacification, fibrosis, and contraction of the anterior capsule [1–3]. In some previous studies, high myopia is the most common risk factor for advanced intracapsular IOL dislocation, with reported incidence ranging from19.7% to 40% [4, 5]. Several studies have reported that this is mostly observed under conditions of zonular weakness and chronic intraocular inflammation [6, 7].

High myopic patients, especially with axial length of >27.0 mm, probably have an enlarged capsular bag with weak zonules and tend to develop cataracts earlier than emmetropic patients [7, 8]. This increases the risk of postoperative intracapsular IOL dislocation and reduces the accuracy of predicting postoperative refractive error. Our previous study, using an ultralong-scan-depth OCT, suggested that weak capsular adhesion and incomplete adhesive capsular bend is increased in high myopic eyes [9]. These factors presumably increase the likelihood of capsular contraction and postoperative refraction deviation. A number of studies have reported that capsular contraction is associated with lens epithelial cell (LEC) proliferation and migration originating underneath the anterior capsule [10–12]. However, anterior capsule polishing remains controversial in the field [11–14]. To the best of our knowledge, no interocular comparison on anterior capsule opening contraction, tilt, and decentration of intraocular lenses in high myopic cataract patients after uneventful phacoemulsification surgery has been conducted. In each patient, we performed phacoemulsification with a 360° anterior capsular polishing in one eye, while the contralateral eye was left unpolished. The surgeon(Z.Y.E) designed an instrument to perform a 360° capsule polishing, featured like a paddle with thin blunt edge, and the tip is approximately 5.0 mm with a diameter of 1.0 mm.

The objective of this study is to determine if the anterior capsule polishing is beneficial to reduce the extent of the anterior capsule contraction and increase the stability of the intraocular lens.

2. Methods

2.1. Patients. This is a prospective patient-masked clinical trial. The study followed the tenets of the Helsinki agreement, and informed consent was obtained from all patients. In this study, 40 eyes from 20 patients were recruited in the Eye Hospital of Wenzhou Medical University. One patient was excluded because of a postoperative retinal tear and did not complete the follow-up protocol. The inclusion criteria included: cataract patients with extremely high myopia (axial length >27 mm); the difference between bilateral eyes was less than 1 mm; and age range from 50 to 75 years. Preoperative assessments included slit-lamp, dilated fundus examination by an ophthalmologist. The same examiner performed noncontact tonometry and optical biometry (IOLMaster 5.0, Carl Zeiss, Germany) measurements. Patients with keratitis, glaucoma, uveitis, retinitis pigmentosa, pseudoexfoliation syndrome, diabetes, or myotonic dystrophy were excluded. Additionally, patients with history of ophthalmic surgery, trauma, severe postoperative inflammatory reactions, or unsuccessful intraoperative continuous circular capsulorhexis (CCC) were excluded.

2.2. Surgical Technique. All surgeries were performed by the same experienced surgeon (Z. Y. E). Phacoemulsification (Alcon infiniti, USA) was performed and a one-piece hydrophilic, square-edged Akreos MI60 IOL with a total length of 11 mm and optical zone diameter length 6.2 mm (Bausch, USA) was implanted. After topical anesthesia, a 2.2 mm corneal incision was made. Ophthalmic viscosurgical devices (OVDs) were used to inflate the anterior chamber, and CCC (diameter range of 5.5 ± 0.2 mm) was performed, ensured the CCC size and shape to expected use of the digital navigation system. Hydrodissection and phacoemulsification were performed, and the cortex was removed with automated irrigation/aspiration. In the polished group, take the left eye for example, after the IOL implantation, a polisher was introduced into the chamber via a side port incision on the temporal to polish the superior and nasal quadrant of the inner surface of the anterior capsule and then via a main incision on the superior to polish the inferior and temporal quadrant capsule. In the unpolished group, the anterior capsule was left unpolished. All posterior capsules were polished.

According to the random number table, one eye was randomly assigned to the polished group, while the other eye was assigned to the unpolished group, and two operations were completed within one week. All cases of postoperative medication were standardized. Immediate application of eye drops occurred after surgery. Levofloxacin (0.5%, Santen, Japan) was administered four times a day for two weeks after surgery. Fluorometholone (0.1%, Santen, Japan) was administered four times a day for 4 weeks after surgery, and the dose was reduced once a week. Bromfenac sodium (0.1%, Stuton, Japan) was administered twice a day for six weeks after surgery.

2.3. Parameters. All patients were examined at one day, one week, and one, three, and six months after surgery. In every follow-up visit, BCVA and intraocular pressure were assessed. Fully dilated fundus exams were also performed. The refractive status and anterior capsule opening size were determined as baseline on the first day after operation. Measured parameters included the area and diameter of the anterior capsule opening (area and D), IOL tilt and decentration, refractive state, and postoperative aqueous depth (PAD). All exams were performed after pupil dilation with tropicamide phenylephrine (Santen, Japan). The investigator acquiring and measuring the data have been masked. Anterior-segmental photography using both diffused light and slit-light across the central visual axis was obtained from each patient. Image J software (2x, National Institutes of Health) was used to determine the anterior capsulorhexis size (Area and D).

The commercially available Scheimpflug imaging system (Pentacam, Oculus) was used to measure the PAD, which is defined as the perpendicular distance from the central corneal endothelium to the anterior surface of IOL. The Pentacam Scheimpflug system also was used to measure IOL tilt and decentration [15, 16] (Figure 1). The pupillary axis was considered to be the center of pupil after mydriasis. Scheimpflug images at 90° and 180° from the pupillary axis were taken to get the best-fit-circle of the anterior and posterior surface of IOL to determine the center line of the IOL using Image Pro Plus(Media Cybernetics, Inc. USA). In order to determine the tilt of the IOL, using the pupillary axis as the baseline, the angle between the axis of optical center of IOL and the baseline was measured. Decentration of IOL was referred to as the difference between horizontal coordinates at the center of the IOL central line and the center of the pupillary axis. Differences were determined to be the change in mean values between examinations.

2.4. Statistical Analysis. Data analysis was performed using SPSS software for Windows (Version 19.0; SPSS Inc., Chicago, IL, U.S.). Kolmogorov–Smirnov tests were used to check the normal distribution of variables. Based on the design of experiment, paired *t*-tests were used for comparison between paired groups. And according to numeric results for paired *t*-tests calculated by SPSS software using

(a)

(b)

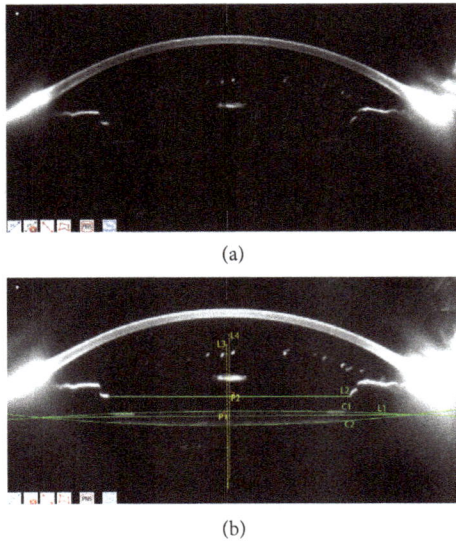

FIGURE 1: Anterior segment of an aphakic eye imaged by the Pentacam Scheimpflug imaging system. L3: axis on the optical center of IOL; L4: axis on the center of pupilla; C1: the best-fit-circle on the anterior surface of IOL; C2: the best-fit-circle on the posterior surface of IOL; L1: horizontal line of IOL; L2: horizontal line of pupilla. The tilt of IOL is defined as the angle between L3 and L4. The decentration of IOL is defined as the distance between horizontal coordinates of P1 and P2.

the number of cases, parameters' means and standard deviation, the sample size was sufficient just need past 6 pairs, a sample of 19 cases was more than adequate for this study. The Wilcoxon rank test was used in cases that data did not have normal distribution. Nominal p values were calculated using t tests, and the level of significance was set at 0.05.

3. Results

A total of 38 eyes (19 patients) with mean age of 60.53 ± 10.18 years were included in this prospective study. No patients received Nd: YAG laser capsulotomy due to serious posterior capsule opacification (PCO) or CCS. There were no significant differences between the polished group and the unpolished group, in terms of the axial length (AL), refraction status, and anterior capsule opening size on the day after surgery (Table 1).

Although the IOL tilt did not show significant differences between groups at one month after operation ($p = 0.065$), it was slightly lower in the polished group. And at the same time, the refraction status and anterior capsule opening size revealed no significant differences (Table 2). At the postoperative three-month visit, both the IOL tilt and decentration in the polished group were significantly lower than those in the unpolished group ($p = 0.047$, $p = 0.045$, respectively) (Table 3). And these differences were prolonged to the six-month follow-up ($p = 0.021$ and 0.021, respectively) (Table 4). With respect to other parameters, no significant differences were found between two groups at both three-month and six-month follow-ups.

TABLE 1: The AL, refraction status, and anterior capsule opening size at the 1st day after surgery.

Parameter ($N = 19$)	Polished	Unpolished	t value	p
AL (mm)	29.90 ± 1.68	29.99 ± 1.86	-0.544	0.583
Refraction status (D)	-3.05 ± 0.91	-2.70 ± 1.06	-1.347	0.195
Area (mm^2)	25.26 ± 1.21	25.46 ± 1.40	-1.008	0.327
Vertical Dia.(mm)	5.45 ± 0.12	5.50 ± 0.10	-1.644	0.118
Horizontal dia. (mm)	5.48 ± 0.10	5.51 ± 0.09	-1.509	0.149

TABLE 2: Cross-sectional comparison between polished and unpolished groups at the 1 month after surgery.

Parameter ($N = 19$)	Polished	Unpolished	t value	p
Refraction status (D)	-3.00 ± 0.77	-2.76 ± 1.12	-1.124	0.276
PAD (mm)	4.79 ± 0.39	4.79 ± 0.39	0.076	0.940
IOL tilt (°)	0.49 ± 0.30	1.06 ± 0.90	-0.364	0.065
IOL decentration (mm)	0.32 ± 0.16	0.38 ± 0.19	-0.973	0.344
Area (mm^2)	23.97 ± 1.34	23.78 ± 2.11	0.495	0.626
Vertical dia. (mm)	5.38 ± 0.17	5.38 ± 0.27	0.026	0.979
Horizontal dia. (mm)	5.37 ± 0.15	5.32 ± 0.22	1.208	0.243

TABLE 3: Cross-sectional comparison between polished and unpolished groups at the 3 months after surgery.

Parameter ($N = 19$)	Polished	Unpolished	t value	p
Refraction status (D)	-2.92 ± 0.74	-2.76 ± 1.03	-0.763	0.455
PAD (mm)	4.86 ± 0.41	4.87 ± 0.40	-0.138	0.891
IOL tilt (°)	0.61 ± 0.41	1.13 ± 1.02	-2.127	0.047^*
IOL decentration (mm)	0.37 ± 0.17	0.49 ± 0.22	-2.154	0.045^*
Area (mm^2)	23.41 ± 1.24	22.97 ± 2.14	1.018	0.322
Vertical dia. (mm)	5.35 ± 0.20	5.32 ± 0.25	0.527	0.605
Horizontal dia.(mm)	5.31 ± 0.16	5.26 ± 0.26	0.773	0.450

*Significant at $p < 0.05$.

TABLE 4: Cross-sectional comparison between polished and unpolished groups at the 6 months after surgery.

Parameter ($N = 19$)	Polished	Unpolished	t value	p
Refraction status (D)	-2.97 ± 0.74	-2.99 ± 1.11	-0.127	0.900
PAD (mm)	4.87 ± 0.47	4.81 ± 0.42	0.645	0.527
IOL tilt (°)	0.69 ± 0.35	1.24 ± 1.00	-2.519	0.021^*
IOL decentration (mm)	0.42 ± 0.14	0.55 ± 0.21	-2.519	0.021^*
Area (mm^2)	23.26 ± 1.24	22.64 ± 1.90	1.636	0.119
Vertical dia. (mm)	5.33 ± 0.18	5.26 ± 0.24	1.452	0.164
Horizontal dia.(mm)	5.28 ± 0.17	5.17 ± 0.25	1.563	0.135

*Significant at $p < 0.05$.

3.1. Longitudinal Comparison between Postoperative Time Points

3.1.1. The Polished Group.
The anterior capsular opening area decreased significantly between each time points (all $p < 0.001$) while the horizontal diameter was significantly reduced ($p = 0.002, 0.017$ and <0.001, respectively). The vertical diameter was significantly reduced only from the three-month visit to the six-month visit ($p = 0.004$). The refraction error and PAD in the polished group showed no significant differences between different postoperative time points (Figures 2 and 3).

3.1.2. The Unpolished Group.
The anterior capsular opening area differed significantly between each time points ($p < 0.001$, < 0.001, and 0.002, respectively). And the horizontal diameter was significantly reduced ($p < 0.001, 0.099$, and 0.005, respectively), while the vertical diameter reduced analogously ($p = 0.059, 0.004$, and <0.001, respectively). The differences of refraction error and PAD in the unpolished group were significant between the three-month and six-month visits ($p = 0.011$ and 0.003, respectively). The IOL tilt between three-month and six-month follow-ups was significantly different ($p = 0.045$), while the IOL decentration between the one-month and three-month follow-ups was also different ($p = 0.018$). (Figures 2 and 3).

4. Discussion

The risk of postoperative complications, such as ACCS, is increased in high myopic patients due to zonular weakness. This is caused by anterior capsular opening shrinkage, zonule elongation, or IOL tilt and decentration. In a previous retrospective analytical study, we demonstrated that the frequency of anterior capsular opening shrinkage and IOL tilt and decentration was significantly higher in cataract eyes with high myopia than that in cataract eyes with a normal axial length [17]. To our knowledge, no study with respect to how to effectively reduce the anterior capsular contraction has been published. Previous studies have reported that LECs play a major role in the pathogenesis of capsule contraction and fibrosis [1, 2, 4, 18]. To this end, we think it is important to ensure residual LECs were eliminated during the operation which can reduce the occurrence of anterior capsular contraction. However, the effectiveness of anterior capsule polishing during phacoemulsification still remains controversial [4,11–14,19]. Most ophthalmic surgeons do not perform anterior capsule polishing during phacoemulsification; however, many surgeons claim that anterior capsule polishing is beneficial. These advocates commonly use the I/A tip or other modified polisher through the main incision to polish the anterior capsule. However, the capsule at the main incision is particularly difficult to polish. With this understanding, we performed an interocular comparison of polished and unpolished capsules as it impacts anterior capsular contraction and intraocular lens stability in high myopic cataract patients. For this procedure, we used a newly designed polisher that is thin and smooth and has a tip that is approximately 5.0 mm long with a diameter of 1.0 mm. The improved instrument can be smoothly inserted through the second incision into the anterior chamber and be positioned 360° the inner surface of the anterior capsule.

No significant difference in the anterior capsule opening formation between the two groups was observed. However, we found the anterior capsule opening area of the two groups similarly contracted after the operation. This is due to myofibrillar contraction of LECs following trans-differentiation [20]. However, the vertical diameter in the polished group had a slight reduction in the early after surgery. Whereas, both vertical diameter and horizontal diameter showed more significant reduction in the unpolished group. Menapace and Di had proved anterior capsule polishing reduced capsulorhexis contraction, and the clinical results were similar by measuring the changes of the capsulorhexis opening [10]. This suggests that anterior capsule polishing can effectively reduce the contraction of anterior capsule and increase the stability of the intraocular lens.

The impact of IOL tilt and decentration on visual quality has been widespread recognized [21, 22]. Several studies suggest that more than 1 mm decentration and a greater than 5° tilt optically impairs visual quality. An average tilt and decentration of 3° and 0.25 mm, respectively, are well below the criteria to affect clinically observable visual acuity [22, 23]. In the present study, both the IOL tilt and decentration in the polished group showed no significant differences between different postoperative time points. By contrast, in the unpolished group, the IOL tilt between the three-month and six-month follow-ups was significantly different, while the IOL decentration between the one-month and three-month follow-ups was also significant different. We speculate that the IOL gradually tilted during the first month and appears statistically significant at three to six months in the unpolished group. The main reason for this is that myofibrillar contraction of the unpolished anterior capsule leads to tilt of the IOL.

In this study, using the Pentacam system to evaluate the PAD, we defined the PAD as the distance from the posterior surface of the corneal to the anterior IOL surface. This reflects the ELP, which has a clinically relevant impact on postoperative refraction [24]. These results indicate that the differences of refraction status and PAD in the unpolished group were significant between the three-month and six-month visits. During three to six months after surgery, the IOL gradually moved forward and the PAD decreased to a statistically significant degree. Due to the change of PAD, myopic shift occurred in 3–6 months after surgery in the unpolished group. This is consistent with the results of our previous retrospective study that showed PAD decreased in high myopic patients, as well as a decrease in the occurrence of a shallow anterior chamber and myopic shift. While the achieved refraction outcome and PAD in the polished group showed no significant differences between different postoperative time points. In conclusion, our results suggest that IOL placement is more stable in polished capsular bags.

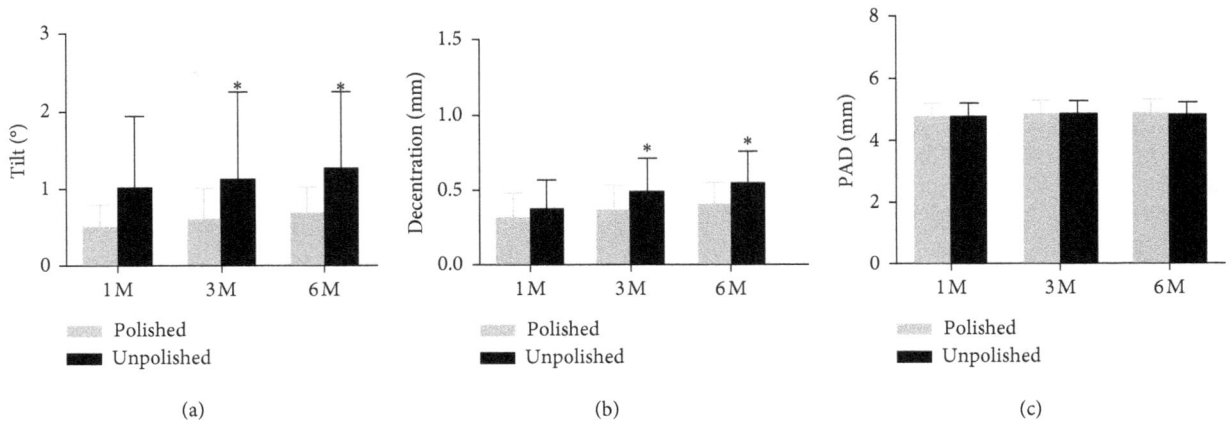

(a)   (b)   (c)

FIGURE 2: The differences in IOL stability between the two groups (*Significant at $p < 0.05$).

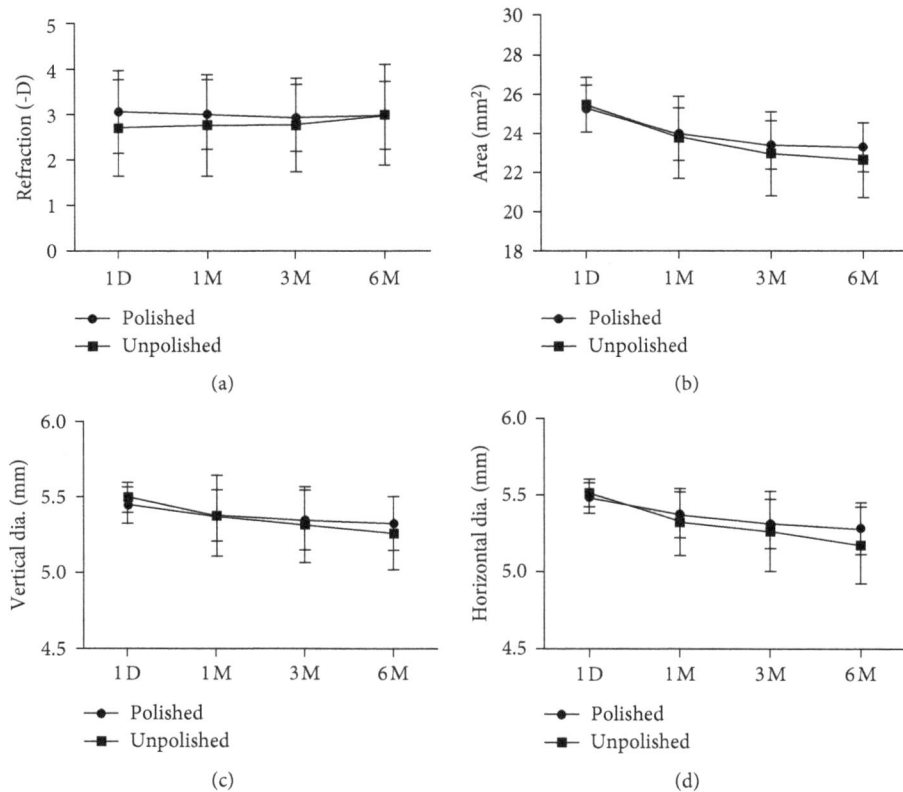

(a)   (b)

(c)   (d)

FIGURE 3: The differences in refraction and anterior capsule opening size between the two groups.

Besides, during the six months follow-up even beyond the experiment, we observed no obvious difference in the incidence of PCO between polished eyes and unpolished eyes which was consistent with the results of the previous study of Liu et al. [14].

The limitation of this study is relatively small sample size and some differences, which has not reached any significant clinical impact in terms of patient symptoms. However, in the present study, all procedures were performed by the same surgeon, and the axial length of our subjects was limited to more than 27; the difference between bilateral eyes was less than 1 mm, and these may minimize influencing factors.

In conclusion, our study suggests that 360° anterior capsule polishing can effectively maintain stability of the position of the IOL-capsule complex.

Additional Points

What Was Known: (i) The risk of postoperative complications, such as capsular contraction syndrome, is increased in high myopic patients due to zonular weakness. (ii) Cataract patients with highly myopia were more likely to experience anterior capsule contraction, particularly during the early postoperative period. (iii) The effectiveness of anterior capsule polishing during phacoemulsification still remains controversial. *What This Paper Adds*: (i) We reported the benefits of using 360° anterior capsule polishing, which can effectively reduce the extent of the anterior capsule contraction and increase the stability of the intraocular lens. (ii) It is worth considering performing 360° anterior capsule polishing during phacoemulsification in cataract patients with highly myopia.

Conflicts of Interest

The authors declare that they have no conflicts of interest.

Authors' Contributions

Dandan Wang and Xiaoyu Yu contributed equally to this work.

Acknowledgments

This study was supported by research grants from the Provincial Construction Project of Zhejiang (Grant no. 201647538), the Innovation Discipline of Zhejiang Province (lens disease in children), and research grants from the Science and Technology Projects of Wenzhou, Zhejiang (Grant no. 20160452).

References

[1] U. Chomanska, P. Krasnicki, E. Proniewska-Skretek, and Z. Mariak, "Anterior capsule contraction syndrome after cataract phacoemulsification surgery," *Klinika Oczna*, vol. 112, no. 7–9, pp. 243–246, 2010.

[2] M. Aose, H. Matsushima, K. Mukai, Y. Katsuki, N. Gotoh, and T. Senoo, "Influence of intraocular lens implantation on anterior capsule contraction and posterior capsule opacification," *Journal of Cataract and Refractive Surgery*, vol. 40, no. 12, pp. 2128–2133, 2014.

[3] S. K. Shah, M. R. Praveen, A. Kaul, A. R. Vasavada, G. D. Shah, and B. R. Nihalani, "Impact of anterior capsule polishing on anterior capsule opacification after cataract surgery: a randomized clinical trial," *Eye*, vol. 23, no. 8, pp. 1702–1706, 2009.

[4] A. Rey, I. Jürgens, A. Dyrda, X. Maseras, and A. Morilla, "Surgical outcome of late in-the-bag intraocular lens dislocation treated with pars plana vitrectomy," *Retina*, vol. 36, no. 3, pp. 576–581, 2016.

[5] R. F. Buenaga, J. L. Alio, A. L. Pérez-Ardoy et al., "Late in-the-bag intraocular lens dislocation requiring explantation: risk factors and outcomes," *Eye*, vol. 27, no. 7, pp. 795–802, 2013.

[6] A. Abbouda, P. Tortorella, L. Restivo, E. Santoro, F. De Marco, and M. La Cava, "Follow-up study of over three years of patients with uveitis after cataract phacoemulsification: outcomes and complications," *Seminars in Ophthalmology*, vol. 31, no. 6, pp. 532–541, 2016.

[7] J. K. Lam, T. C. Chan, A. L. Ng, V. W. Chow, V. W. Wong, and V. Jhanji, "Outcomes of cataract operations in extreme high axial myopia," *Graefe's Archive for Clinical and Experimental Ophthalmology*, vol. 254, no. 9, pp. 1811–1817, 2016.

[8] S. Cetinkaya, N. O. Acir, Y. F. Cetinkaya, Z. Dadaci, H. İ. Yener, and F. Saglam, "Phacoemulsification in eyes with cataract and high myopia," *Arquivos Brasileiros De Oftalmologia*, vol. 78, no. 5, p. 286, 2015.

[9] Y. Zhao, J. Li, W. Lu et al., "Capsular adhesion to intraocular lens in highly myopic eyes evaluated in vivo using ultralong-scan-depth optical coherence tomography," *American Journal of Ophthalmology*, vol. 155, no. 3, pp. 484–491, 2013.

[10] R. Menapace and N. S. Di, "Aspiration curette for anterior capsule polishing: laboratory and clinical evaluation," *Journal of Cataract and Refractive Surgery*, vol. 32, no. 12, pp. 1997–2003, 2006.

[11] Y. Gao, G. F. Dang, X. Wang, L. Duan, and X. Y. Wu, "Influences of anterior capsule polishing on effective lens position after cataract surgery: a randomized controlled trial," *International Journal of Clinical and Experimental Medicine*, vol. 8, no. 8, pp. 13769–13775, 2015.

[12] S. Sacu, R. Menapace, M. Wirtitsch, W. Buehl, G. Rainer, and O. Findl, "Effect of anterior capsule polishing on fibrotic capsule opacification: three-year results," *Journal of Cataract and Refractive Surgery*, vol. 30, no. 11, pp. 2322–2327, 2004.

[13] R. Baile, M. Sahasrabuddhe, S. Nadkarni, V. Karira, and J. Kelkar, "Effect of anterior capsular polishing on the rate of posterior capsule opacification: a retrospective analytical study," *Saudi Journal of Ophthalmology*, vol. 26, no. 1, pp. 101–104, 2012.

[14] X. Liu, B. Cheng, D. Zheng, Y. Liu, and Y. Liu, "Role of anterior capsule polishing in residual lens epithelial cell proliferation," *Journal of Cataract and Refractive Surgery*, vol. 36, no. 2, pp. 208–214, 2010.

[15] A. de Castro, P. Rosales, and S. Marcos, "Tilt and decentration of intraocular lenses in vivo from Purkinje and Scheimpflug imaging," *Journal of Cataract and Refractive Surgery*, vol. 33, no. 3, pp. 418–429, 2007.

[16] P. Rosales, A. De Castro, I. Jimenez-Alfaro, and S. Marcos, "Intraocular lens alignment from purkinje and Scheimpflug imaging," *Clinical and Experimental Optometry*, vol. 93, no. 6, pp. 400–408, 2010.

[17] D. Wang, Y. Zheng, and X. YU, "Study on the anterior capsular changes and intraocular lenses stability of super high myopiceyes cataract after phacoem ulsification," *Zhejiang Medical Journal*, vol. 38, no. 17, pp. 1397–1400, 2016.

[18] K. M. Spang, J. M. Rohrbach, and E. G. Weidle, "Complete occlusion of the anterior capsular opening after intact capsulorhexis: clinicopathologic correlation," *American Journal of Ophthalmology*, vol. 127, no. 3, pp. 343–345, 1999.

[19] R. J. Hanson, A. Rubinstein, S. Sarangapani, L. Benjamin, and C. K. Patel, "Effect of lens epithelial cell aspiration on postoperative capsulorhexis contraction with the use of the AcrySof intraocular lens: randomized clinical trial," *Journal of Cataract and Refractive Surgery*, vol. 32, no. 10, pp. 1621–1626, 2006.

[20] P. J. McDonnell, M. A. Zarbin, and W. R. Green, "Posterior capsule opacification in pseudophakic eyes," *Ophthalmology*, vol. 90, no. 12, pp. 1548–1553, 1983.

[21] J. B. Ale, "Intraocular lens tilt and decentration: a concern for contemporary IOL designs," *Nepalese Journal of Ophthalmology*, vol. 3, no. 1, pp. 68–77, 2011.

[22] T. Eppig, K. Scholz, A. Loffler, A. Messner, and A. Langenbucher, "Effect of decentration and tilt on the image quality of aspheric intraocular lens designs in a model eye," *Journal of Cataract and Refractive Surgery*, vol. 35, no. 6, pp. 1091–1100, 2009.

[23] D. L. Guyton, H. Uozato, and H. J. Wisnicki, "Rapid determination of intraocular lens tilt and decentration through the undilated pupil," *Ophthalmology*, vol. 97, no. 10, pp. 1259–1264, 1990.

[24] T. Olsen, "Calculation of intraocular lens power: a review," *Acta Ophthalmologica Scandinavica*, vol. 85, no. 5, pp. 472–485, 2007.

19

Clinical Results of Diffractive, Refractive, Hybrid Multifocal, and Monofocal Intraocular Lenses

Agnieszka Dyrda ⓘ,[1,2] Ana Martínez-Palmer,[1] Daniel Martín-Moral,[1] Amanda Rey,[2] Antonio Morilla,[2] Miguel Castilla-Martí ⓘ,[3] and Janny Aronés-Santivañez[1]

[1]Department of Ophthalmology, Hospital Universitario del Mar and Hospital de la Esperanza, Pompeu and Fabra University, Barcelona, Spain
[2]Institut Català de Retina, Barcelona, Spain
[3]Valles Ophthalmology Research, Hospital General de Catalunya, Barcelona, Spain

Correspondence should be addressed to Agnieszka Dyrda; agnieszkaannadyrda@wp.pl

Academic Editor: David P. Piñero

Purpose. To present the outcomes of hybrid multifocal and monofocal intraocular lenses (IOLs) and to compare with refractive and diffractive multifocal IOLs (MFIOLs). *Methods.* Three hundred twenty eyes (160 patients) underwent cataract surgery with randomized IOLs bilateral implantation. Changes in uncorrected and distance-corrected logMAR distance, intermediate and near (UNVA and DCNVA) visual acuity (VA), contrast sensitivity (CS), presence of dysphotopsia, spectacle independence, and patient satisfaction were analyzed. *Results.* Postoperative VA in the hybrid (OptiVis) group was improved in all distances ($p < 0.001$). OptiVis acted superiorly to monofocal IOLs in UNVA and DCNVA ($p < 0.001$ for both) and to refractive ones in DCNVA ($p < 0.005$). Distance, mesopic, without glare CS in OptiVis was lower than in the monofocal group and similar to other MFIOLs. No differences in dysphotopsia pre- and postoperatively and spectacle independence in near for OptiVis and refractive MFIOLs were detected. OptiVis patients were more satisfied than those with monofocal IOLs ($p = 0.015$). *Conclusions.* After cataract surgery, patients with OptiVis improved VA in all distances. Near and intermediate VA was better than monofocal, and DCNVA was better than the refractive group. CS was lower in OptiVis than in the monofocal group, but there was no difference between MFIOLs. Patient satisfaction was higher in OptiVis than in the monofocal group. This trial is registered with NCT03512626.

1. Introduction

Nowadays, cataract surgery is a refractive procedure. Although monofocal intraocular lenses (IOLs) ensure excellent distance acuity, patients require spectacles for near and intermediate vision [1]. Multifocal IOLs (MFIOLs) have different depth of focus capabilities within the optical zone and effectively achieve good visual acuity (VA) for far and near distances, guaranteeing spectacle independence. MFIOLs use a refractive, a diffractive, or a combination of both designs. One of the main disadvantages of refractive multifocal IOLs is their pupil dependence, while the loss of energy is the main drawback of the diffractive design. Studies showed that MFIOLs had increased dysphotopsia and decreased contrast sensitivity (CS) compared with monofocal IOLs [1, 2]. These side effects can limit visual function and reduce patient's quality of life [3]. Comparison of aspheric and spherical IOLs showed superior visual performance of aspheric IOLs, especially in CS [4, 5]. The OptiVis™ MFIOL (Aaren Scientific, Inc., Ontario, CA, USA) offers several advantages, as it is a real multifocal hybrid design. The lens is distance dominant and has a central progressive refractive zone within 1.5 mm surrounded by a diffractive zone from 1.5 mm to 3.8 mm of diameter that allows far and near vision in a full range of pupil sizes. The progressive power refractive zone allows far and intermediate vision, and the apodized diffractive design minimizes light loss outside and reduces halos in the far focus. Additionally, aspheric lens periphery improves image contrast in large pupils for different corneal asphericities [6]. Binocular implantation of MFIOLs is preferred to monocular implantation [7].

The purpose of this study was to compare the visual outcomes after cataract surgery with bilateral implantation of a hybrid (refractive-diffractive) multifocal IOL (OptiVis, Aaren Scientific) and a monofocal IOL (AR40e, AMO) and to compare with our previous study of refractive and diffractive multifocal IOLs.

2. Patients and Methods

This prospective, randomized, controlled study was conducted at the Ophthalmology Department of the Hospital de la Esperanza, Barcelona, Spain. Institutional review board approval was obtained, and the study adhered to the Declaration of Helsinki. Written informed consent was obtained from all patients. Eligibility was determined based on a complete ophthalmologic examination. Inclusion criteria were senile cataract with Snellen VA ≤ 0.5 and motivation for spectacle independence for near vision. As the study was conducted in the Spanish public health care system, entering the study was the only option to get multifocal lens, as they are not provided by public health care, and the patients were conscious of the possibility of randomization to the monofocal group. Exclusion criteria were corneal astigmatism ≥ 1.10 diopters (D), irregular astigmatism, axial length <21.5 or ≥ 25 mm, pupillary diameter in mesopic conditions in distance vision ≤ 2.5 mm and ≥ 6 mm, age ≥ 80 years, ocular pathology that could affect the visual function and/or IOL centering, and intraoperative or postoperative complications. Highly demanding patients and those whose profession could be affected by a multifocal design (professional drivers, jewelers, etc.) were also excluded, as in the Spanish public health care system's secondary procedures needed to satisfy patients' expectation, such as LRIs, LASIK, and PRKs, are not available. Patients were randomly assigned to have bilateral implantation with either a monofocal IOL (AR40e, AMO-Abbott 30 Laboratories Inc., Abbott Park, Illinois, USA) or multifocal IOL (OptiVis, Aaren Scientific, Inc., Ontario, CA, USA).

We used the previously unpublished results of a randomized, controlled study, performed in the same center with the same protocol and methodology, to compare performance of a refractive-diffractive multifocal IOL (OptiVis, Aaren Scientific, Inc., Ontario, CA, USA) with refractive (M-Flex, Rayner Intraocular Lenses Limited, Hove, UK; ReZoom, AMO-Abbott 30 Laboratories Inc., Abbott Park, Illinois, USA) and diffractive (ReSTOR +4, Alcon Laboratories, Inc., Fort Worth, USA) IOLs. Since OptiVis is a hybrid multifocal lens, it is assumed to offer the advantages of both designs.

2.1. Preoperative Assessment. Preoperatively, all patients had a full ophthalmologic examination including uncorrected distance visual acuity (UDVA), corrected distance visual acuity (CDVA) at 6 m, uncorrected intermediate visual acuity (UIVA), distance-corrected intermediate visual acuity (DCIVA) at 60 cm (in the OptiVis group only, as they were supposed to provide intermediate distance vision in contrary to the other studied lenses), uncorrected near visual acuity (UNVA), distance-corrected near visual acuity (DCNVA) at 33 cm (all measured using Snellen acuity charts under photopic conditions), refraction, slit lamp biomicroscopy, Goldmann applanation tonometry, and fundoscopy. Monocular and binocular CS were measured in mesopic conditions, without glare at spatial frequencies of 1.5, 3, 6, 12, and 18 cycles per degree (cpd) using the functional acuity contrast test (FACT, OPTEC 6500®, Stereo Optical Co. Inc.). Pupil diameter in distance vision was evaluated using a "Rosenbaum pocket-card." Spectacle dependence, determined by questionnaire (Do you wear glasses for distance/near vision?), and presence of dysphotopsia (halos, glare), spontaneously mentioned or elicited in response to questioning were also assessed preoperatively. The IOL power was calculated using the SRK/T with an A-constant of 118.4 for AR40e and 118.1 for OptiVis using partial coherence interferometry (IOLMaster 500, Carl Zeiss Meditec AG). Postoperative target refraction was emmetropia. Table 1 shows the patient demographics.

2.2. Intraocular Lenses. The IOLs used in our study are presented in Table 2.

2.3. Surgical Technique. The same experienced surgeon (AMP) performed all the surgeries under topical anesthesia using a standard phacoemulsification procedure with Infiniti Vision System (all from Alcon Laboratories, Inc., Fort Worth, TX) and with IOL implantation in the capsular bag through a 2.75 mm clear corneal incision. The incision was performed in the steepest meridian. Both eyes were operated on within 1–4 weeks.

2.4. Postoperative Examination. Routine postoperative examinations were performed 1 day, 1 month, and 3 months after surgery. The main and secondary outcomes were assessed at the last follow-up visit, and included UDVA, CDVA, UIVA, DCIVA, UNVA and DCNVA, refraction, CS, pupil diameter, spectacle dependence, and presence of dysphotopsia, as described in the preoperative examination. Patient satisfaction was also assessed with the VF-14 test, consisting of 14 questions evaluating various patient activities (Figure 1). The validity and reproducibility of this test have already been reported [8, 9].

2.5. Statistical Analysis

2.5.1. Sample Size. Sixty-four eyes (32 patients) were required per group to detect a statistically significant difference of at least 0.15 in VA between the two groups with statistical power of 80% and an alpha error of 0.05.

Patients were assigned randomly to the multifocal or monofocal group using a 1 : 1 block randomization scheme.

Table 1: Patient demographics and clinical information.

Parameter	Group 1 OptiVis	Group 2 AR40e	Group 3 M-Flex	Group 4 ReZoom	Group 5 ReSTOR	p value between groups
Number of patients	32	32	32	32	32	
Number of eyes	64	64	64	64	64	
Age (y)						1 versus 2 0.004[†]
Mean ± SD	67.0 ± 4.9	72.31 ± 3.26	70.3 ± 5.0	68.2 ± 6.1	69.2 ± 6.9	1 versus 3 0.184[†]
						1 versus 4 0.929[†]
Range	55; 74	63; 77	57; 76	52; 78	49; 77	1 versus 5 0.593[†]
Sex (F)						1 versus 2 0.296[*]
						1 versus 3 0.196[*]
Percentage	72%	59%	56%	66%	56%	1 versus 4 0.593[*]
						1 versus 5 0.196[*]
UDVA (logMAR)						1 versus 2 0.029[*]
Mean ± SD	0.75 ± 0.36	0.55 ± 0.30	0.56 ± 0.25	0.61 ± 0.33	0.52 ± 0.28	1 versus 3 0.051[*]
						1 versus 4 0.124[*]
Range	1.30; 0.22	1.30; 0.15	1.00; 0.15	1.30; 0.22	1.30; 0.15	1 versus 5 0.072[*]
CDVA (logMAR)						1 versus 2 0.003[*]
Mean ± SD	0.39 ± 0.21	0.24 ± 0.11	0.26 ± 0.11	0.21 ± 0.10	0.24 ± 0.12	1 versus 3 0.020[*]
						1 versus 4 0.000[*]
Range	1.00; 0.15	0.52; 0.05	0.52; 0.10	0.52; 0.05	0.52; 0.05	1 versus 5 0.003[*]
UNVA (logMAR)						1 versus 2 0.030[*]
Mean ± SD	0.67 ± 0.36	0.50 ± 0.34	0.64 ± 0.44	0.58 ± 0.47	0.59 ± 0.41	1 versus 3 0.395[*]
						1 versus 4 0.058[*]
Range	1.30; 0.10	1.30; 0.00	1.30; 0.00	2.00; 0.10	1.30; 0.00	1 versus 5 0.204[*]
DCNVA (logMAR)						1 versus 2 0.000[*]
Mean ± SD	0.49 ± 0.15	0.15 ± 0.12	0.17 ± 0.14	0.14 ± 0.11	0.16 ± 0.12	1 versus 3 0.000[*]
						1 versus 4 0.000[*]
Range	0.80; 0.10	0.40; 0.00	0.52; 0.00	0.30; 0.00	0.40; 0.00	1 versus 5 0.000[*]
SE (D) RE						1 versus 2 0.876[*]
Mean ± SD	−0.74 ± 2.66	−0.77 ± 2.12	−0.09 ± 1.77	−0.41 ± 2.50	0.20 ± 1.92	1 versus 3 0.427[*]
						1 versus 4 0.604[*]
Range	−6.00; 3.75	−4.75; 3.75	−4.50: 3.75	−5.50; 3.00	−4.00; 3.25	1 versus 5 0.189[*]
SE (D) LE						1 versus 2 0.755[*]
Mean ± SD	−0.50 ± 2.65	−0.20 ± 2.04	0.03 ± 1.94	−0.44 ± 2.70	−0.02 ± 2.58	1 versus 3 0.406[*]
						1 versus 4 0.859[*]
Range	−6.00; 4.00	−5.25; 3.5	−4.75; 3.75	−5.75; 3.75	−10.00; 3.75	1 versus 5 0.350[*]

[†]ANOVA post hoc; [*]Mann–Whitney; y, years; SD, standard deviation; F, female; UDVA, uncorrected distance visual acuity; CDVA, corrected distance visual acuity; UNVA, uncorrected near visual acuity; DCNVA, distance-corrected near visual acuity; SE, spherical equivalent; D, diopters; RE, right eye; LE, left eye.

All data were collected in an Excel database (Office 2010, Microsoft Corporation), and statistical analyses were performed using SPSS for Windows software (version 22, SPSS Inc., Chicago, IL).

Normality of all data was evaluated using the Kolmogorov–Smirnov test. When parametric analysis was not possible, the differences between preoperative and postoperative data were evaluated with the Mann–Whitney U test. The test was also used for comparison of OptiVis with other types of IOL individually for all the parameters except age and CS, which were compared with ANOVA post hoc. The Kruskal–Wallis test was used to detect differences among all groups.

The results are presented as linear diagrams, where the medians are connected and the standard deviation (SD) of each median is presented as a vertical line, and by box plot diagrams, where the bottom and top of the box correspond to the first and third quartiles, and the band inside the box corresponds to the second quartile (the median);

the point outside the box is the value between 1.5 and 3 box lengths, while the asterisk represents a value greater than 3 lengths.

Demographic data were used to check whether the preoperative characteristics of the groups differed statistically. The results are expressed as mean ± SD. For all statistical tests, a p value of less than 0.05 was considered as statistically significant.

3. Results

Each IOL group comprised 64 eyes of 32 patients. All patients completed the 3-month follow-up. No eye was excluded from analysis because of intraoperative or postoperative complications. Although significant differences between OptiVis and AR40e were observed, we assumed that this was aleatory, as it was a randomized clinical trial (Table 1). There was no significant difference in any parameter, except initial

TABLE 2: Characteristics of IOLs implanted in 160 patients who underwent cataract surgery.

Data	OptiVis	AR40e	M-Flex	ReZoom	ReSTOR
Manufacturer	Aaren Scientific	AMO	Rayner	AMO-Abbott	Alcon
Material	Hydrophilic acrylic, single piece	Hydrophobic acrylic with PMMA modified C haptic, three piece	Hydrophilic acrylic, single piece	Hydrophobic acrylic with PMMA modified C haptic, three piece	Hydrophobic acrylic, single piece
Optics	Hybrid (refractive and diffractive properties) multifocal, biconvex, aspheric	Monofocal, biconvex, aspheric	Refractive multifocal anterior surface, aspheric	Refractive multifocal anterior surface, aspheric	Diffractive multifocal
Near add spectacle plane	+2.80 D	0 D	+2.25 D	+2.50 D	+3.20 D
Light distribution	2 mm pupil diameter: 33% near, 38% intermediate, 27% far focus 5 mm pupil diameter: 20% near, 6% intermediate, 60% far focus	100% far focus	2 mm pupil diameter: 18% near, 17% intermediate, 64% far focus 5 mm pupil diameter: 29% near, 10% intermediate, 60% far focus	2 mm pupil diameter: 0% near, 17% intermediate, 80% far focus 5 mm pupil diameter: 30% near focus, 9% intermediate, 60% far focus	2 mm pupil diameter: 38% near, 40% far focus 5 mm pupil diameter: 10% near, 84% far focus
Pupil dependence	Yes	No	Yes	Yes	Yes
Dimensions	Total diameter 11 mm; optic diameter 6 mm	Total diameter 13 mm; optic diameter 6 mm	Total diameter 12.5 mm; optic diameter 6.25 mm	Total diameter 13 mm; optic diameter 6 mm	Total diameter 13 mm; optic diameter 6 mm
Available powers	+10.00 D ÷ +30.00 D in 0.50 D increment	+10.00 D ÷ +30.00 D in 0.50 D increment	+14.00 D ÷ +25.00 D in 0.50 D increment	+6.00 D ÷ +30.00 D in 0.50 D increment	+10.00 D ÷ +30.00 D in 0.50 D increment

IOL, intraocular lens; mm, millimeter; D, diopter.

CDVA and DCNVA between groups of previously studied MFIOLs (M-Flex, ReZoom, and ReSTOR) and OptiVis (Table 1), so comparison was possible.

3.1. Visual Acuity and Refraction. Postoperative VA improved after implantation of OptiVis and AR40e IOLs. Significant differences were found when postoperative and preoperative results were compared for all distance and near uncorrected and corrected VA in the OptiVis group ($p < 0.001$), while this difference was not observed in UNVA in the AR40e group ($p = 0.321$). When postoperative results were compared between these studied groups, differences were detected for all VA, except distance VA, as seen in Table 3.

VA was contrasted between all MFIOLs at the final visit and presented in Table 3. No differences in UDVA and CDVA were noticed. Diffractive IOL performed significantly better than OptiVis in UNVA ($p < 0.009$), but this difference became insignificant in DCNVA. While in DCNVA, OptiVis acted significantly better than M-Flex and ReZoom ($p < 0.001$, 0.004, resp.), as noted in Table 3. Figure 2 shows pre- and postoperative visual performance (UDVA and UNVA) of all five IOLs.

As OptiVis was supposed to provide good intermediate VA, we checked the outcomes in this group. The preoperative mean ± SD logMAR UIVA and DCIVA were 0.8 ± 0.33 and 0.23 ± 0.22, respectively, and postoperatively were 0.54 ± 0.31

and 0.04 ± 0.06, respectively. As shown in Figure 3, post-operative UIVA and DCIVA gain were significant ($p < 0.001$ for both).

The predictability of the refractive outcome was good with postoperative mean ± SD spherical equivalent (SE) of 0.17 ± 0.58 and SE within ±0.50 D of the attempted spherical correction in 26 eyes (80%) and within ±1.00 D in 30 eyes (94%) in the OptiVis group. SE was slightly hyperopic in the OptiVis and ReSTOR groups and slightly myopic in the M-Flex and ReZoom groups (Table 3).

3.2. Contrast Sensitivity. After cataract surgery in both studied IOLs, multifocal (OptiVis) and monofocal (AR40e), CS at all frequencies: 1.5, 3, 6, 12, and 18 cpd, improved significantly ($p < 0.001$). Under mesopic conditions without glare, distance CS with the multifocal IOL was significantly lower than with the monofocal IOL at any tested frequencies (1.5 cpd, $p < 0.001$; 3 cpd, $p = 0.004$; 6 cpd, $p = 0.022$; 12 cpd, $p = 0.012$; and 18 cpd, $p = 0.017$, Kruskal–Wallis), as seen in Figure 4. There was no significant difference between MFIOLs performance after surgery, as presented in Table 4.

3.3. Spectacle Independence Evaluation, Dysphotopic Phenomena, and Visual Function. The participants used

Patient name: _____ DOB: _____ Date of visit: _____

VF-14 QOL questionnaire

Because of your vision, how much difficulty do you have with the following activities?
Check the box that best describes how much difficulty you have, even with glasses.
If you do not perform the activity for reasons unrelated to your vision, circle "n/a"

Activity		None	A little	Moderate	Great deal	Unable to do
1. Reading small print, such as medicine bottle labels, a telephone book, or food labels	n/a	☐	☐	☐	☐	☐
2. Reading a newspaper or a book	n/a	☐	☐	☐	☐	☐
3. Reading a large-print book or large-print newspaper or numbers on a telephone	n/a	☐	☐	☐	☐	☐
4. Recognizing people when they are close to you	n/a	☐	☐	☐	☐	☐
5. Seeing steps, stairs or curbs	n/a	☐	☐	☐	☐	☐
6. Reading traffic signs, street signs or store signs	n/a	☐	☐	☐	☐	☐
7. Doing fine handwork like sewing, knitting, crocheting, carpentry	n/a	☐	☐	☐	☐	☐
8. Writing checks or filling out forms	n/a	☐	☐	☐	☐	☐
9. Playing games such as bingo, dominos, card games, or mahjong	n/a	☐	☐	☐	☐	☐
10. Taking part in sports like bowling, handball, tennis, golf	n/a	☐	☐	☐	☐	☐
11. Cooking	n/a	☐	☐	☐	☐	☐
12. Watching television	n/a	☐	☐	☐	☐	☐
13. Driving during the day	n/a	☐	☐	☐	☐	☐
14. Driving at night	n/a	☐	☐	☐	☐	☐

Patient signature: _____

Office use only: (C) # checked boxes in column _____

(F) factored amounts   X4 = ____   X3 = ____   X2 = ____   X1 = ____   0

C = total number of checked boxes in column

F = sum of the factored amounts   Final score: (F _____ / C _____) × 25 = V

V = Final V-14 score   V= [   ]

VF-14 QOL questionnaire_10-28-09   MD signature: _____

FIGURE 1

spectacles less often after surgery ($p < 0.001$); 16% and 9% of patients declared spectacle independence for far distance in the OptiVis and AR40e groups ($p = 0.436$), and 50% and 13% for near distance, respectively, with significantly less spectacle dependence for near in the OptiVis group ($p = 0.001$). In general, there were no differences in spectacle independence between MFIOLs at tested distances, except for ReZoom at far distance ($p = 0.021$) and ReSTOR at near distance ($p = 0.004$) when compared with OptiVis (Table 5).

There were no differences in dysphotopsia spontaneously mentioned in the pre- and postoperative assessment ($p = 0.796$) or in the questionnaire ($p = 0.802$) in the OptiVis group. There were also no differences between MFIOLs (Table 5).

Visual function evaluation by VF-14 questionnaire showed that patients with bilateral OptiVis implantation

TABLE 3: Postoperative binocular visual acuity results at 3-month follow-up.

Parameter	Group 1 OptiVis	Group 2 (AR40e)	Group 3 M-Flex	Group 4 ReZoom	Group 5 ReSTOR	p value* between groups
Number of patients	32	32	32	32	32	
Number of eyes	64	64	64	64	64	
UDVA (logMAR)						1 versus 2 0.076
Mean ± SD	0.13 ± 0.12	0.08 ± 0.08	0.13 ± 0.11	0.09 ± 0.07	0.12 ± 0.10	1 versus 3 0.800 / 1 versus 4 0.091
Range	0.52; 0.00	0.30; 0.00	0.40; 0.00	0.30; 0.00	0.40; 0.00	1 versus 5 0.864
CDVA (logMAR)						1 versus 2 0.094
Mean ± SD	0.07 ± 0.05	0.04 ± 0.05	0.09 ± 0.09	0.07 ± 0.06	0.08 ± 0.07	1 versus 3 0.198 / 1 versus 4 0.989
Range	0.30; 0.00	0.15; 0.00	0.15; 0.00	0.30; 0.00	0.30; 0.00	1 versus 5 0.501
UNVA (logMAR)						1 versus 2 0.000
Mean ± SD	0.20 ± 0.14	0.43 ± 0.27	0.23 ± 0.16	0.17 ± 0.13	0.12 ± 0.13	1 versus 3 0.269 / 1 versus 4 0.437
Range	0.52; 0.00	1.30; 0.00	0.70; 0.00	0.52; 0.00	0.40; 0.00	1 versus 5 0.009
DCNVA (logMAR)						1 versus 2 0.000
Mean ± SD	0.09 ± 0.06	0.43 ± 0.27	0.25 ± 0.17	0.18 ± 0.13	0.11 ± 0.13	1 versus 3 0.000 / 1 versus 4 0.004
Range	0.22; 0.00	1.30; 0.00	0.70; 0.00	0.40; 0.00	0.40; 0.00	1 versus 5 0.824
SE (D) RE						1 versus 2 0.001
Mean ± SD	0.21 ± 0.59	−0.26 ± 0.49	−0.19 ± 0.39	−0.10 ± 0.28	0.04 ± 0.47	1 versus 3 0.002 / 1 versus 4 0.011
Range	−1.50; 1.00	−1.75; 0.75	−1.00; 0.75	−1.00; 0.25	−1.50; 1.00	1 versus 5 0.296
SE (D) LE						1 versus 2 0.005
Mean ± SD	0.14 ± 0.65	−0.28 ± 0.58	−0.13 ± 0.39	−0.08 ± 0.31	0.20 ± 0.50	1 versus 3 0.026 / 1 versus 4 0.054
Range	−1.25; 2.00	−2.75; 0.5	−1.00; 0.75	−1.00; −0.50	−1.25; 1.25	1 versus 5 0.420

*Mann–Whitney; SD, standard deviation; UDVA, uncorrected distance visual acuity; CDVA, corrected distance visual acuity; UNVA, uncorrected near visual acuity; DCNVA, distance-corrected near visual acuity; SE, spherical equivalent; D, diopter; RE, right eye; LE, left eye.

were more satisfied than monofocal users ($p = 0.015$). As shown in Figure 5, patients' satisfaction was high after the multifocal procedure. OptiVis and ReSTOR had the highest scores in the VF-14 survey: 89.28 ± 11.11 and 89.51 ± 14.85, respectively, but the results were not statistically different from other MFIOLs (Table 5).

4. Discussion

MFIOLs provide spectacle independence after cataract surgery. The classic design (refractive or diffractive) allows bifocality with good visual function at distance and near but with poor intermediate vision. More recent models were designed to have lower near addition to improve intermediate vision. However, these IOLs still provide only average visual results for intermediate distances or improve intermediate vision at the expense of near VA [10], so better solutions are sought. A new idea was to fuse two classical designs in one MFIOL. OptiVis, a hybrid MFIOL, currently unique on the market to our knowledge, has three different zones: (1) a progressive power refractive zone within central diameter of 1.5 mm that allows far and intermediate vision, (2) a diffractive apodized bifocal zone with a diameter of 1.5–3.8 mm that allows far and near vision for a full range of pupil sizes and less halos, and (3) aspheric distance periphery to improve CS. We compared the visual performance of

OptiVis to monofocal IOL (AR40e) in a clinical setting. We also compared the results of this clinical trial with our previously unpublished study, as we considered it interesting to assess the superiority of a hybrid model over refractive (M-Flex, Rayner, ReZoom, and AMO) and diffractive (ReSTOR and Alcon) MFIOLs. As we know, ReZoom and ReSTOR have been for years the reference in refractive and diffractive design, with which the new multifocal lens models were usually compared.

As expected, there were no significant differences in UDVA and CDVA between all studied MFIOLs and monofocal IOLs ($p = 0.131$, Kruskal–Wallis), but MFIOLs performed much better in UNVA and DCNVA ($p < 0.001$ for both, Kruskal–Wallis). Randomized, controlled trials (RCTs) [11–15] and meta-analyses of RCTs [1, 16, 17] comparing the results of multifocal and monofocal IOLs concluded that uncorrected near vision is improved by implantation of a multifocal IOL, resulting in lower spectacle dependence for near tasks without compromising distance VA [18, 19], as shown in our study: OptiVis patients were less spectacle dependent for near vision than AR40e patients ($p = 0.001$). No statistical differences were found in distance VA between different MFIOLs [20], as in our study.

After 3-month follow-up, VA of 0.3 logMAR in UDVA, UIVA, and UNVA was achieved by 93.75%, 93.75%, and

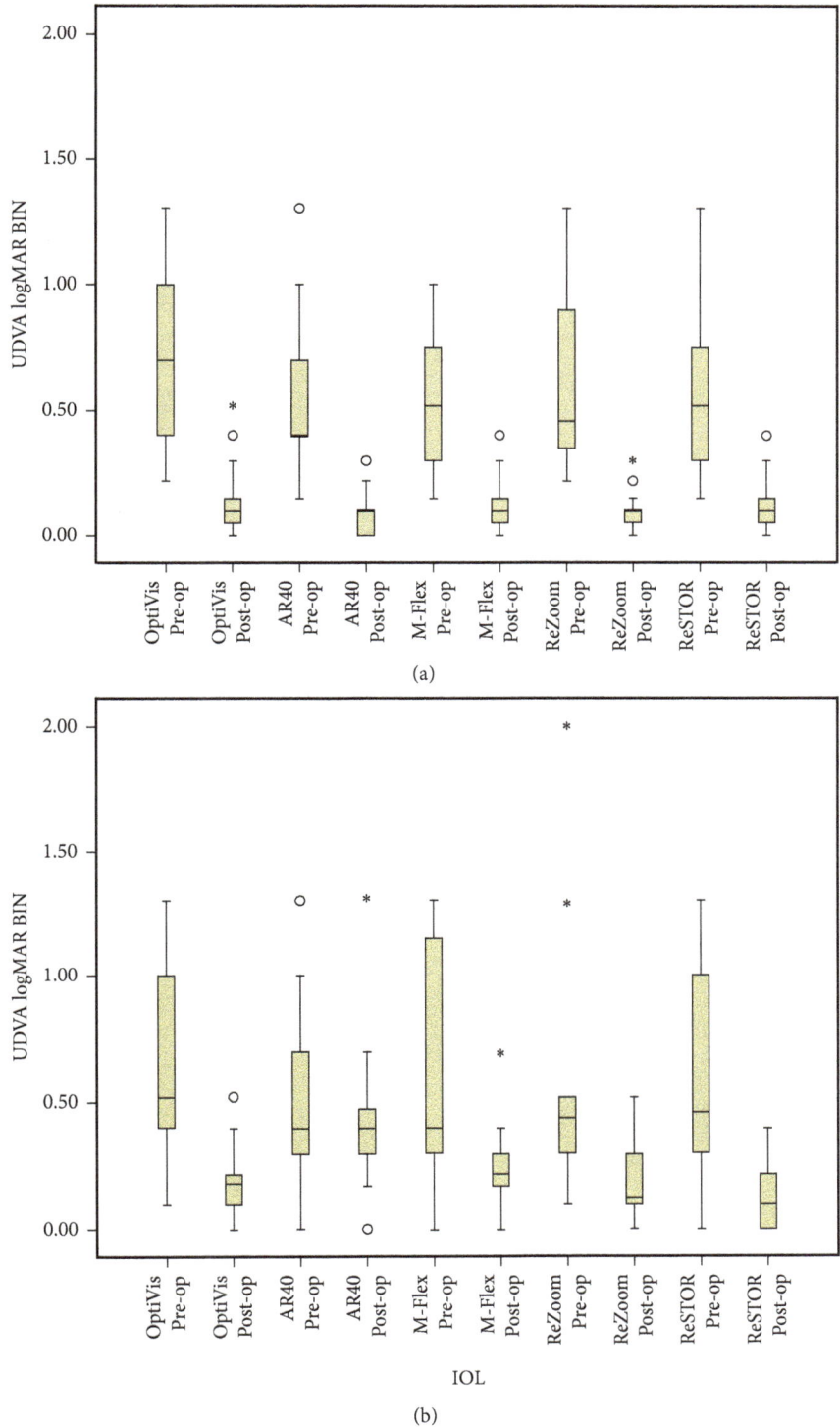

FIGURE 2: Pre- and postoperative visual performance of (a) UDVA and (b) UNVA of all five IOLs. UDVA BIN: binocular uncorrected distance visual acuity; UNVA BIN: binocular uncorrected near visual acuity; IOL: intraocular lens.

81.25% of OptiVis patients, respectively, compared to 3-month outcomes after bilateral OptiVis implantation in the study by Piovella and Bosc [6] 96.8%, 71.3%, and 92.6%, respectively. The difference between our study and Piovella's [6] in UIVA and UNVA might be caused by a choice of distinct measures in

intermediate (60 cm versus 70 cm, resp.) and near distance (33 cm versus 40 cm, resp.). The choice of 60 and 33 cm was dictated by distance measurements in our previously conducted study in order to be able to compare OptiVis with refractive and diffractive IOLs as we wanted to assess the superiority of the

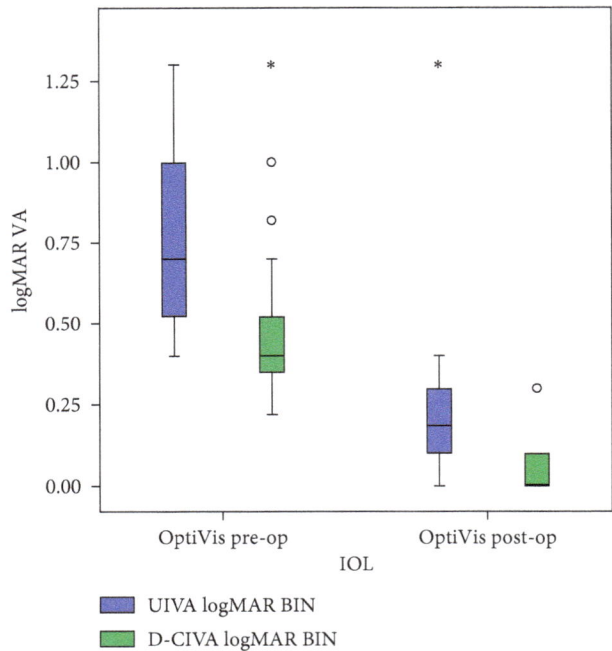

FIGURE 3: Binocular UIVA and DCIVA pre- and postoperative results in the OptiVis group. UIVA BIN: binocular uncorrected intermediate visual acuity; DCIVA BIN: binocular distance-corrected intermediate visual acuity; IOL: intraocular lens.

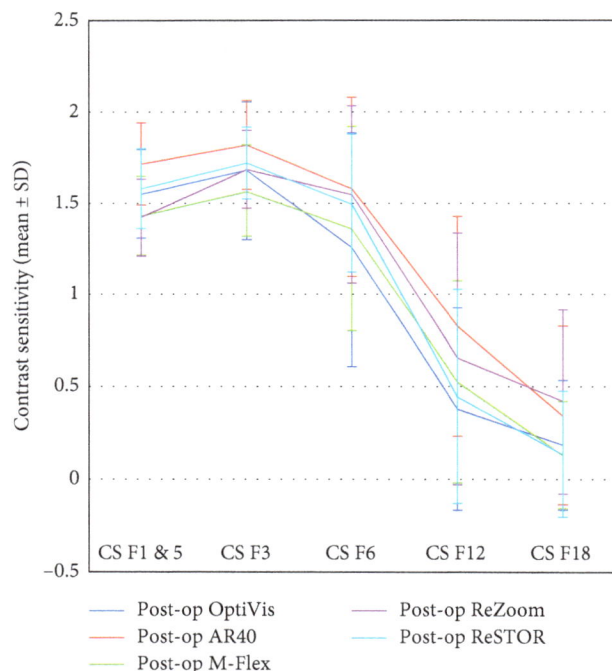

FIGURE 4: Postoperative mesopic log contrast sensitivity function at far distances without glare in all five IOLs. IOL: intraocular lens; SD: standard deviation; CS: contrast sensitivity; spatial frequencies of 1.5, 3, 6, 12, and 18 cycles per degree.

hybrid model. Moreover, as far as we know, 60 and 33 cm are used frequently in literature in order to check visual outcomes. On the contrary, we could not expect that other studies using OptiVis with perhaps other distances would not be published.

Bilateral OptiVis implantation after cataract extraction provided useful UIVA and DCIVA to our patients. Mean logMAR VA in DCIVA was much higher in our study (0.04 ± 0.06) than in the spherical diffractive (0.38 ± 0.14) and aspheric diffractive MFIOLs (0.14 ± 0.17) at the 60 cm distance [10]. Binocular UIVA was significantly better in the refractive MFIOLs than in the diffractive MFIOLs [21] and was similar to OptiVis results. In the study by Chiam et al. [22], UIVA was 0.24 ± 0.1 in the ReZoom group, similar to the results obtained for the OptiVis group (0.23 ± 0.22).

MFIOLs, as we know, provide good vision in wide range of distances, but intermediate vision might be insufficient for daily life. That is why MFIOL design is currently evolving. Progress towards trifocal IOLs with useful third focus for intermediate vision is a good example. According to many studies, trifocal IOLs improved intermediate vision when compared with bifocal IOLs, without impairing distance and near vision [23–25], but another study reported that bifocal IOLs provide similar UIVA [26]. To our knowledge, there are only 2 systematic reviews and meta-analysis published [27, 28]. Unfortunately, none included OptiVis. In both studies, the quality of the evidence in terms of intermediate VA was very low, as there was a limited number of studies [24, 26, 29] included, and heterogeneity was high. Mean UIVA in the trifocal group was insignificantly better than that in the bifocal group, but when analyzing the defocus curves, trifocal IOLs had significantly better performance [27, 28]. The mean UIVA in the trifocal group was 0.33 ± 0.10 (70 cm, Finevision Micro F, PhysIOL S.A.) [26], 0.06 ± 0.07 (66 cm, AT LISA Tri 839 MP, Carl Zeiss Meditec, Dublin, CA) [29], and 0.07 ± 0.05 (66 cm, Finevision Micro F) [24]. As seen, our results (0.23 ± 0.22) were better than the ones of Jonker et al. [26] but clearly worse than two other studies included in the meta-analysis [24, 29]. Although the meta-analysis did not support superiority of trifocal IOLs in intermediate VA, there are increasing number of studies providing excellent results of trifocal IOLs as the one of Bilbao-Calabuig et al. [30] where binocular mean UIVA measured at 80 cm in 4282 eyes (AT LISA Tri 839 MP) and 5802 eyes (Finevision Micro F) was -0.05 ± 0.14 and -0.05 ± 0.12, respectively.

Extended depth of focus (EDOF) IOLs are the latest variation. Tecnis Symfony IOL (Abbott Medical Optics, Inc.) differs from multifocal IOLs, as it provides a continuous range of vision by spreading out light along a range, instead of splitting it between two distinct points. By minimizing chromatic aberration, the lens is maximizing image quality and contrast. Its weakness is suboptimal VA in near distance. Although there are still only few studies published, EDOF IOLs provided successful visual restoration after cataract surgery with excellent visual outcomes across all distances [31]. UIVA mean values are similar to or better than those obtained for different types of multifocal IOLs, including diffractive bifocal and trifocal IOLs [11, 24, 32–36]. Cochener et al. [31] noted mean binocular UIVA of 0.13 ± 0.16 (70 cm), while Pedrotti et al. [36] noted mean binocular UIVA of 0.10 ± 0.09 (60 cm), much better than intermediate VA outcomes in OptiVis patients. In Pedrotti's study [36], UIVA of 20/32 (in Snellen) was reached by 100% of patients with Tecnis Symfony IOL (60 cm), whereas only by 40.6% of our OptiVis (60 cm) and 44.3% of Piovella's patients (70 cm) [6].

TABLE 4: Mesopic log contrast sensitivity function at far distances without glare in multifocal intraocular lenses at 3-month follow-up.

Parameter	Group 1 OptiVis	Group 3 M-flex	Group 4 ReZoom	Group 5 ReSTOR	p value*
Number of patients	32	32	32	32	
Number of eyes	64	64	64	64	
CS at 1.5 cpd					1 versus 3 0.288
Mean ± SD	1.56 ± 0.25	1.43 ± 0.22	1.42 ± 0.21	1.58 ± 0.22	1 versus 4 0.222
					1 versus 5 0.996
CS at 3 cpd					1 versus 3 0.560
Mean ± SD	1.68 ± 0.38	1.57 ± 0.25	1.68 ± 0.21	1.72 ± 0.19	1 versus 4 1.000
					1 versus 5 0.986
CS at 6 cpd					1 versus 3 0.968
Mean ± SD	1.26 ± 0.66	1.36 ± 0.56	1.56 ± 0.49	1.50 ± 0.38	1 versus 4 0.293
					1 versus 5 0.503
CS at 12 cpd					1 versus 3 0.909
Mean ± SD	0.38 ± 0.54	0.53 ± 0.55	0.66 ± 0.68	0.45 ± 0.57	1 versus 4 0.482
					1 versus 5 0.994
CS at 18 cpd					1 versus 3 0.986
Mean ± SD	0.19 ± 0.34	0.13 ± 0.29	0.48 ± 0.49	0.14 ± 0.34	1 versus 4 0.240
					1 versus 5 0.994

*ANOVA post hoc; CS, contrast sensitivity; spatial frequencies of 1.5, 3, 6, 12, and 18 cycles per degree; SD, standard deviation.

TABLE 5: Visual function in multifocal IOLs at 3-month follow-up.

Parameter	Group 1 OptiVis	Group 3 M-Flex	Group 4 ReZoom	Group 5 ReSTOR	p value*
Number of patients	32	32	32	32	
Number of eyes	64	64	64	64	
Spectacle dependence (far)	16	3	0	6	1 versus 3 0.089
					1 versus 4 0.021
					1 versus 5 0.223
Spectacle dependence (near)	50	44	44	16	1 versus 3 0.619
					1 versus 4 0.619
					1 versus 5 0.004
Presence of dysphotopsia (spontaneously mentioned)	34	25	41	25	1 versus 3 0.415
					1 versus 4 0.608
					1 versus 5 0.415
Presence of dysphotopsia (by questionnaire)	59	53	59	38	1 versus 3 0.617
					1 versus 4 1.000
					1 versus 5 0.082
Visual function					1 versus 3 0.286
Mean ± SD	89.28 ± 11.11	84.62 ± 13.91	87.73 ± 11.19	89.51 ± 14.85	1 versus 4 0.686
Range	50.00; 100.00	55.36; 100.00	58.93; 100.00	37.50; 100.00	1 versus 5 0.300

*Mann–Whitney; SD, standard deviation.

The four MFIOLs studied (OptiVis, M-Flex, ReZoom, and ReSTOR) were compared for near vision. OptiVis and ReSTOR had better DCNVA than refractive models, but OptiVis performed worse than diffractive MFIOL in UNVA and equal to refractive MFIOLs. Our results in UNVA are similar to those presented by Piovella and Bosc [6]. Cumulative UNVA of 20/25 or better (in Snellen) was achieved by 37.4% of our patients and by 40.4% of Piovella's patients [6]. Diffractive IOL performed better in UNVA, as it has higher addition (+4.0 D) [37]. Moreover, in the hybrid lens, intermediate focus is potentiated at the expense of near focus. This was reflected in significantly less spectacle dependence for near vision in ReSTOR, but such strong addition impaired intermediate VA and led to a really short reading distance

[38]. This was the reason for lowering addition to +3 D in a newer model of ReSTOR. Moreover, slightly hyperopic postoperative SE was observed in the OptiVis group, and this could also partially prejudice the UNVA (Table 3).

Despite the benefits of uncorrected VA at various distances, MFIOLs are associated with certain disadvantages. Firstly, they provide lower CS when compared with monofocal IOLs [11, 13, 39], especially in mesopic conditions [40], as confirmed by our findings. Although CS in individuals with multifocal IOLs is diminished, it is generally within the normal range of contrast in age-matched phakic individuals [41]. Patients in our study did not have a reduction in CS after implantation of the OptiVis. Moreover, they improved significantly ($p < 0.001$) in low

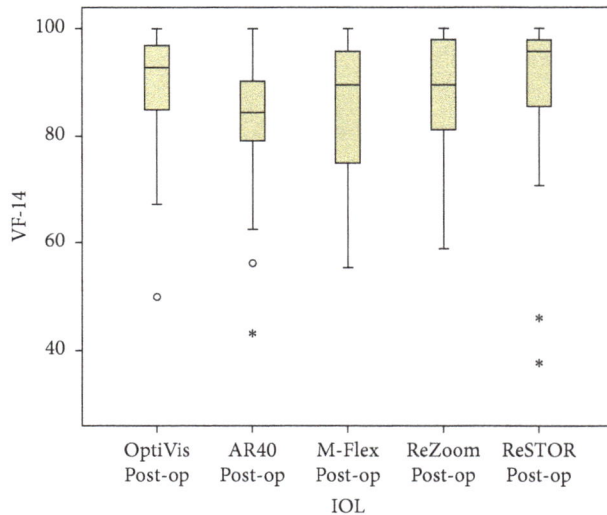

FIGURE 5: Visual function (VF-14) results in multifocal intraocular lens. VF-14: visual function test; IOL: intraocular lens.

cpd and gained significantly ($p = 0.003$) in the high frequencies (12 and 18 cpd) due to cataract surgery. These results were comparable to a previously published report by Hohberger et al. [42], who evaluated CS in normal subjects in a similar age cohort. Our results could not be compared to those reported by Piovella and Bosc [6], as they studied CS in photopic and scotopic conditions after glare. Although diffractive MFIOLs cause light energy dispersion among the secondary orders of diffraction, they appear to be comparable to refractive multifocal IOLs in terms of CS [43, 44], as seen in our study.

Secondly, halos and glare are more often reported with a multifocal IOL than with a monofocal lens [1]. Nevertheless, OptiVis patients did not complain, as no differences were observed in the incidence of dysphotopsia before and after surgery ($p = 0.796$ for dysphotopsia spontaneously mentioned and $p = 0.802$ when asked). Fifty-nine percent of OptiVis patients reported dysphotopsia postoperatively, similar to the 54% of patients in the study by Piovella and Bosc [6] We did not observe differences between MFIOL groups (Kruskal–Wallis test: $p = 0.458$ for dysphotopsias spontaneously mentioned and $p = 0.254$ when asked), although the literature suggests that refractive MFIOLs are associated with more dysphotopic phenomena than diffractive MFIOLs [11]. However, Cochener et al. [2] did not find any significant differences in the incidence of halos with different types of multifocal IOLs, which is consistent with our findings.

Patients demonstrate high satisfaction with bilateral cataract surgery. According to a meta-analysis by de Silva et al. [1], there were no significant differences in visual function in far distance reported by patients with multifocal and monofocal implantation, but MFIOLs obtained a better score in visual function when evaluating tasks at near distance [11, 13, 14]. Satisfaction was higher in the OptiVis group than in the AR40e group ($p = 0.015$). VF-14 mean ± SD score was 89.3 ± 11.1 in OptiVis patients, comparable to the 89.5 ± 12.6 found in the study by Nijkamp et al. [14].

Patients' comfort with MFIOLs was high and similar to previously published studies [1].

In summary, patients with bilateral implantation of OptiVis were satisfied, although uncorrected intermediate and near VA were not optimal. As mentioned, intermediate VA of our patients with OptiVis was similar to the previously published results with refractive MFIOLs and better than ReSTOR outcomes but worse than with trifocal and EDOF IOLs. DCNVA was better than with refractive MFIOLs, but UNVA was slightly worse than with diffractive MFIOL.

Although the idea seemed good in principle, VA should be better. Consequently, the emergence of trifocal IOLs and the search for new accommodative solutions are justified by the need to improve the quality of vision at all distances.

Conflicts of Interest

The authors declare that there are no conflicts of interest regarding the publication of this article.

Acknowledgments

The authors wish to thank Vladimir Poposki, MD for his help in the production of the manuscript.

References

[1] S. R. de Silva, J. R. Evans, V. Kirthi, M. Ziaei, and M. Leyland, "Multifocal versus monofocal intraocular lenses after cataract extraction," *Cochrane Database of Systematic Reviews*, vol. 12, p. CD003169, 2016.

[2] B. Cochener, A. Lafuma, B. Khoshnood, L. Courouve, and G. Berdeaux, "Comparison of outcomes with multifocal intraocular lenses: a meta-analysis," *Clinical Ophthalmology*, vol. 5, pp. 45–56, 2011.

[3] J. C. Javitt and R. F. Steinert, "Cataract extraction with multifocal intraocular lens implantation: a multinational clinical trial evaluating clinical, functional, and quality-of-life outcomes," *Ophthalmology*, vol. 107, no. 11, pp. 2040–2048, 2000.

[4] T. Kohnen, O. K. Klaproth, and J. Bühren, "Effect of intraocular lens asphericity on quality of vision after cataract removal: an intraindividual comparison," *Ophthalmology*, vol. 116, no. 9, pp. 1697–1706, 2009.

[5] P. F. Tzelikis, L. Akaishi, F. C. Trindade, and J. E. Boteon, "Spherical aberration and contrast sensitivity in eyes implanted with aspheric and spherical intraocular lenses: a comparative study," *American Journal of Ophthalmology*, vol. 145, no. 5, pp. 827–833, 2008.

[6] M. Piovella and J.-M. Bosc, "Clinical evaluation of the OptiVis™ multifocal intraocular lens," *Advances in Therapy*, vol. 28, no. 11, pp. 1012–1020, 2011.

[7] R. J. Cionni, R. H. Osher, M. E. Snyder, and M. L. Nordlund, "Visual outcome comparison of unilateral versus bilateral implantation of apodized diffractive multifocal intraocular lenses after cataract extraction: prospective 6-month study," *Journal of Cataract & Refractive Surgery*, vol. 35, no. 6, pp. 1033–1039, 2009.

[8] E. P. Steinberg, J. M. Tielsch, O. D. Schein et al., "National study of cataract surgery outcomes. Variation in 4-month postoperative outcomes as reflected in multiple outcome

measures," *Ophthalmology*, vol. 101, no. 6, pp. 1131–1140, 1994.

[9] S. D. Cassard, D. L. Patrick, A. M. Damiano et al., "Reproducibility and responsiveness of the VF-14. An index of functional impairment in patients with cataracts," *Archives of Ophthalmology*, vol. 113, no. 12, pp. 1508–1513, 1995.

[10] J. F. Alfonso, L. Fernández-Vega, C. Puchades, and R. Montés-Micó, "Intermediate visual function with different multifocal intraocular lens models," *Journal of Cataract & Refractive Surgery*, vol. 36, no. 5, pp. 733–739, 2010.

[11] S. Cillino, A. Casuccio, F. Di Pace et al., "One-year outcomes with new-generation multifocal intraocular lenses," *Ophthalmology*, vol. 115, no. 9, pp. 1508–1516, 2008.

[12] F. E. Harman, S. Maling, G. Kampougeris et al., "Comparing the 1CU accommodative, multifocal, and monofocal intraocular lenses: a randomized trial," *Ophthalmology*, vol. 115, no. 6, pp. 993–1001, 2008.

[13] G. Zhao, J. Zhang, Y. Zhou, L. Hu, C. Che, and N. Jiang, "Visual function after monocular implantation of apodized diffractive multifocal or single-piece monofocal intraocular lens. Randomized prospective comparison," *Journal of Cataract & Refractive Surgery*, vol. 36, no. 2, pp. 282–285, 2010.

[14] M. D. Nijkamp, M. G. T. Dolders, J. de Brabander, B. van den Borne, F. Hendrikse, and R. M. M. A. Nuijts, "Effectiveness of multifocal intraocular lenses to correct presbyopia after cataract surgery: a randomized controlled trial," *Ophthalmology*, vol. 111, no. 10, pp. 1832–1839, 2004.

[15] M. Zeng, Y. Liu, X. Liu et al., "Aberration and contrast sensitivity comparison of aspherical and monofocal and multifocal intraocular lens eyes," *Clinical & Experimental Ophthalmology*, vol. 35, no. 4, pp. 355–360, 2007.

[16] M. Leyland and E. Zinicola, "Multifocal versus monofocal intraocular lenses in cataract surgery," *Ophthalmology*, vol. 110, no. 9, pp. 1789–1798, 2003.

[17] D. Calladine, J. R. Evans, S. Shah, and M. Leyland, "Multifocal versus monofocal intraocular lenses after cataract extraction," *Cochrane Database of Systematic Reviews*, vol. 9, p. CD003169, 2012.

[18] N. E. de Vries and R. M. M. A. Nuijts, "Multifocal intraocular lenses in cataract surgery: literature review of benefits and side effects," *Journal of Cataract & Refractive Surgery*, vol. 39, no. 2, pp. 268–278, 2013.

[19] S. Shah, C. Peris-Martinez, T. Reinhard, and P. Vinciguerra, "Visual outcomes after cataract surgery: multifocal versus monofocal intraocular lenses," *Journal of Refractive Surgery*, vol. 31, no. 10, pp. 658–666, 2015.

[20] J. Lan, Y.-S. Huang, Y.-H. Dai, X.-M. Wu, J.-J. Sun, and L.-X. Xie, "Visual performance with accommodating and multifocal intraocular lenses," *International Journal of Ophthalmology*, vol. 10, no. 2, pp. 235–240, 2017.

[21] X. Xu, M.-M. Zhu, and H.-D. Zou, "Refractive versus diffractive multifocal intraocular lenses in cataract surgery: a meta-analysis of randomized controlled trials," *Journal of Refractive Surgery*, vol. 30, no. 9, pp. 634–644, 2014.

[22] P. J. T. Chiam, J. H. Chan, S. I. Haider, N. Karia, H. Kasaby, and R. K. Aggarwal, "Functional vision with bilateral ReZoom and ReSTOR intraocular lenses 6 months after cataract surgery," *Journal of Cataract & Refractive Surgery*, vol. 33, no. 12, pp. 2057–2061, 2007.

[23] K. G. Gundersen and R. Potvin, "Comparison of visual outcomes and subjective visual quality after bilateral implantation of a diffractive trifocal intraocular lens and blended implantation of apodized diffractive bifocal intraocular lenses," *Clinical Ophthalmology*, vol. 10, pp. 805–811, 2016.

[24] P. Mojzis, L. Kukuckova, K. Majerova, K. Liehneova, and D. P. Piñero, "Comparative analysis of the visual performance after cataract surgery with implantation of a bifocal or trifocal diffractive IOL," *Journal of Refractive Surgery*, vol. 30, no. 10, pp. 666–672, 2014.

[25] A. B. Plaza-Puche and J. L. Alio, "Analysis of defocus curves of different modern multifocal intraocular lenses," *European Journal of Ophthalmology*, vol. 26, no. 5, pp. 412–417, 2016.

[26] S. M. R. Jonker, N. J. C. Bauer, N. Y. Makhotkina, T. T. J. M. Berendschot, F. J. H. M. van den Biggelaar, and R. M. M. A. Nuijts, "Comparison of a trifocal intraocular lens with a +3.0 D bifocal IOL: results of a prospective randomized clinical trial," *Journal of Cataract & Refractive Surgery*, vol. 41, no. 8, pp. 1631–1640, 2015.

[27] Z. Xu, D. Cao, X. Chen, S. Wu, X. Wang, and Q. Wu, "Comparison of clinical performance between trifocal and bifocal intraocular lenses: A meta-analysis," *PLoS One*, vol. 12, no. 19, article e0186522, 2017.

[28] Z. Shen, Y. Lin, Y. Zhu, X. Liu, J. Yan, and K. Yao, "Clinical comparison of patient outcomes following implantation of trifocal or bifocal intraocular lenses: a systematic review and meta-analysis," *Scientific Reports*, vol. 7, p. 45337, 2017.

[29] B. Cochener, "Prospective clinical comparison of patient outcomes following implantation of trifocal or bifocal intraocular lenses," *Journal of Refractive Surgery*, vol. 32, no. 3, pp. 146–151, 2016.

[30] R. Bilbao-Calabuig, A. Llovet-Rausell, J. Ortega-Usobiaga et al., "Visual outcomes following bilateral implantation of two diffractive trifocal intraocular lenses in 10 084 eyes," vol. 179, no. 29, pp. 55–66, 2017.

[31] B. Cochener, "Clinical outcomes of a new extended range of vision intraocular lens: International Multicenter Concerto Study," *Journal of Cataract & Refractive Surgery*, vol. 42, no. 9, pp. 1268–1275, 2016.

[32] FT. A. Kretz, M. Gerl, R. Gerl, M. Müller, G. U. Auffarth, and ZKB00G Studyroup, "Clinical evaluation of a new pupil independent diffractive multifocal intraocular lens with a +2.75 D near addition: a European multicentre study," *British Journal of Ophthalmology*, vol. 99, no. 12, pp. 1655–1659, 2015.

[33] B. Cochener, J. Vryghem, P. Rozot et al., "Clinical outcomes with a trifocal intraocular lens: a multicenter study," *Journal of Refractive Surgery*, vol. 30, no. 11, pp. 762–768, 2014.

[34] J. F. Alfonso, C. Puchades, L. Fernández-Vega, R. Montés-Micó, B. Valcárcel, and T. Ferrer-Blasco, "Visual acuity comparison of 2 models of bifocal aspheric intraocular lenses," *Journal of Cataract & Refractive Surgery*, vol. 35, no. 4, pp. 672–676, 2009.

[35] T. Kohnen, C. Titke, and M. Böhm, "Trifocal intraocular lens implantation to treat visual demands in various distances following lens removal," *American Journal of Ophthalmology*, vol. 161, pp. 71–77.e1, 2016.

[36] E. Pedrotti, E. Bruni, E. Bonacci, R. Badalamenti, R. Mastropasqua, and G. Marchini, "Comparative analysis of the clinical outcomes with a monofocal and an extended range of vision intraocular lens," *Journal of Refractive Surgery*, vol. 32, no. 7, pp. 436–442, 2016.

[37] U. Unsal and G. Baser, "Evaluation of different power of near addition in two different multifocal intraocular lenses," *Journal of Ophthalmology*, vol. 2016, Article ID 1395302, 4 pages, 2016.

[38] M. R. Santhiago, S. E. Wilson, M. V. Netto et al., "Visual performance of an apodized diffractive multifocal intraocular lens with +3.00-D addition: 1-year follow-up," *Journal of Refractive Surgery*, vol. 27, no. 12, pp. 899–906, 2011.

[39] M. A. Gil, C. Varón, G. Cardona, F. Vega, and J. A. Buil, "Comparison of far and near contrast sensitivity in patients symmetrically implanted with multifocal and monofocal IOLs," *European Journal of Ophthalmology*, vol. 24, no. 1, pp. 44–52, 2014.

[40] J. F. Alfonso, C. Puchades, L. Fernández-Vega, C. Merayo, and R. Montés-Micó, "Contrast sensitivity comparison between AcrySof ReSTOR and Acri.LISA aspheric intraocular lenses," *Journal of Refractive Surgery*, vol. 26, no. 7, pp. 471–477, 2010.

[41] R. Montés-Micó, E. España, I. Bueno, W. N. Charman, and J. L. Menezo, "Visual performance with multifocal intraocular lenses: mesopic contrast sensitivity under distance and near conditions," *Ophthalmology*, vol. 111, no. 1, pp. 85–96, 2004.

[42] B. Hohberger, R. Laemmer, W. Adler, A. G. M. Juenemann, and F. K. Horn, "Measuring contrast sensitivity in normal subjects with OPTEC 6500: influence of age and glare," *Graefe's Archive for Clinical and Experimental Ophthalmology*, vol. 245, no. 12, pp. 1805–1814, 2007.

[43] C. Mesci, H. H. Erbil, A. Olgun, N. Aydin, B. Candemir, and A. A. Akçakaya, "Differences in contrast sensitivity between monofocal, multifocal and accommodating intraocular lenses: long-term results," *Clinical & Experimental Ophthalmology*, vol. 38, no. 8, pp. 768–777, 2010.

[44] A. Martínez Palmer, P. Gómez Faíña, A. España Albelda, M. Comas Serrano, D. Nahra Saad, and M. Castilla Céspedes, "Visual function with bilateral implantation of monofocal and multifocal intraocular lenses: a prospective, randomized, controlled clinical trial," *Journal of Refractive Surgery*, vol. 24, no. 3, pp. 257–264, 2008.

20

Clinical Outcomes of Sequential Intrastromal Corneal Ring Segments and an Extended Range of Vision Intraocular Lens Implantation in Patients with Keratoconus and Cataract

C. Lisa,[1] R. Zaldivar,[2] A. Fernández-Vega Cueto,[3] R. M. Sanchez-Avila ⓘ,[1] D. Madrid-Costa,[4] and J. F. Alfonso ⓘ[1]

[1]*Fernández-Vega Ophthalmological Institute, Oviedo, Spain*
[2]*Instituto Zaldivar, Mendoza, Argentina*
[3]*Centro de Oftalmología Barraquer, Barcelona, Spain*
[4]*Optics II Department, Faculty of Optics and Optometry, Universidad Complutense de Madrid, Madrid, Spain*

Correspondence should be addressed to J. F. Alfonso; j.alfonso@fernandez-vega.com

Academic Editor: Biju B. Thomas

Purpose. To evaluate efficacy, safety, and predictability of sequential Ferrara-type intrastromal corneal ring segments (ICRS) and an extended range of vision intraocular lens (IOL) implantation in patients with keratoconus and cataract. *Methods*. This study comprised patients with keratoconus and cataract that had ICRS implantation followed 6 months later by extended range of vision IOL implantation. The uncorrected distance visual acuity (UDVA), corrected distance visual acuity (CDVA), and residual refractive errors, analysed using vector analysis, were recorded preoperatively, 6 months after ICRS implantation, and 6 months after IOL implantation, respectively. *Results*. The study enrolled 17 eyes (11 patients). The mean UDVA (logMAR scale) was 1.15 ± 0.67 preoperatively, 0.88 ± 0.69 six months after ICRS implantation ($P = 0.005$), and 0.27 ± 0.18 six months after IOL implantation ($P < 0.0001$). The CDVA changed from 0.26 ± 0.15 (logMAR) before surgery to 0.17 ± 0.08 six months after Ferrara-type ICRS implantation ($P = 0.002$) and to 0.07 ± 0.06 six months after IOL implantation ($P < 0.0001$). The spherical equivalent and the refractive cylinder declined steeply after IOL implantation ($P < 0.001$). The magnitude of depth of focus was 2.60 ± 1.02 D. There were no statistically significant differences in visual acuity for a defocus range from +0.50 D to −0.50 D ($P > 0.1$). *Conclusion*. Sequential Ferrara-type ICRS and an extended range of vision IOL implantation provided good visual and refractive outcomes, being an effective, safe, and predictable procedure for the treatment of selected cases of patients with keratoconus and cataract. In addition, this approach provides an increase of tolerance to defocus.

1. Introduction

The most common human ocular afflictions are presbyopia and cataract [1]. Both presbyopia and cataract developments contribute to further decreased visual quality of keratoconic patients. Furthermore, it has been suggested that patients affected by keratoconus tend to develop cataracts sooner than others [2]. Several options have been proposed for replacement of the lens (either by refractive lens exchange or cataract removal). Toric intraocular lens (IOL) implantation has shown to be an effective and safe option to improve the uncorrected distance visual acuity (UDVA), corrected distance visual acuity (CDVA), and refractive error [3–10]. Multifocal toric IOL implantation has shown encouraging outcomes [11–13]. The main problem for these IOLs is that the corneal irregularities are still present after IOL implantation, and it could restrict the visual rehabilitation. In fact, it has been reported that keratoconic patients with more regular corneas obtained higher improvement in UDVA after cataract surgery and toric IOL implantation [8]. Another important challenge is the IOL power calculation. A combined procedure, instrastromal corneal ring segments (ICRS) implantation followed by cataract surgery with IOL implantation, has also been proposed [14, 15]. This approach could have a double benefit. By one way, ICRS implantation improves the corneal shape and consequently the visual quality; on the other hand, improving the corneal shape could help the IOL estimation [14]. Basing on this previous experience, we currently present a case series of patients affected by cataract and keratoconus who underwent ICRS implantation followed by an extended range of vision IOL implantation. By means of increasing the depth of focus, this approach has a two-fold objective: one is to improve the visual acuity from far to intermediate distances and the other is to increase the tolerance to defocus, making the IOL calculation a little less important.

2. Patients and Methods

This study was a retrospective longitudinal analysis of the visual and refractive results of sequential implantation of the Ferrara-type ICRS (AJL Ophthalmic, Spain) and an extended range of vision IOL implantation in eyes with keratoconus and cataract. It was carried out at Fernández-Vega Ophthalmological Institute, Oviedo, Spain. The tenets of the Declaration of Helsinki were followed, and full ethical approval from the institute was obtained. After receiving a full explanation of the nature and possible consequences of the study and surgery, all patients signed the informed consent.

The presence of keratoconus and cataract, contact lens intolerance, and a clear cornea, along with a minimum corneal thickness over 400 μm at the optical zone involved in the implantation (a general criterion for surgery), constituted the criteria for inclusion in the study. In addition, the keratoconus had to be stage I, II, or III according to the Amsler-Krumeich keratoconus classification. Keratoconus was diagnosed by combining computerised videokeratography of the anterior and posterior corneal surfaces (Sirius, CSO, Italy), K readings, and corneal pachymetry [16–18]. Contact lens use was discontinued 1 month prior to corneal topography.

The exclusion criteria defined for the study were previous corneal or intraocular surgery, history of herpetic keratitis, diagnosed autoimmune disease, systemic connective tissue disease, endothelial cell density < 2000 cells/mm², history of glaucoma or retinal detachment, macular degeneration or retinopathy, neuroophthalmic diseases, and history of ocular inflammation.

All eyes in this study received Ferrara-type ICRS (AJL Ophthalmic, Spain). These Ferrara-type ICRS are poly(-methyl methacrylate) with a triangular cross section that induces a prismatic effect on the cornea. The apical diameter of ICRS is 5.0 mm (AFR5) (the flat basis width is 0.6 mm) or 6.0 mm (AFR6) (the flat basis width is 0.8 mm), with variable thickness (0.15 mm to 0.30 mm with 0.05 mm steps) and arc lengths (90, 120, 150, and 210 degrees). The Ferrara-type ICRS were implanted following the nomogram used in previous studies [19–22]. The same surgeon (JFA) performed all the procedures using topical anaesthesia and following the standard procedure as previously described [19–22].

Postoperative treatment consisted of the combination of antibiotic (tobramycin, 3 mg/mL) and steroid (dexamethasone, 1 mg/mL) eye drops (Tobradex, Alcon Laboratories Inc., Fort Worth, Texas, USA) administered three times daily for 2 weeks.

TABLE 1: Patient demographics. Age, pre-ICRS implantation manifest refraction (spherical equivalent (SE), refractive sphere and cylinder) and prekeratometry (K) readings shown as mean ± standard deviation (SD) and range.

Characteristic	Value
Eyes (n)	17
Age (years)	59 ± 12.8
Mean SE (D)	−5.35 ± 5.09
Range	(+2.50 to −14.00)
Mean refractive sphere (D)	−3.97 ± 4.98
Range	(+3.50 to −13.00)
Mean refractive cylinder (D)	−2.77 ± 1.04
Range	(−1.50 to −5.00)
Mean minimum K (D)	47.06 ± 3.71
Range	(42.5 to 55.5)
Mean maximum K (D)	48.79 ± 3.69
Range	(45 to 57.75)

Cataract extraction with IOL implantation was performed 6 months after ICRS implantation. The IOL implanted was an extended range of vision IOL (Tecnis Symfony, Abbott Alb Inc.). The posterior surface of this IOL incorporates a 5.5 mm diffractive area which is aimed at compensating the eye's chromatic aberration and increasing the depth of focus. All surgeries in this study were performed by an experienced surgeon (JFA) using peribulbar anaesthesia and a 2.2 mm to 3.2 mm axis incision in order to reduce the preexisting astigmatism. Phacoemulsification was performed with the INFINITI vision system (Alcon Laboratories, Fort Worth, Texas). Phacoemulsification was followed by irrigation and aspiration of the cortex and IOL implantation in the capsular bag using the injector developed for the specific IOL.

Axial length and anterior segment size were measured with the IOLMaster biometer (Carl Zeiss Meditec, Germany, software version 5.4). We chose the SRK/T formula for IOL power calculation. In order to reduce the astigmatism, axis incisions were performed. In eyes with astigmatism less than 1.25 D, one axis incision (2.2 mm) was performed on the steepest meridian. In eyes with astigmatism higher than 1.50 D, two opposite axis incisions (3.2 mm) were created on the steepest meridian, as what previous authors have done in phacoemulsification [14, 15]. All incisions were performed with a bevel-up steel blade (Equipsa S.A., Madrid, Spain).

All patients had a complete ophthalmologic examination preoperatively, 6 months after ICRS implantation (before cataract surgery), and 6 months after IOL implantation.

The clinical measurement taken primarily included corneal topography (Sirius, CSO, Italy), anterior segment optical coherence tomography (Visante Zeiss Meditec, Germany), uncorrected (UDVA) and best-corrected (CDVA) distance visual acuity (ETDRS charts), and manifest and cycloplegic refractions. The Thibos and Horner [23] power method was used to assess presurgery and postsurgery refraction findings. Furthermore, through-focus monocular logMAR visual acuity (defocus curve) was also measured 6 months after IOL implantation. Patients observed a distance ETDRS chart through lenses that increased from +2.00

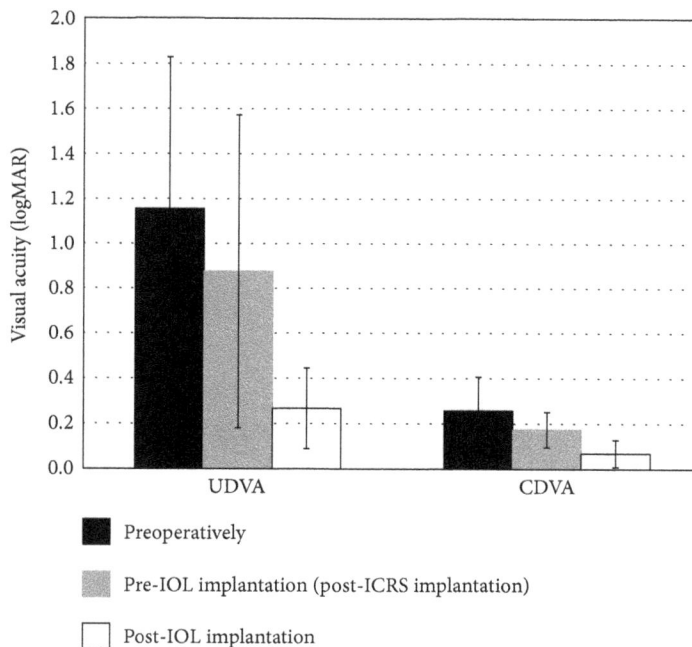

FIGURE 1: The uncorrected distance visual acuity (UDVA) and corrected distance visual acuity (CDVA) before surgery, 6 months after intrastromal corneal ring segments (ICRS) implantation, and 6 months after intraocular lens (IOL) implantation (efficacy).

to −5.00 D in 0.50 D steps. The magnitude of depth of focus depends on how it is defined, and for our study, we used the criterion that depth of focus is the range of focussing error for which the visual acuity does not decrease below two lines of CDVA.

Data analysis was performed using SPSS for Windows, version 14.0 (SPSS Inc., Chicago, IL). Normality was checked by the Kolmogorov-Smirnov test, and a repeated measures analysis of variance (ANOVA) was performed to compare outcomes. Differences were considered to be statistically significant when the P value was <0.01.

3. Results

This study comprised 17 eyes of 11 patients with a mean age of 59 ± 12.8 years old. Table 1 shows the patient's demographics.

Figure 1 shows the efficacy of the ICRS and IOL procedures. UDVA and CDVA (logMAR scale) rose significantly after both surgeries ($P < 0.0001$). The mean UDVA (logMAR) varied from the preoperative 1.15 ± 0.67 to 0.88 ± 0.69 six months after ICRS implantation (before IOL implantation) ($P = 0.005$) and 0.27 ± 0.18 six months after IOL implantation ($P < 0.0001$). The mean CDVA was 0.26 ± 0.15 (logMAR) before ICRS implantation, 0.17 ± 0.08 six months after ICRS implantation ($P = 0.002$), and 0.07 ± 0.06 six months after IOL implantation ($P < 0.0001$). The efficacy index (mean postoperative UDVA/mean preoperative CDVA) 6 months after ICRS implantation was 0.50 and 6 months after IOL implantation was 0.85. There were no statistically significant differences between UDVA after the whole procedure (ICRS + IOL implantation) and the preoperative CDVA ($P = 0.4$), which provided an efficacy index of 1.00.

None of the patients lost lines of CDVA after any of the surgeries (see Figure 2). By six months after ICRS implantation, 7 had no change of CDVA, 6 eyes gained one line, and 4 eyes gained two lines or more. The safety index 6 months after ICRS implantation (ratio of postoperative and preoperative monocular CDVA) was 1.18. By six months after IOL implantation, all eyes gained CDVA, 7 eyes gained one line, and 10 eyes gained two lines or more of CDVA. The safety index 6 months after IOL implantation was 1.17. The safety index of the whole procedure (ICRS + IOL implantation) was 1.26.

Table 2 shows the distribution of manifest refraction error (power vector method) preoperatively, 6 months after ICRS implantation, and 6 months after IOL implantation. There was a large reduction in M value (spherical equivalent) and B value (blur strength) after surgery ($P < 0.0001$). Six months after IOL implantation, the spherical equivalent was ≤ 1.00 D in 86.7% of the eyes. Figure 3 shows the astigmatism component of the power vector represented by a two-dimensional vector (J_0, J_{45}). The origin of the graph (0, 0) represents an eye free of astigmatism. The spread of the post-ICRS implantation data from the origin is more concentrated than the spread of the preoperative data. The spread in the post-ICRS implantation data was converted into a concentrated data set around the origin after IOL implantation. The percentage of eyes with a refractive cylinder ≤ -1.5 D increased from 17.6% preoperatively to 100% six months after IOL implantation (Figure 3, red circle), while the percentage of eyes with a refractive cylinder ≤ -1.0 D varied from 0% to 76.5% (13 eyes) (Figure 3, blue circle).

Figure 4 shows the defocus curve for each group separately. The magnitude of depth of focus was 2.60 ± 1.02 D. There were no statistically significant differences in visual acuity for a defocus range from +0.50 D to −0.50 D ($P > 0.1$)

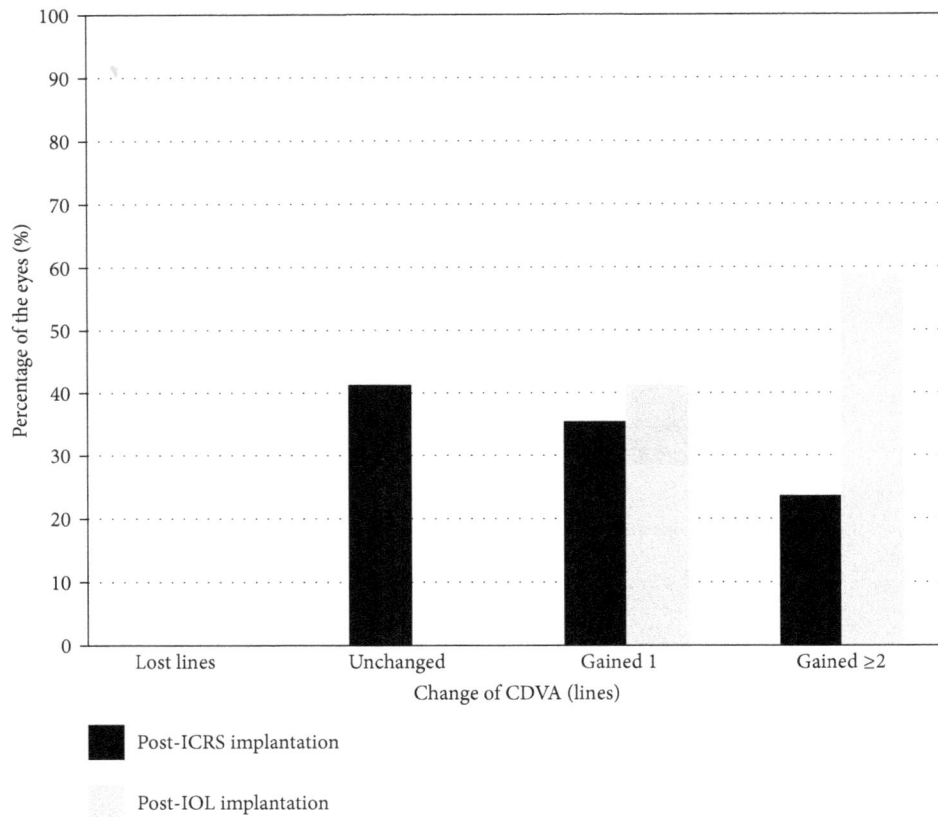

FIGURE 2: Change in corrected distance visual acuity (CDVA) 6 months after intrastromal corneal ring segments (ICRS) implantation and 6 months after intraocular lens (IOL) implantation (safety).

TABLE 2: Summary of distribution of manifest refractive errors before surgery, 6 months after ICRS implantation, and 6 months after IOL implantation, following the power vector method.

	Preoperatively	After ICRS implantation	After IOL implantation	P value
M	$-5.35 \pm 5.09^{*}$	$-3.45 \pm 3.88^{**}$	-0.59 ± 0.80	<0.0001
J_0	$-0.40 \pm 0.92^{*}$	$-0.32 \pm 0.63^{**}$	-0.07 ± 0.40	$P = 0.009$
J_{45}	0.17 ± 1.13	$0.23 \pm 0.40^{**}$	-0.09 ± 0.57	$P = 0.02$
B	$6.28 \pm 4.08^{*}$	$4.17 \pm 3.15^{**}$	0.94 ± 0.74	<0.0001

Data are shown as mean ± standard deviation. Manifest refraction in conventional script notation (S (sphere), C (cylinder) × ϕ (axis)), were converted to power vector coordinates and overall strength blur by the following formulas: $M = S + C/2$; $J_0 = (-C/2) \cos (2\phi)$; $J_{45} = (-C/2) \sin (2\phi)$; $B = (M^2 + J_0^2 + J_{45}^2)^{1/2}$. *Statistically significant between before Keraring ICRS insertion and after IOLs implantation. **Statistically significant between after Keraring ICRS implantation and after IOLs implantation.

4. Discussion

Earlier studies [3–15] have assessed several alternatives for replacement of the lens in keratoconic patients. The most studied approach has been the replacement of the lens by a toric IOL. The first three studies [3–5] were case reports, which showed encouraging results. Subsequent case series studies [6–10] (from 12 to 23 eyes) reported a significant improvement in UDVA, CDVA, and refractive error. The visual and refractive outcomes of multifocal toric IOL have been also evaluated. Montano et al. [11] described two cases, a "forme fruste" keratoconus and a stable keratoconus. Farideh et al. [12] evaluated the clinical results of toric intraocular trifocal IOL in 10 eyes (5 patients) with mild keratoconus. Both studies concluded that multifocal toric IOL provides satisfactory results in mild and stable keratoconus.

Despite these encouraging outcomes for visual quality restoring in patients with cataract and keratoconus, all these approaches should face two challenges: the first challenge is that the corneal abnormalities may lessen the optimal restoration of the visual quality and the second challenge is the IOL power estimation. Regarding the first challenge, a previous study [8] reported that patients with more regular corneas obtained higher improvement of UDVA after surgery. A previous study [14] from our research group reported the visual and refractive outcomes of a combined procedure (ICRS + monofocal IOL implantation). This sequential procedure is aimed at providing the higher level of visual rehabilitation in patients with keratoconus and cataract by improving the corneal shape and removing cataract and refractive error. In this previous study, both the UDVA and CDVA improved after each procedure. The UDVA and CDVA (logMAR scale) six months after IOL implantation were 0.44 ± 0.29 and 0.11 ± 0.16, respectively. In the current study, the UDVA

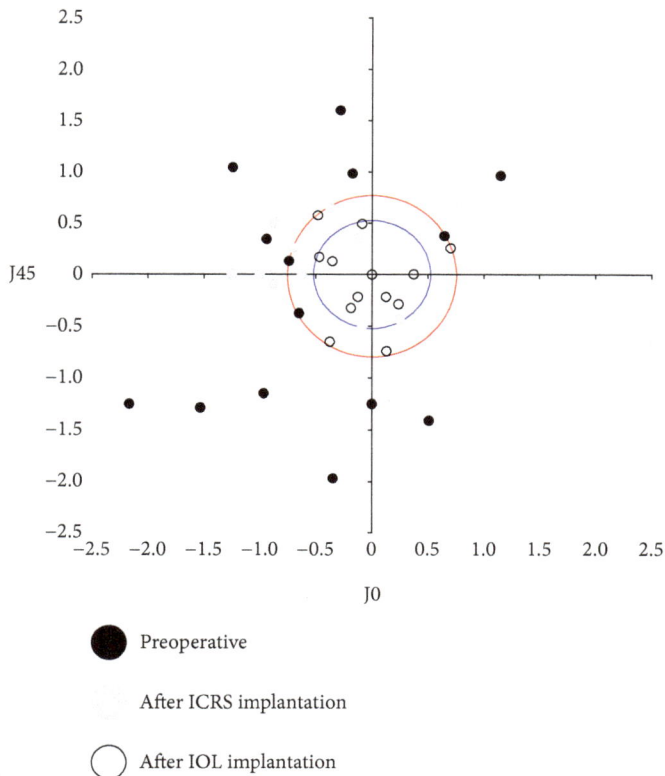

FIGURE 3: Representation of the astigmatic vector (J0 and J45) before surgery, 6 months after intrastromal corneal ring segments (ICRS) implantation, and 6 months after intraocular lens (IOL) implantation.

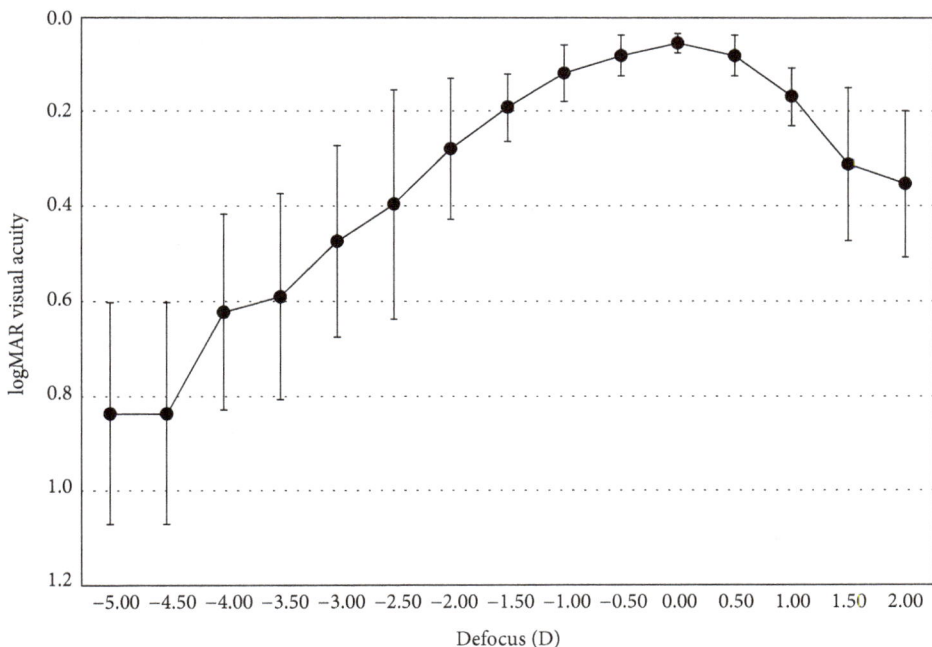

FIGURE 4: Mean high-contrast monocular logMAR acuity with best correction for distance as a function of the lens defocus (D).

and CDVA also improved after each procedure (ICRS implantation and an extended range of vision IOL implantation). The CDVA improvement after the whole procedure was greater in the previous study. However, in the current study the UDVA improvement was greater than those reported in the previous one (from 1.15 ± 0.67 (logMAR) to

0.27 ± 0.18 and from 1.08 ± 0.24 to 0.44 ± 0.29, resp.). The difference in the spherical equivalent between the two studies after the whole procedure was less than a quarter of dioptre. The difference in the CDVA and UDVA results can be attributed to the IOL implanted (monofocal versus extended range of vision IOL). A monofocal IOL provides a better CDVA than an extended range of vision IOL; while, as explained below, the residual refractive errors can be better tolerated with an extended range of vision IOLs.

Choosing the IOL power may be a challenge in keratoconic patients. Leccisotti [24] reported that refractive exchange in keratoconic eyes is a predictable procedure to correct myopia. However, 32% of the cases required an IOL exchange due to inaccurate IOL power calculation. Thebpatiphat et al. [2] compared the SRKI, SRKII, and SRK/T IOL formulas in patients with keratoconus and suggested that the SRKII formula might provide the most accurate IOL power in patients with mild keratoconus. However, in moderate and severe keratoconus, IOL calculations were less accurate and no differences in calculation formulas were found. A source of error for IOL power calculation in keratoconic patients is the determination of the optical power of the cornea. Usually, the power of cornea is estimated by considering only the radius of the anterior surface and a simulated refractive keratometric index. This estimation could lead to inaccuracies in the calculation of total corneal power in keratoconic eyes, where both the anterior and posterior surfaces of the cornea can be affected. ICRS implantation before cataract surgery could help to regularize the corneal shape and consequently minimize the inaccuracies in the determination of optical power of the cornea. An earlier study [14] found that the spherical equivalent after sequential implantation of the Ferrara-type ICRS and IOL implantation was −0.82 ± 0.91 D. The refractive outcome results of the current study are in accordance with the previous one. Six months after IOL implantation, the mean spherical equivalent was −0.59 ± 0.80 and 86.7% of eyes had a spherical equivalent ≤ 1.00 D. In addition to the predictability of the refractive outcomes, an important aspect is the impact of the residual refractive error on the visual acuity outcomes, in other words, the tolerance to defocus. In the current study, an extended range of vision IOL was implanted which is aimed at increasing the tolerance to defocus. Analysing the defocus curve shown in Figure 4, there were no statistically significant differences in visual acuity for a defocus range from +0.50 D to −0.50 D. These findings could suggest that some residual refractive errors can be tolerated after this combined procedure (ICRS + an extended range of vision IOL implantation). In addition, the magnitude of depth of focus was 2.60 ± 1.02 D, which provide an optimal visual acuity at intermediate distance (Figure 4).

The success of this sequential procedure requires knowledge of the risk of progression of keratoconus, because the progression of keratoconus can lead to refraction change and it could be a problem after IOL implantation. A previous study from our research group [14] showed that sequential Ferrara-type ICRS and IOL implantation provides stable visual and refractive outcomes. In the current study, the only difference was the IOL implanted; hence, it seems logical to think that the visual and refractive outcomes will be stable too. However, further long-term studies should be carried out to confirm this hypothesis and to assess whether small corneal changes could have more impact after an extended range of vision IOL implantation than a monofocal IOL implantation.

In conclusion, our outcomes suggest that sequential Ferrara-type ICRS and extended range of vision IOL implantation provides good visual and refractive outcomes, being an effective, safe, and predictable procedure for the treatment of selected cases of patients with keratoconus and cataract. In addition, this approach provides an increase of tolerance to defocus.

Conflicts of Interest

The authors have no proprietary interest in any of the materials mentioned in this article.

References

[1] A. G. Abraham, N. G. Condon, and E. West Gower, "The new epidemiology of cataract," *Ophthalmology Clinics of North America*, vol. 19, no. 4, pp. 415–425, 2006.

[2] N. Thebpatiphat, K. M. Hammersmith, C. J. Rapuano, B. D. Ayres, and E. J. Cohen, "Cataract surgery in keratoconus," *Eye & Contact Lens*, vol. 33, no. 5, pp. 244–246, 2007.

[3] G. Sauder and J. B. Jonas, "Treatment of keratoconus by toric foldable intraocular lenses," *European Journal of Ophthalmology*, vol. 13, no. 6, pp. 577–579, 2018.

[4] A. Navas and R. Suárez, "One-year follow-up of toric intraocular lens implantation in forme fruste keratoconus," *Journal of Cataract and Refractive Surgery*, vol. 35, no. 11, pp. 2024–2027, 2009.

[5] N. Visser, S. T. J. M. Gast, N. J. C. Bauer, and R. M. M. A. Nuijts, "Cataract surgery with toric intraocular lens implantation in keratoconus: a case report," *Cornea*, vol. 30, no. 6, pp. 720–723, 2011.

[6] M. Jaimes, F. Xacur-García, D. Alvarez-Melloni, E. O. Graue-Hernández, T. Ramirez-Luquín, and A. Navas, "Refractive lens exchange with toric intraocular lenses in keratoconus," *Journal of Refractive Surgery*, vol. 27, no. 9, pp. 658–664, 2011.

[7] M. A. Nanavaty, D. B. Lake, and S. M. Daya, "Outcomes of pseudophakic toric intraocular lens implantation in keratoconic eyes with cataract," *Journal of Refractive Surgery*, vol. 28, no. 12, pp. 884–890, 2012.

[8] J. L. Alió, P. Peña-García, F. Abdulla Guliyeva, F. A. Soria, G. Zein, and S. K. Abu-Mustafa, "MICS with toric intraocular lenses in keratoconus: outcomes and predictability analysis of postoperative refraction," *The British Journal of Ophthalmology*, vol. 98, no. 3, pp. 365–370, 2014.

[9] H. Hashemi, S. Heidarian, M. A. Seyedian, A. Yekta, and M. Khabazkhoob, "Evaluation of the results of using toric IOL in the cataract surgery of keratoconus patients," *Eye & Contact Lens*, vol. 41, no. 6, pp. 354–358, 2015.

[10] K. Kamiya, K. Shimizu, and T. Miyake, "Changes in astigmatism and corneal higher-order aberrations after phacoemulsification with toric intraocular lens implantation for mild keratoconus with cataract," *Japanese Journal of Ophthalmology*, vol. 60, no. 4, pp. 302–308, 2016.

[11] M. Montano, K. P. López-Dorantes, A. Ramirez-Miranda, E. O. Graue-Hernández, and A. Navas, "Multifocal toric intraocular lens implantation for forme fruste and stable keratoconus," *Journal of Refractive Surgery*, vol. 30, no. 4, pp. 282–285, 2014.

[12] D. Farideh, S. Azad, N. Feizollah et al., "Clinical outcomes of new toric trifocal diffractive intraocular lens in patients with cataract and stable keratoconus: six months follow-up," *Medicine*, vol. 96, no. 12, article e6340, 2017.

[13] M. Ouchi and S. Kinoshita, "Implantation of refractive multifocal intraocular lens with a surface-embedded near section for cataract eyes complicated with a coexisting ocular pathology," *Eye*, vol. 29, no. 5, pp. 649–655, 2015.

[14] J. F. Alfonso, C. Lisa, L. Fernández-Vega Cueto, A. Poo-López, D. Madrid-Costa, and L. Fernández-Vega, "Sequential intrastromal corneal ring segment and monofocal intraocular lens implantation for keratoconus and cataract: long-term follow-up," *Journal of Cataract and Refractive Surgery*, vol. 43, no. 2, pp. 246–254, 2017.

[15] J. F. Alfonso, L. Fernández-Vega Cueto, D. Madrid-Costa, and R. Montés-Micó, "Intrastromal corneal ring segment and intraocular lens implantation in patients with keratoconus and cataract," *Journal of Emmetropia: Journal of Cataract, Refractive and Corneal Surgery*, vol. 3, pp. 193–200, 2012.

[16] N. Maeda, S. D. Klyce, and M. K. Smolek, "Comparison of methods for detecting keratoconus using videokeratography," *Archives of Ophthalmology*, vol. 113, no. 7, pp. 870–874, 1995.

[17] Y. S. Rabinowitz, K. Rasheed, H. Yang, and J. Elashoff, "Accuracy of ultrasonic pachymetry and videokeratography in detecting keratoconus," *Journal of Cataract & Refractive Surgery*, vol. 24, no. 2, pp. 196–201, 1998.

[18] H. B. Fam and K. L. Lim, "Corneal elevation indices in normal and keratoconic eyes," *Journal of Cataract and Refractive Surgery*, vol. 32, no. 8, pp. 1281–1287, 2006.

[19] J. F. Alfonso, L. Fernández-Vega Cueto, B. Baamonde, J. Merayo-Lloves, D. Madrid-Costa, and R. Montés-Micó, "Inferior intrastromal corneal ring segments in paracentral keratoconus with no coincident topographic and coma axis," *Journal of Refractive Surgery*, vol. 29, no. 4, pp. 266–272, 2013.

[20] L. F.-V. Cueto, C. Lisa, A. Poo-López, D. Madrid-Costa, J. Merayo-Lloves, and J. F. Alfonso, "Intrastromal corneal ring segment implantation in 409 paracentral keratoconic eyes," *Cornea*, vol. 35, no. 11, pp. 1421–1426, 2016.

[21] C. Lisa, L. Fernández-Vega Cueto, A. Poo-López, D. Madrid-Costa, and J. F. Alfonso, "Long-term follow-up of intrastromal corneal ring segments (210-degree arc length) in central keratoconus with high corneal asphericity," *Cornea*, vol. 36, no. 11, pp. 1325–1330, 2017.

[22] L. F.-V. Cueto, C. Lisa, D. Madrid-Costa, J. Merayo-Lloves, and J. F. Alfonso, "Long-term follow-up of intrastromal corneal ring segments in paracentral keratoconus with coincident corneal keratometric, comatic and refractive axes: stability of the procedure," *Journal of Ophthalmology*, vol. 2017, Article ID 4058026, 9 pages, 2017.

[23] L. N. Thibos and D. Horner, "Power vector analysis of the optical outcome of refractive surgery," *Journal of Cataract and Refractive Surgery*, vol. 27, no. 1, pp. 80–85, 2001.

[24] A. Leccisotti, "Refractive lens exchange in keratoconus," *Journal of Cataract and Refractive Surgery*, vol. 32, no. 5, pp. 742–746, 2006.

21

Comparative Analysis of the Safety and Functional Outcomes of Anterior versus Retropupillary Iris-Claw IOL Fixation

Paolo Mora ⓘ,[1] Giacomo Calzetti,[1] Stefania Favilla,[2] Matteo Forlini,[1] Salvatore Tedesco,[1] Purva Date ⓘ,[3] Viola Tagliavini,[1] Arturo Carta,[1] Rino Frisina,[4] Emilio Pedrotti ⓘ,[5] and Stefano Gandolfi[1]

[1]Ophthalmology Unit, University Hospital of Parma, Parma, Italy
[2]Independent Researcher, Parma, Italy
[3]Aditya Jyot Eye Hospital, Wadala, Mumbai, India
[4]Department of Ophthalmology, University of Padova, Padova, Italy
[5]Eye Clinic, Department of Neurosciences, Biomedicine and Movement Sciences, University of Verona,
  AOUI-Policlinico G. B. Rossi, Verona, Italy

Correspondence should be addressed to Paolo Mora; paolo.mora@unipr.it

Academic Editor: Tamer A. Macky

Purpose. To compare the functional and clinical outcomes of the iris-claw intraocular lens (IOL) placed on the anterior versus posterior surface of the iris. *Patients and Methods.* A multicenter, retrospective study. Data on eyes that underwent anterior or retropupillary iris-claw IOL implantation because of inadequate capsular support secondary to complicated cataract surgery, trauma, and dislocated/opacified IOLs since January 2015 were analyzed. For study inclusion, evaluation results had to be available in the medical records both preoperatively and at 1 and 12 months after implantation. The following parameters were compared between the groups: best-corrected distance visual acuity (BCDVA), spherical and cylindrical refractive error, endothelial cell density (ECD), central macular thickness (CMT), and percentage and type of postoperative complications. *Results.* In total, 60 eyes of 60 patients aged 73 ± 13 years were included: 28 eyes (47%) involved anterior, and 32 eyes (53%) retropupillary, iris-claw IOL fixations. Preoperatively, the groups were similar in all parameters except for a significantly higher proportion of retropupillary fixations in patients who had previously experienced a closed-globe trauma ($p = 0.03$). The groups showed comparable improvements in BCDVA after surgery (final BCDVA: 0.34 ± 0.45 vs. 0.37 ± 0.50 logMAR in the anterior and retropupillary placement groups, respectively). During follow-up, no group difference was observed in refractive error or CMT. Both groups experienced similarly marked ECD loss and showed similar incidence of postoperative complications, with cystoid macular edema being the most common complication. Multivariable linear regression showed that BCDVA at 1 month was the best predictor of the final BCDVA. *Conclusions.* Anterior chamber and posterior chamber iris-claw IOL fixations proved equally effective and safe for aphakic correction in eyes with inadequate capsular support.

1. Introduction

Management of intraocular lens (IOL) implantation in eyes with inadequate capsular support is challenging. Inadequate capsular support precluding the availability of the natural bag or of the sulcus can result from complicated cataract surgery, luxation of the crystalline lens, or from dislocation or opacification of a previous conventional IOL. Various methods of surgical correction have been described, including placement of specialized IOLs supported by the anterior chamber (AC) angle or iris or of scleral-fixated IOLs [1–3]. Iris-fixated IOLs secured to the anterior surface of the iris using a claw-shaped haptic device were initially used for correction of aphakia [4]. Although this type of IOL was used extensively in the past, it is no longer recommended because of relatively high complication rates and suboptimal visual outcomes [5, 6]. However, anterior iris-claw IOLs have since undergone significant design changes, including vault modifications, which have enabled their use for refractive correction of high myopia in phakic eyes. These advances, along with the ease of surgical insertion, have led to the reintroduction of anterior iris-claw IOLs for correction of aphakia without a capsular support [7, 8]. Iris-claw IOLs can also be securely fixed to the posterior surface of the iris, to maintain the physiological position of the diaphragm in the posterior chamber (PC) of the eye and thus reduce the potential for the complications associated with AC IOLs. Many investigators have reported relatively large series, both prospective and retrospective, demonstrating the midterm safety and efficacy of this procedure [9–12]. Both AC and PC iris-claw IOLs were also found to be safe and effective for visual rehabilitation in young patients [13, 14]. Iris-claw fixation, both anterior and retropupillary, is technically less demanding than scleral fixation and is now used in routine practice by many surgeons. Only one study has prospectively compared the visual outcomes between the anterior and retropupillary approaches for fixation of iris-claw IOLs, wherein no difference was noted [15]. However, the study was limited by a small sample size and short follow-up. The present study aimed to supplement the available data by retrospectively investigating long-term safety and visual outcomes in a larger cohort of eyes implanted with either AC or PC iris-claw IOLs.

2. Methods

This was a three-center retrospective study of patients who received AC or PC iris-claw IOL implants from January 2015. Informed consent was obtained from all patients, and all procedures adhered to the tenets of the Declaration of Helsinki. The inclusion criteria were (a) uneventful implantation (i.e., absence of intraoperative complications such as iridodialysis, iris bleeding, or intraoperative disenclavation) of an Artisan® (Ophtec, Groningen, The Netherlands) iris-claw IOL, inserted due to a lack of capsule support; and (b) medical records showing the results of complete eye examinations (as detailed below), preoperatively and at 1 and 12 months after surgery. Windows of ±1 and ±4 weeks were allowed for the evaluations at 1 and 12 months, respectively. The exclusion criterion was any severe media opacity precluding examination of the ocular structures. Complete examination results had to be available within the medical records, including an up-to-date medical history; refraction assessment; best-corrected distance visual acuity (BCDVA; assessed by the standard Early Treatment of Diabetic Retinopathy Study chart); slit lamp examination, fundus evaluation, and intraocular pressure (IOP) results; corneal endothelial cell density (ECD) count; and macular optical coherence tomography (OCT) data. Included eyes (one per patient) were divided into two groups according to the implant position: anterior (group A) or posterior (group B) (Figure 1). The following parameters were compared between the groups: BCDVA (given by the logarithm of the minimum angle of resolution, logMAR), the spherical and cylindrical refractive error (considered separately after conversion to positive cylinders), ECD, central macular thickness (CMT), and the percentage and type of postoperative complications and/or anomalies. These data were collected by an experienced clinician; either an ophthalmologist or a certified ophthalmic technician. ECD was expressed as the number of cells per mm^2 and was measured in all patients with a specular microscope (SP-2000P; Topcon America, Paramus, NJ, USA) using the "center-dot" cell counting method. CMT was assessed in all patients, according to the central subfield thickness, via "macular cube 512×128" OCT scans performed with the Cirrus HD-OCT 4000 instrument (Carl Zeiss Meditec, Dublin, CA, USA).

2.1. Surgical Techniques. An Artisan® (Ophtec) IOL was used during the surgery; Artisan® is a rigid poly(methyl methacrylate) IOL 8.5 mm in length and with a maximum height of 1.04 mm and an optical zone width of 5.4 mm. The IOL power was calculated using the SRK/T formula. The IOL targeted emmetropia in all patients. An A-constant of 115.0, as per the manufacturer's recommendation, was used for anterior implantation, while an A-constant of 116.5 was used for retropupillary fixation. Anesthesia was either general or peribulbar. Whenever indicated, the surgical procedure was combined with lens/IOL removal or pars plana vitrectomy (PPV). Surgeons selected either AC or PC placement depending on their individual experience and the characteristics of the specific surgical procedure, in particular the presence/necessity of a vitreous access which could allow to handle the implant even from behind by a vitreous pick as a rescue measure in the case of unsuitable retropupillary iris hooking. The same standardized surgical technique was applied in both procedures. Two side ports were made at the 3 and 9 o'clock positions. Anterior vitrectomy was performed as required. Miosis was achieved using intracameral carbachol, and a viscoelastic agent was injected into the anterior chamber. A 5.5 mm superior limbal corneal incision was made, and the IOL (with the vault facing up and down for the anterior clawed lens and retropupillary lens, respectively) was inserted into the AC. The IOL was rotated such that the haptics were lined at the 3 and 9 o'clock positions. Thereafter, the IOL optic plate was held in place with Artisan lens forceps (Ophtec); for AC implantation, iris was enclavated at midperiphery between claw haptics using a special enclavation microspatula introduced through the ipsilateral side port. For retropupillary fixation, after positioning one haptic of the IOL behind the iris, it was enclavated using the microspatula, followed by enclavation of the other haptic. Superior peripheral iridectomy was performed only for AC implantations. Finally, the corneal incision was sutured using noncontinuous 10-0 nonabsorbable nylon sutures, which were removed at a minimum of 6 weeks after surgery. Postoperative therapy included antibiotic and nonsteroidal anti-inflammatory eye drops for 1 month.

2.2. Statistical Analysis. Continuous variables were expressed as means ± standard deviation (SD) or as medians with the interquartile range (IQR), while categorical variables were presented as proportions. Differences between groups in the preoperative characteristics (Table 1)

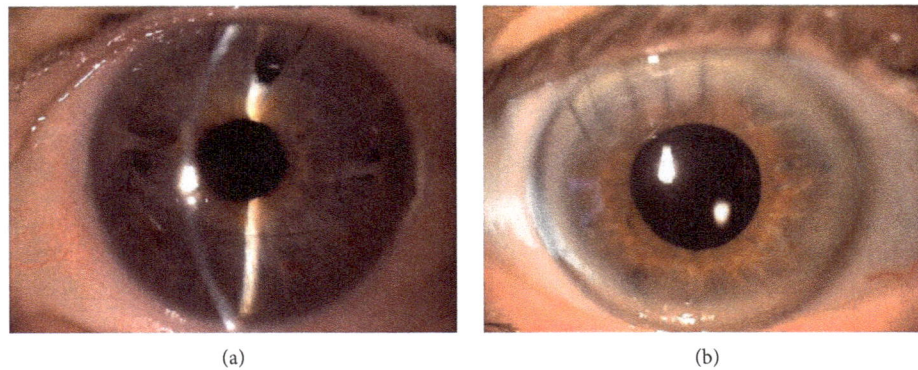

(a)   (b)

FIGURE 1: Slit-lamp photographs of iris-claw IOLs implanted in the anterior chamber (a) and in the posterior chamber (b).

TABLE 1: Demographic and baseline characteristics in the two groups.

Patients' characteristics	Group A ($n = 28$)	Group B ($n = 32$)	p value
Age, years	72.7 ± 13.5	73.8 ± 13.4	N.S.
Males, n (%)	20 (71%)	21 (66%)	N.S.
Right eyes, n (%)	17 (61%)	14 (44%)	N.S.
IOP, mmHg	15.7 ± 5.1	16.2 ± 4.3	N.S.
Preexistent corneal pathology, n (%)	3 (11%)	4 (12.5%)	N.S.
Preexistent macular pathology, n (%)	2 (7%)	2 (6%)	N.S.
Preexistent retinal pathology, n (%)	8 (29%)	11 (34%)	N.S.
Prior closed-globe trauma, n (%)	3 (11%)	11 (34%)	0.03
Prior open-globe trauma, n (%)	2 (7%)	5 (16%)	N.S.
Prior cataract surgery, n (%)	18 (64%)	17 (53%)	N.S.
Preoperative lens status			
Subluxated cataract, n (%)	5 (18%)	4 (12.5%)	
Dislocated nucleus, n (%)	5 (18%)	11 (34%)	
Subluxated IOL, n (%)	6 (21%)	5 (16%)	N.S.
Dislocated IOL, n (%)	1 (3.5%)	4 (12.5%)	
Opacified IOL, n (%)	1 (3.5%)	0 (0%)	
Aphakia, n (%)	10 (36%)	8 (25%)	

Continuous variables are presented as means ± standard deviation. n: number; IOP: intraocular pressure; IOL: intraocular lens; N.S.: not significant, $p > 0.05$.

TABLE 2: Cumulative incidence of postoperative complications in the two groups over 12 months after surgery.

Postoperative complication	Group A	Group B	p value
Cystoid macular edema (%)	33	25	N.S.
Transiently raised IOP (%)	32	22	N.S.
Pseudophakic bullous keratopathy (%)	7	16	N.S.
Epiretinal membrane (%)	7	16	N.S.
Persistent IOP elevation (%)	18	3	N.S. (0.08)
IOL tilting or decentration (%)	11	3	N.S.
Iritis (%)	7	3	N.S.
Retinal detachment (%)	0	3	N.S.
Endophthalmitis (%)	0	0	
IOL disenclavation, subluxation, or dislocation (%)	0	0	

IOP: intraocular pressure; IOL: intraocular lens; N.S.: not significant, $p > 0.05$.

and in postoperative complications (Table 2) were analyzed using Student's t-test for continuous variables and the chi-squared test or Fisher's exact test for categorical variables. The study outcomes BCDVA, CMT, and ECD loss were analyzed with a two-way ANOVA model (main effect: Group and Time) with interaction term (Group ∗ Time). The program R cran, ver. 3.4.0 was used to perform the analyses. For post hoc analysis, we used a Fisher's Least Significant Difference (LSD) test (95% family-wise confidence level). Univariate and multivariable linear regression analyses were performed to evaluate factors influencing the final BCDVA. Covariates significant at $p < 0.1$ in univariate analyses were included in the multivariable analyses, as were those showing variance inflation ≤10 or having

TABLE 3: Outcomes variables at different time points in the two groups.

	Group A ($n = 28$)	Group B ($n = 32$)	p value
Preop. BCDVA (logMAR)	0.66 ± 0.60	0.80 ± 0.66	
1-month postop. BCDVA (logMAR)	0.35 ± 0.30	0.50 ± 0.50	N.S.
1-year postop. BCDVA (logMAR)	0.34 ± 0.45	0.37 ± 0.50	
p value (preop. to 1 month, preop. to 1 year, 1 month to 1 year)	0.019, <0.001, N.S.		
Refractive components	$n = 28$	$n = 32$	
1-year postop. Sphere, D	-0.46 ± 0.65	-1.02 ± 1.51	N.S.
1-year postop. Cylinder, D	1.02 ± 1.51	1.08 ± 0.43	N.S.
CMT	$n = 21$	$n = 27$	
Preop. CMT (μm)	227 ± 64	214 ± 54	
1-month postop. CMT (μm)	229 ± 61	233 ± 99	N.S.
1-year postop. CMT (μm)	273 ± 158	229 ± 79	
p value (any time interval)	N.S.		
ECD	$n = 25$	$n = 25$	
Preop. ECD, number of cells (mm^2)	2043 ± 647	2047 ± 489	
1-month postop. ECD, number of cells (mm^2)	1721 ± 566	1605 ± 521	N.S.
1-year postop. ECD, number of cells (mm^2)	1512 ± 588	1395 ± 380	
p value (preop. to 1-month, preop. to 1-year, 1-month to 1-year)	<0.01, <0.01, N.S.		

Continuous variables are presented as means ± standard deviation. n: number; BCDVA: best-corrected distance visual acuity; D: diopter; CMT: central macular thickness; ECD: endothelial cell density; N.S.: not significant, $p > 0.05$.

clinical relevance for the study (e.g., anterior vs. posterior implantation). Best-fit regression models were created based on stepwise forward and backward methods. Correlations between continuous variables are described by LOWESS curves and Pearson's correlation coefficients. All data were entered into Excel software (Microsoft Corp., Redmond, WA, USA) and analyzed using Stata software (ver. 12.0; Stata Corp., Fort Worth, TX, USA). A p value of <0.05 was considered statistically significant.

3. Results

Sixty eyes of sixty subjects (41 males and 19 females; mean age, 73 ± 13 years) were included in the study. In total, 28 eyes (47%) with anterior iris-claw IOL fixation were assigned to group A, and 32 eyes (53%) with retropupillary fixation were assigned to group B. The demographic and preoperative characteristics of the two groups are listed in Table 1. The groups were similar on all parameters, except for a significantly higher proportion of retropupillary fixations in patients who had previously experienced a closed-globe trauma ($p = 0.03$). Iris-claw IOL fixation directly followed lens removal in 25 eyes (42% of cases): the indications were complicated cataract surgery in 15 patients and lens dislocation because of trauma or pseudoexfoliative syndrome in 10 patients; the remaining cases were secondary implantations in aphakic eyes (18 cases, 30%) or conventional IOL exchanges because of subluxation/dislocation or opacification (17 cases, 28%). Overall, PPV was performed in combination with iris-claw IOL fixation in 38 eyes (no difference in the rate of performance between the two groups). According to the within-group analysis shown in Table 3, BCDVA significantly improved after surgery in both groups, without significant difference between the two groups. The post hoc analysis showed that the improvement was

statistically significant in the time intervals: preop.: 1 month, and preop.: 12 months. At 12 months, spherical and cylindrical refractive errors were also comparable between the two groups. Preoperative OCT data were available, and of suitable quality, in 48 patients (21 in group A and 27 in group B): CMT data and the incidence of CME referred to this subgroup of patients accordingly; the CMT did not significantly change after surgery in either group (Table 3). To determine the ECDs, ten eyes (seven in group B) were excluded from the analysis because of a prior corneal surgery (corneal transplantation or corneal wound suture) or because they developed corneal decompensation during the follow-up. Compared with the preoperative assessments, the ECDs were significantly reduced in both groups after surgery, without a significant intergroup difference (Table 3); at the 1-month postoperative visit, the median losses were 194 cells/mm^2 (IQR: 65–554 cells/mm^2) and 203 cells/mm^2 (IQR: 93–755 cells/mm^2) in groups A and B, respectively, with no intergroup difference ($p = 0.51$). The ECD showed a further decrease at the final evaluation; the median losses between 1 and 12 months were 90 cells/mm^2 (IQR: 7–221 cells/mm^2) and 109 cells/mm^2 (IQR: 15–209 cells/mm^2) in groups A and B, respectively, with no intergroup difference ($p = 0.89$) (Figure 2). Again, the post hoc analysis showed that the loss was statistically significant in the time intervals: preop.: 1 month, and preop.: 12 months. The most frequent complications in both groups throughout the postoperative follow-up were cystoid macular edema (CME) (Figure 3) and transiently increased IOP. CME was detected in 5 subjects at the 1-month visit (1 patient in group A and 4 in group B). At the 1-year visit, CME was detected in 10 subjects (6 in group A and 4 in group B), with one patient in group B showing CME at both the postoperative visits. The cumulative incidence of CME over 12 months after surgery was not significantly different between the two groups. CME occurred in 6 patients

(a)

(b)

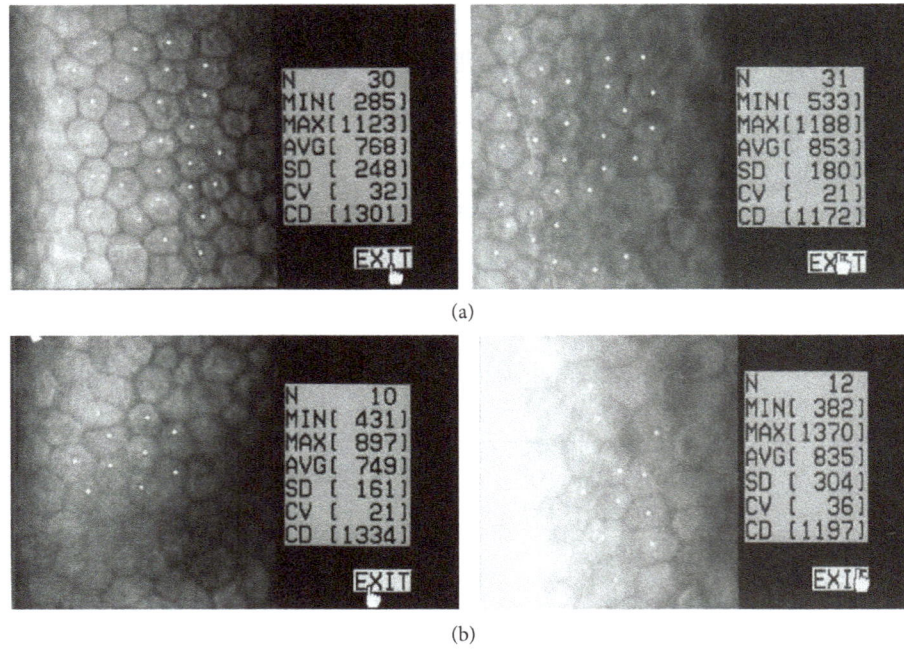

FIGURE 2: Corneal specular microscopy pictures for both groups. (a) On the left, preoperative endothelial cell density (ECD) and on the right, ECD of the same patient in group A 1 month after surgery. (b) Same sequence in a patient in group B.

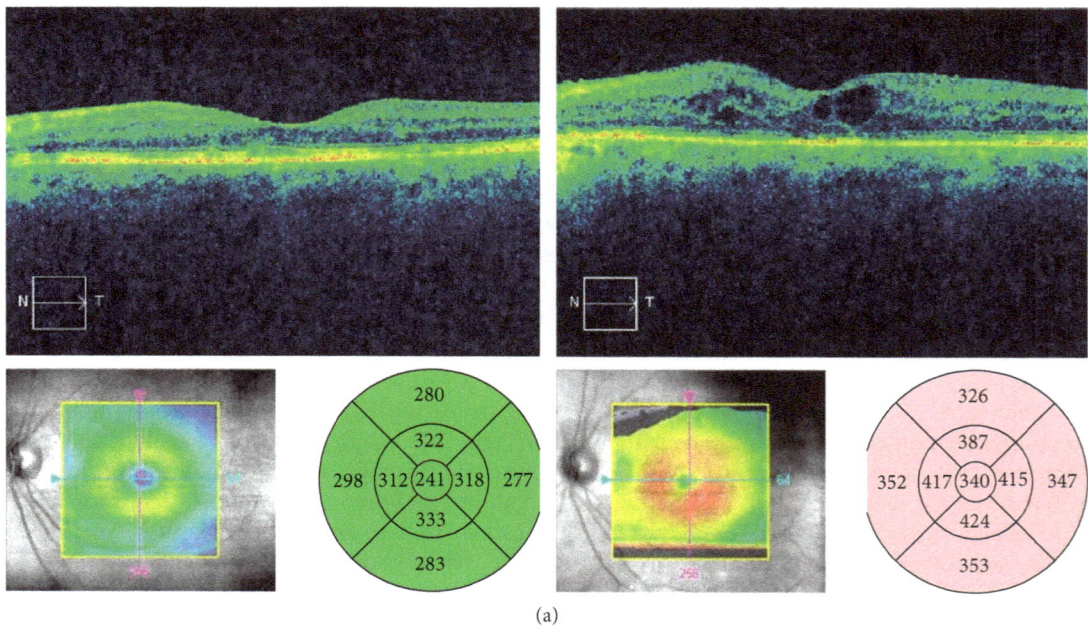

(a)

FIGURE 3: Continued.

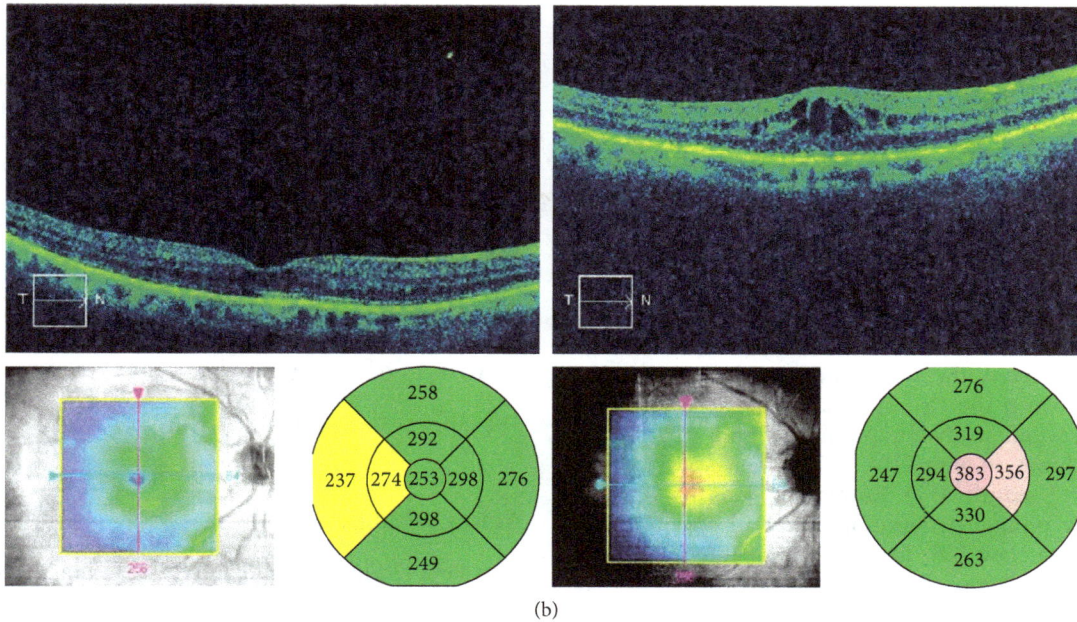

(b)

FIGURE 3: Optical coherence tomography (OCT) scans of cystoid macular edema (CME). (a) OCT scans of a patient in group A at the preoperative visit (left) and at the 1-year postoperative visit, when CME was detected. (b) OCT scans of a patient in group B showing normal foveal thickness at the preoperative visit and CME at the 1-month postoperative visit.

TABLE 4: Univariate and multivariable regression analysis showing factors influencing final BCDVA.

Covariate	Interval	Univariate analysis		Multivariable analysis	
		β coeff	95% CI	β coeff	95% CI
Age	1 year increment	0.06	−0.02–0.16	—	
Gender	Female vs. male	0.32	0.07–0.57	0.14	−0.05–0.34
Iris-claw IOL placement	AC vs. PC	0.02	−0.22–0.27	−0.07	−0.26–0.11
Prior trauma	Vs. no prior trauma	0.01	−0.08–1.1	—	
Previous surgery	Vs. no surgery	0.13*	0.05–0.20	0.08*	0.02–0.14#
Preexistent corneal pathology	Vs. no preexistent corneal pathology	0.24	−0.13–0.62	—	
Preexistent macular pathology	Vs. no preexistent macular pathology	0.68*	0.22–1.14	0.21	−0.16–0.59
Preexistent retinal pathology	Vs. no preexistent retinal pathology	0.11	−0.15–0.37	—	
Postop. CME	Vs. no postop. CME	0.07	−0.19–0.35	—	
Postop. PBK	Vs. no postop. PBK	0.25	−0.12–0.63	—	
Postop. complication†	Vs. no postop. complications	0.25*	0.01–0.49	—	
BCDVA at 1 month	0.1 logMAR increment	0.70*	0.48–0.92	0.63*	0.42–0.84#

* $p < 0.05$; † = excluded from multivariable model due to variance inflation; # = β-coefficient based on stepwise regression model for best fit. $R^2 = 0.57$; IOL: intraocular lens; CME: cystoid macular edema; PBK: pseudophakic bullous keratopathy; BCDVA: best-corrected distance visual acuity; AC: anterior chamber; PC: posterior chamber; CI: confidence interval.

who underwent PPV and in 8 without PPV. The treatment of CME included nonsteroidal anti-inflammatory eye drops in seven cases, prednisolone eye drops in one case, and subtenon injection of steroid in two cases (one was followed by intravitreal dexamethasone implant a few months later). Table 2 shows the cumulative incidence of all complications over 12 months after surgery. Notably, there were no cases of endophthalmitis, IOL disenclavation, subluxation, or dislocation, while IOL tilting or decentration was reported in four eyes (three in group A). The incidence of each type of complication was comparable between the two groups. Univariate and multivariable stepwise linear regression analyses were performed on the final BCDVA, which was predicted most strongly by the BCDVA at 1 month after

surgery. The final BCDVA did not show an association with the IOL placement type (anterior vs. retropupillary; Table 4).

4. Discussion

Although some previous studies described using iris-claw IOL implantations, very few compared the AC and PC positions [15–17]. The need for a thorough comparison including variables such as ECD and CMT prompted us to perform the present study [18], where we assessed long-term functional and safety outcomes in a large group of eyes that underwent AC or PC iris-claw IOL implantation. We found that both positions afforded significant BCDVA improvement at early (1 month) and long-term

(12 months) follow-ups, with final visual and refractive outcomes being similar between the two groups. Concerning safety, CMT, ECD loss, and type and percentage of postoperative complications were comparable between the groups. At the end of follow-up, the CMT was not significantly different from the preoperative value in either group, which was consistent with previous studies [11, 12]. We analyzed ECD loss at 1 and 12 months; loss at the first time point is assumed to mainly reflect intraoperative cellular loss, while ECD loss occurring between 1 month and 12 months is attributable to the presence of the IOL. As expected, the ECD loss rate at 1 month was approximately twice that observed thereafter; however, there was no difference between the two groups in the ECD loss over time. In a previous study comparing AC and PC iris-claw IOLs in combination with PPV, no difference in ECD loss was found at 3 months [17]. Conversely, another study in patients undergoing penetrating keratoplasty, IOL removal, and iris-claw IOL fixation documented a greater ECD loss between 6 months and 12 months after surgery in case of AC IOL placement [16]. The cumulative incidence of all other recorded postoperative complications was similar between the two groups although there was a trend toward a higher proportion of chronic IOP elevation in the AC versus PC IOL position ($p = 0.08$). Previous studies evaluating long-term outcomes of iris-claw IOLs reported variable postoperative complication rates [7, 8, 10, 11]. To understand this variability, the surgical procedures performed in conjunction with IOL implantation should be considered, such as complicated cataract surgery or PPV. The relatively high incidence of complication of our groups was comparable to those in a study evaluating iris-claw IOL fixation in conjunction with PPV and lens/IOL removal [17]. Similarly, in our study, the majority of the surgeries (70%) were performed in combination with lens or conventional IOL removal. The elder age of our patients might also have contributed to the increased proportion of complications.

Multivariable analysis of the whole cohort indicated that the BCDVA at 1 month predicted the final BCDVA (i.e., that at the 12-month follow-up). Assuming that variables such as irregular astigmatism, perioperative complications, and preexistent macular or corneal anomalies may influence visual acuity at both 1 and 12 months after surgery, it was expected that good visual acuity at 1 month would persist to 12 months. Notably, the majority of the eyes in our study still had corneal sutures after 1 month. Therefore, we suggest that, for optimal outcomes, astigmatism control should be ensured during application of the corneal suture, irrespective of whether an AC or PC iris-claw IOL is used. The major weakness of our study lays in its retrospective design and the consequent lack of randomization to IOL placement groups or standardization of data collection.

5. Conclusion

The present study compared AC and PC iris-claw IOL implantation outcomes over a 12-month follow-up period.

Our results showed that the procedures were equally effective and safe for managing cases of aphakia with inadequate capsular support. Future studies should include ultrasound biomicroscopy assessments of the anatomy of AC and PC structures after implantation. Furthermore, in cases of posterior luxation of the lens during cataract surgery, primary iris-claw IOL implantation and a two-step procedure including correction of aphakia at a later and quieter stage should be compared.

Conflicts of Interest

The authors declare that there are no conflicts of interest.

Acknowledgments

We thank Dr. Lucia Di Stefano for her valuable assistance in data collection.

References

[1] M. Saleh, A. Heitz, T. Bourcier et al., "Sutureless intrascleral intraocular lens implantation after ocular trauma," *Journal of Cataract and Refractive Surgery*, vol. 39, no. 1, pp. 81–86, 2013.

[2] T. Ohta, H. Toshida, and A. Murakami, "Simplified and safe method of sutureless intrascleral posterior chamber intraocular lens fixation: Y-fixation technique," *Journal of Cataract and Refractive Surgery*, vol. 40, no. 1, pp. 2–7, 2014.

[3] W. Jing, L. Guanlu, Z. Qianyin et al., "Iris-claw intraocular lens and scleral-fixated posterior chamber intraocular lens implantations in correcting aphakia: a meta-analysis," *Investigative Opthalmology and Visual Science*, vol. 58, no. 9, pp. 3530–3536, 2017.

[4] C. D. Binkhorst, "Results of implantation of intraocular lenses in unilateral aphakia. With special reference to the pupillary or iris clip lens–a new method of fixation," *American Journal of Ophthalmology*, vol. 49, no. 4, pp. 703–710, 1960.

[5] J. S. Wigton, "Review of the literature on intraocular lenses 1976–1977," *Optometry and Vision Science*, vol. 55, no. 11, pp. 780–791, 1978.

[6] J. L. Pearce and T. Ghosh, "Surgical and postoperative problems with Binkhorst 2- and 4-loop lenses," *Transactions of the Ophthalmological Societies of the United Kingdom*, vol. 97, no. 1, pp. 84–90, 1977.

[7] S. R. De Silva, K. Arun, M. Anandan, N. Glover, C. K. Patel, and P. Rosen, "Iris-claw intraocular lenses to correct aphakia in the absence of capsule support," *Journal of Cataract and Refractive Surgery*, vol. 37, no. 9, pp. 1667–1672, 2011.

[8] J. L. Güell, P. Verdaguer, D. Elies et al., "Secondary iris-claw anterior chamber lens implantation in patients with aphakia without capsular support," *British Journal of Ophthalmology*, vol. 98, no. 5, pp. 658–663, 2014.

[9] J. Gonnermann, M. K. Klamann, A. K. Maier et al., "Visual outcome and complications after posterior iris-claw aphakic intraocular lens implantation," *Journal of Cataract and Refractive Surgery*, vol. 38, no. 12, pp. 2139–2143, 2012.

[10] A. Anbari and D. B. Lake, "Posteriorly enclavated iris claw intraocular lens for aphakia: long-term corneal endothelial

safety study," *European Journal of Ophthalmology*, vol. 25, no. 3, pp. 208–213, 2015.

[11] G. Jayamadhury, S. Potti, K. V. Kumar et al., "Retropupillary fixation of iris-claw lens in visual rehabilitation of aphakic eyes," *Indian Journal of Ophthalmology*, vol. 64, no. 10, pp. 743–746, 2016.

[12] N. M. Jare, A. G. Kesari, S. S. Gadkari et al., "The posterior iris-claw lens outcome study: 6-month follow-up," *Indian Journal of Ophthalmology*, vol. 64, no. 12, pp. 878–883, 2016.

[13] M. Brandner, S. Thaler-Saliba, S. Plainer, B. Vidic, Y. El-Shabrawi, and N. Ardjomand, "Retropupillary fixation of Iris-claw intraocular lens for aphakic eyes in children," *PLoS One*, vol. 10, no. 6, Article ID e0126614, 2015.

[14] J. Català-Mora, D. Cuadras, J. Díaz-Cascajosa, M. Castany-Aregall, J. Prat-Bartomeu, and J. García- Arumí, "Anterior iris-claw intraocular lens implantation for the management of nontraumatic ectopia lentis: long-term outcomes in a paediatric cohort," *Acta Ophthalmologica*, vol. 95, no. 2, pp. 170–174, 2017.

[15] S. Helvaci, S. Demirduzen, and H. Oksuz, "Iris-claw intraocular lens implantation: anterior chamber versus retropupillary implantation," *Indian Journal of Ophthalmology*, vol. 64, no. 1, pp. 45–49, 2016.

[16] J. J. Gicquel, S. Guigou, R. A. Bejjani, B. Briat, P. Ellies, and P. Dighiero, "Ultrasound biomicroscopy study of the Verisyse aphakic intraocular lens combined with penetrating keratoplasty in pseudophakic bullous keratopathy," *Journal of Cataract and Refractive Surgery*, vol. 33, no. 3, pp. 455–464, 2007.

[17] E. Labeille, C. Burillon, and P. L. Cornut, "Pars plana vitrectomy combined with iris-claw intraocular lens implantation for lens nucleus and intraocular lens dislocation," *Journal of Cataract and Refractive Surgery*, vol. 40, no. 9, pp. 1488–1497, 2014.

[18] S. J. Lee and M. Kim, "Han SB comment to: iris-claw intraocular lens implantation: anterior chamber versus retropupillary implantation," *Indian Journal of Ophthalmology*, vol. 64, no. 6, pp. 478-479, 2016.

22

Short-Term Clinical Results of Ab Interno Trabeculotomy using the Trabectome with or without Cataract Surgery for Open-Angle Glaucoma Patients of High Intraocular Pressure

Handan Akil,[1,2] **Vikas Chopra,**[1,2] **Alex S. Huang,**[1,2] **Ramya Swamy,**[1,2] **and Brian A. Francis**[1,2]

[1]*Doheny Image Reading Center, Doheny Eye Institute, Los Angeles, CA, USA*
[2]*Department of Ophthalmology, David Geffen School of Medicine, Los Angeles, CA, USA*

Correspondence should be addressed to Brian A. Francis; bfrancis@doheny.org

Academic Editor: Chelvin Sng

Purpose. To assess the safety and efficacy of Trabectome procedure in patients with preoperative intraocular pressure (IOP) of 30 mmHg or higher. *Methods.* All patients who had underwent Trabectome stand-alone or Trabectome combined with phacoemulsification were included. Survival analysis was performed by using Kaplan-Meier, and success was defined as IOP $\leq$ 21 mmHg, 20% or more IOP reduction from baseline for any two consecutive visits after 3 months, and no secondary glaucoma surgery. *Results.* A total of 49 cases were included with an average age of 66 (range: 13–91). 28 cases had Trabectome stand-alone and 21 cases had Trabectome combined with phacoemulsification. Mean IOP was reduced from a baseline of 35.6 ± 6.3 mmHg to 16.8 ± 3.8 mmHg at 12 months ($p < 0.01^*$), while the number of medications was reduced from 3.1 ± 1.3 to 1.8 ± 1.4 ($p < 0.01^*$). Survival rate at 12 months was 80%. 9 cases required secondary glaucoma surgery, and 1 case was reported with hypotony at day one, but resolved within one week. *Conclusion.* Trabectome seems to be safe and effective in patients with preoperative IOP of 30 mmHg or greater. Even in this cohort with high preoperative IOP, the end result is a mean IOP in the physiologic range.

1. Introduction

Glaucoma is a progressive disease which causes irreversible damage to the optic nerve [1]. The main goal of treatment is to lower intraocular pressure (IOP) to a level which is safe for the optic nerve head. Although trabeculectomy or episcleral aqueous drainage implants demonstrated a permanent IOP reduction, they may have a high risk profile regarding the intraoperative and postoperative complications [2]. This has influenced the development of a less invasive surgical technique, trabeculotomy by internal approach with the Trabectome (NeoMedix Corp., Tustin, CA), which works on the trabecular meshwork and inner wall of Schlemm's canal to reduce outflow resistance [3, 4]. This surgical approach provides a postoperatively stable eye without damaging the conjunctiva and can be further combined with cataract surgery easily with low incidence of intraoperative and postoperative complications.

Results of Trabectome in various types of open-angle glaucoma patients with preoperative IOP of less than 30 mmHg have been shown to be favorable with fewer rates of complication compared to those of traditional trabeculectomy, giving the surgeons hope of an effective and safe treatment option for patients with higher preoperative IOPs [2–4].

The study was conducted to report the success rate of ab interno trabeculotomy within a single-surgeon single-

TABLE 1: Demographics and descriptive statistics of all the patients with IOP ≥ 30 mmHg.

	$n = 49$
Age	
Mean ± SD	66 ± 18
Range	18–91
Gender	
Female	19 (39%)
Male	30 (61%)
Race	
African American	2 (4%)
Asian	5 (10%)
Caucasian	31 (63%)
Hispanics	7 (14%)
Others	4 (8%)
Diagnosis	
POAG	24 (49%)
Pseudoexfoliation glaucoma	12 (24%)
ACG	2 (4%)
Pigment dispersion	5 (10%)
Ocular hypertension	2 (4%)
Secondary glaucoma	2 (4%)
Others	2 (4%)
Preop Snellen acuity	
20/20–20/40	22 (45%)
20/50–20/70	9 (18%)
20/80–20/100	4 (8%)
20/200–20/400	8 (16%)
<20/400	1 (2%)
NR	5 (10%)
VF	
Mild	4 (8%)
Moderate	12 (24%)
Advanced	3 (6%)
MD/others	30 (61%)
Disc C/D	
<0.7	13 (27%)
0.7 to 0.8	17 (35%)
>0.8	11 (22%)
NR	8 (16%)
Lens status	
Phakic	39 (80%)
Pseudophakic	8 (16%)
Aphakic	0 (0%)
NR	2 (4%)
Shaffer grade	
I	0 (0%)
II	2 (4%)
III	11 (22%)
IV	5 (10%)
NR	31 (63%)

TABLE 1: Continued.

	$n = 49$
Prior surgeries	
SLT	17 (35%)
ALT	4 (8%)
Trabeculectomy	1 (2%)
Trabectome	2 (4%)
YAG	1 (2%)
Combined surgeries	
Trabectome + Phaco	21 (43%)
Trabectome only	28 (57%)

center cohort of patients with a preoperative IOP of 30 mmHg or higher.

2. Patient and Methods

This is a nonrandomized prospective analysis of patients treated by a single experienced surgeon (BAF). The study followed the tenets of the Declaration of Helsinki and the Health Insurance Portability and Accountability Act and had the Institutional Review Board approval. Cohort comparison was studied between patients with open-angle glaucoma-receiving Trabectome combined with phacoemulsification cataract extraction and intraocular lens (IOL) and patients receiving Trabectome alone.

The inclusion criteria for both the combined Trabectome group and Trabectome-alone group were as follows: open-angle glaucoma (as defined by glaucomatous optic nerve appearance with or without glaucomatous visual field damage)—an unobstructed view of the angle, age greater than or equal to 18, a visually significant cataract, and follow-up of at least 2 years. The severity of visual fields was graded according to the Hodapp-Anderson-Parrish (HAP) classification and visual field index (VFI) score [5]. Exclusion criteria were as follows: angle closure, uveitic or neovascular glaucoma, previous glaucoma surgery, and no clear view of the nasal angle.

A total number of 49 eyes of 49 patients were included in the study. Twenty-one eyes underwent combined Trabectome surgery and 28 eyes underwent Trabectome-alone surgery. In each group, patient demographics, preoperative cup-to-disc ratio, preoperative and postoperative visual acuity, IOP, and medications were recorded. Postoperative data at day one and months 1, 3, 6, and 12 were collected.

The surgical procedure has been described in detail elsewhere [2–4]. Briefly, the surgery was performed with the Trabectome® system, including the single-use handpiece with an irrigation-aspiration (I/A) system (Neomedix Inc., Tustin, USA). In combined surgery, the Trabectome surgery was performed prior to phacoemulsification. The head and microscope were tilted to give a gonioscopic view of the angle. The goniosurgical lens (a modified Swann-Jacobs lens)

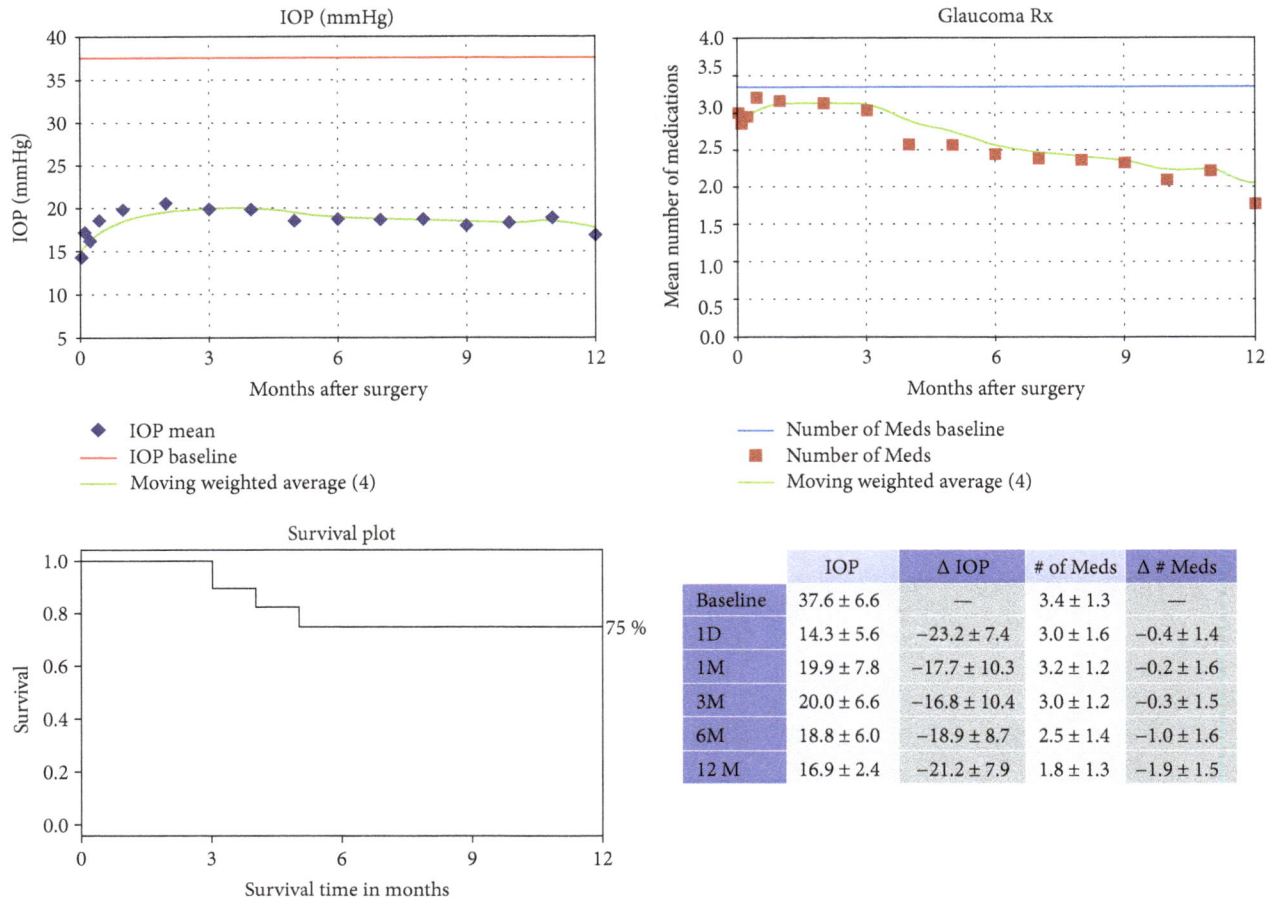

FIGURE 1: Intraocular pressure (IOP) and number of glaucoma medications data with survival rate over time from all the eyes with IOP > 30 mmHg and having undergone Trabectome surgery with or without cataract extraction. Kaplan-Meier survival curve of the success of the procedure defined as decrease in IOP of 20% or more or a decrease in glaucoma medications with no need for additional medications or glaucoma procedures.

was placed on the cornea to visualize the angle structures. A 1.7 mm keratome was used to create a temporal corneal incision. An ophthalmic viscosurgical device (OVD) was injected to form the anterior chamber. The Trabectome handpiece was inserted and advanced along the meshwork, ablating and removing between 90 and 150 degrees of the nasal trabecular meshwork and inner wall of Schlemm's canal. The power was adjusted up or down depending on the desire to ablate a wider strip of trabecular meshwork or to minimize burning of tissue, respectively. Irrigation and aspiration were then used to remove any remaining blood, viscoelastic, or cellular material.

Postoperative care is varied according to clinical presentation but routinely includes topical steroids four times per day tapered over 8 weeks, topical antibiotics four times per day for 7 days, and pilocarpine 1% three to four times per day tapering over two to eight weeks. Typically, the patients were advised to continue preoperative glaucoma medications after surgery if needed.

The estimated cumulative success rate was obtained by Kaplan-Meier life-table analyses using the following criteria: Kaplan-Meier survival curve of the success of the procedure

defined as a decrease in IOP of 20% or more or a decrease in glaucoma medications with no need for additional medications or glaucoma procedures.

3. Statistical Analysis

One-way repeated-measures analysis of variance (ANOVA) test was used for the baseline and postoperative values for each group. The difference in IOP and number of antiglaucoma medications between groups were assessed by an unpaired t-test. Pearson's χ^2 test was used for subgroup comparison of sex and lens status before surgery. We estimated the cumulative percentages of success as well as the failure rates over time with the Kaplan-Meier method. Statistical significance was assumed for $p \leq 0.05$.

4. Results

Demographic data and descriptive statistics of 49 cases were included into the study (Table 1). The mean age of the study population was 66 ± 18 and 39% were females. The proportion of Caucasians was higher (63%) and the proportion of

TABLE 2: Demographics and descriptive statistics of the patients with IOP $\geq$ 30 mmHg and having undergone combined Trabectome surgery.

	$n = 21$
Age	
Mean ± SD	72 ± 17
Range	23–88
Gender	
Female	12 (57%)
Male	9 (43%)
Race	
African American	1 (5%)
Asian	3 (14%)
Caucasian	12 (57%)
Hispanics	5 (24%)
Diagnosis	
POAG	6 (29%)
Pseudoexfoliation glaucoma	9 (43%)
ACG	2 (10%)
Ocular hypertension	1 (5%)
Secondary glaucoma	1 (5%)
Others	2 (10%)
Preop Snellen acuity	
20/20–20/40	5 (24%)
20/50–20/70	6 (29%)
20/80–20/100	3 (14%)
20/200–20/400	6 (29%)
<20/400	0 (0%)
NR	1 (5%)
VF	
Mild	1 (5%)
Moderate	4 (19%)
Advanced	0 (0%)
MD/others	16 (76%)
Disc C/D	
<0.7	5 (24%)
0.7 to 0.8	9 (43%)
>0.8	5 (24%)
NR	2 (10%)
Lens status	
Phakic	20 (95%)
Pseudophakic	0 (0%)
Aphakic	0 (0%)
NR	1 (5%)
Shaffer grade	
I	0 (0%)
II	1 (5%)
III	4 (19%)
IV	1 (5%)
NR	15 (71%)

TABLE 2: Continued.

	$n = 21$
Prior surgeries	
SLT	9 (43%)
ALT	1 (5%)
Trabeculectomy	1 (5%)

African American patients was lower (4%) in the study group. The mean preoperative IOP was 35.6 ± 6.3 mmHg. By postoperative month 12, the average IOP was 16.8 ± 3.8 (55.3% decrease) ($p < 0.01$). The average number of glaucoma medication use was significantly decreased from 3.1 ± 1.3 to 1.8 ± 1.3 at month 12 ($p < 0.01$). Primary open-angle glaucoma (POAG) was the major diagnosis (49%) in the study group and it was followed by pseudoexfoliation glaucoma (24%). Nine patients (18%) needed secondary surgery one year after the surgery and 1 case was reported with hypotony at postoperative 1st day but resolved within one week. The overall survival rate was 80% by postoperative month 12. Figure 1 shows the IOP and glaucoma medication trend with the survival rate of the procedure during the postoperative follow-up.

Twenty-eight cases had Trabectome-alone surgery and 21 cases had combined Trabectome phacoemulsification surgery. There were some statistically significant differences found between the two groups. The preoperative IOP was significantly lower in the combined Trabectome group (33.0 ± 4.9 mmHg) compared to that in the Trabectome-alone group (37.6 ± 6.6 mmHg) ($p = 0.01$). The Trabectome only group had a better preoperative visual acuity, which reflects the presence of the cataract in the combined Trabectome group. The mean age of the combined Trabectome group was 72 ± 17 and 57% were female. However, the mean age of the Trabectome-alone group was 62 ± 18 and 75% were male ($p = 0.06$). The study reported a higher proportion of Caucasians and lower proportion of Asian patients in both groups. The Trabectome-alone group showed a higher proportion of severe visual field defects compared to the combined Trabectome group. Tables 2 and 3 give the demographic data of each group.

5. Combined Trabectome Group

The mean preoperative IOP was 33.0 ± 4.9 mmHg (Figure 2) and by postoperative month 1, it has dropped to 18.5 ± 6.4 (44.2% decrease). By postoperative month 12, the average IOP was even lower at 16.6 ± 4.8 (51.8% decrease) ($p < 0.01$). Figure 2 shows the IOP and glaucoma medication trend with the survival rate during the postoperative follow-up. The average number of glaucoma medications use in the group was 2.7 ± 1.1. By postoperative month 12, it has significantly decreased to 1.8 ± 1.5 ($p < 0.01$). Survival rate at 12 months of follow-up was 86%. One eye (5%) needed secondary surgery to control IOP one year after the surgery. Hypotony, aqueous misdirection, wound leak, and postoperative infection were not reported in any of the patients. There was no clinically significant bleeding which may require intervention.

TABLE 3: Demographics and descriptive statistics of the patients with IOP ≥ 30 mmHg and having undergone Trabectome-alone surgery.

	n = 28
Age	
Mean ± SD	62 ± 18
Range	30–91
Gender	
Female	7 (25%)
Male	21 (75%)
Race	
African American	1 (4%)
Asian	2 (7%)
Caucasian	19 (68%)
Hispanics	2 (7%)
Other	4 (14%)
Diagnosis	
POAG	18 (64%)
Pseudoexfoliation glaucoma	3 (11%)
Pigment dispersion	5 (18%)
Ocular hypertension	1 (4%)
Secondary glaucoma	1 (4%)
Preop Snellen acuity	
20/20–20/40	17 (61%)
20/50–20/70	3 (11%)
20/80–20/100	1 (4%)
20/200–20/400	2 (7%)
<20/400	1 (4%)
NR	4 (14%)
VF	
Mild	3 (11%)
Moderate	8 (29%)
Advanced	3 (11%)
MD/others	14 (50%)
Disc C/D	
<0.7	8 (29%)
0.7 to 0.8	8 (29%)
>0.8	6 (21%)
NR	6 (21%)
Lens status	
Phakic	19 (68%)
Pseudophakic	8 (29%)
NR	1 (4%)
Shaffer grade	
I	0 (0%)
II	1 (4%)
III	7 (25%)
IV	4 (14%)
NR	16 (57%)

TABLE 3: Continued.

	n = 28
Prior surgeries	
SLT	3 (29%)
ALT	3 (11%)
Trabectome	2 (7%)
YAG	1 (4%)

6. Trabectome-Alone Group

The mean preoperative IOP was 37.6 ± 6.6 mmHg (Figure 3) and on postoperative day 1, it has decreased to 14.3 ± 5.6 mmHg (61.7% decrease). But by postoperative month 1, IOP increased to 19.9 ± 7.8 (47.1% decrease). By postoperative month 12, the IOP was stable at 16.9 ± 2.4 (56.9% decrease). The average number of glaucoma medications used in the group was 3.4 ± 1.3. By postoperative month 12, it has significantly decreased to 1.8 ± 1.3 ($p < 0.01$). Figure 3 shows the IOP and glaucoma medication trend with the survival rate during the postoperative follow-up. Eight cases required secondary surgery. Hypotony (IOP < 5 mmHg) at postoperative day one was observed in one patient (4%) and resolved later.

7. Discussion

The Trabectome seems to be a favorable method of minimal invasive glaucoma surgery with or without cataract surgery in patients with preoperative IOP of 30 mmHg or greater. The current data also suggests the effectiveness of Trabectome-alone surgery in reducing IOP and postoperative number of medications compared to combined Trabectome surgery.

The baseline IOP in our study was 33.0 ± 4.9 mmHg in the combined Trabectome group and 37.6 ± 6.6 in the Trabectome-alone group which is higher than the values in the studies by Francis [3] (22 mmHg). Minckler et al. [4] (25.7 mmHg), Jea et al. [6] (28.1 mmHg), or Trabectome-alone surgery significantly reduced the postoperative IOP in our study patients as well as combined Trabectome surgery. The IOPs at 1 year after surgery were significantly reduced from baseline to mid teens (16.9 ± 2.4 mmHg and 16.6 ± 4.8 mmHg, resp.) which is similar to those previously reported [2–6]. These results suggest that Trabectome surgery with or without cataract extraction may offer a clinically useful control on IOP levels. Some studies reported IOPs as 16.1 mmHg [4], 17.4 mmHg [6], and 16.6 mmHg [7] after 1 year of Trabectome surgery. Moreover, in this study, the number of medications were significantly reduced after both surgeries similar to other studies [3, 4, 8]. The success rate after Trabectome surgery has been reported to be about 30%–50% in the literature [2–4, 6–8]. In our study, the success rate for IOP decrease was 55% in the overall study population, 51.8% in the combined group, and 56.8% in the Trabectome-alone group. Mizoguchi et al. [9] reported that their Trabectome failure rate was higher in the eyes with a preoperative IOP <18 mmHg and lower in those with a preoperative IOP of 18–22 mmHg, and they concluded that the

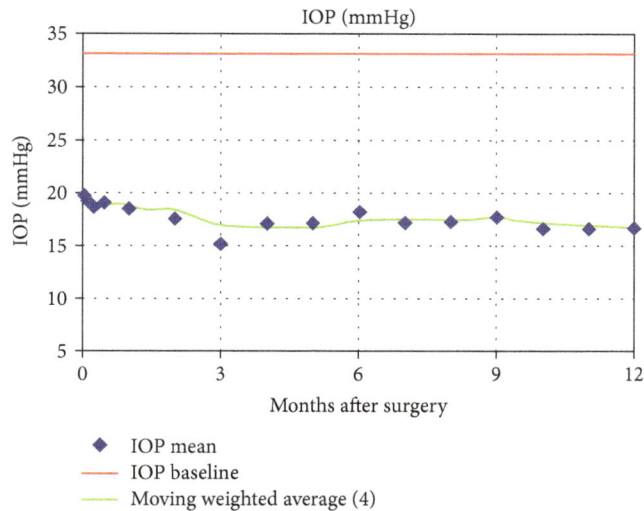

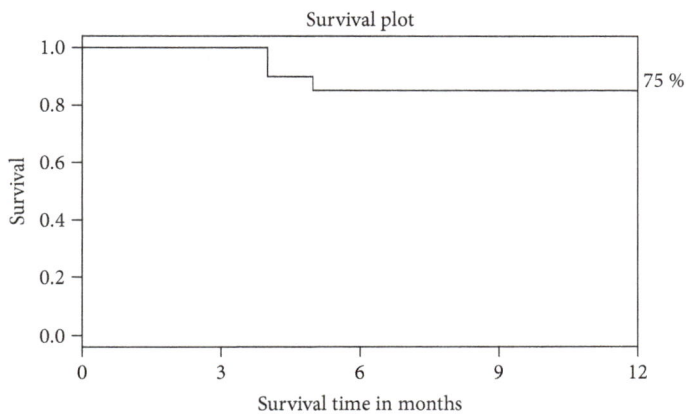

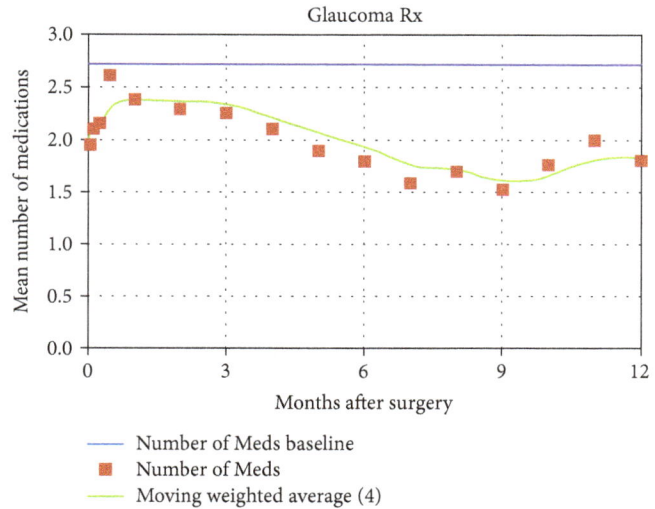

FIGURE 2: Intraocular pressure (IOP) and number of glaucoma medications data with survival rate over time from the eyes with IOP > 30 mmHg and having undergone combined Trabectome surgery. Kaplan-Meier survival curve of the success of the procedure defined as decrease in IOP of 20% or more or a decrease in glaucoma medications with no need for additional medications or glaucoma procedures.

results of Trabectome surgery may differ according to baseline IOP. Although the relationship of the surgical success and preoperative IOP level has not been established yet, our study showed that Trabectome surgery can be effective and safe at baseline IOP levels around 35.6 (±6.3) mmHg. Markedly high and low baseline IOPs have been reported as risk factors for poor surgical outcomes [6, 7].

The current study had a control group of glaucoma patients having Trabectome surgery alone; therefore, it was possible to determine to what extent Trabectome trabeculotomy or cataract extraction contributed to the lowering of IOP and medications. The IOP was lowered by 17.7 ± 7.7 mmHg (51.8% decrease) in the combined Trabectome group and 21.2 ± 7.9 mmHg (56.9% decrease) in the Trabectome-alone group by postoperative month 12. It has been generally suggested that phacoemulsification cataract extraction alone may lower IOP in glaucoma patients as well as in nonglaucomatous individuals, with the amount of 2–4 mmHg [10, 11]. Our study showed that there is a decrease to the normal physiologic level in IOP after a Trabectome procedure. Although a higher proportion of IOP decrease was reported

in the Trabectome-alone group, it may be caused by higher baseline IOP levels compared to that in the combined Trabectome group.

In a prospective interventional study [12], patients with open-angle glaucoma underwent combined Trabectome surgery. Mean preoperative IOP was 20.0 ± 6.3 mmHg, and mean postoperative IOP was 15.5 ± 2.9 mmHg, with a 1.4 ± 1.3 mean number of glaucoma medications after one year of follow-up. Nine patients needed additional glaucoma procedures.

Another study with a large number of case series evaluated the outcomes of Trabectome-alone versus combined procedures with phacoemulsification [4]. At 24 months, IOP decreased by 40% from 25.7 ± 7.7 mmHg preoperatively to 16.6 ± 4.0 mmHg in the Trabectome-alone group compared to 30% from 20.0 ± 6.2 mmHg to 14.9 ± 3.1 mmHg in the combined Trabectome group. Mean number of medications decreased from 2.9 to 1.2 in the Trabectome group and from 2.6 to 1.5 in the combined group. A total of 14% of patients were considered failure cases from the Trabectome-alone group.

IOP (mmHg) chart — IOP mean, IOP baseline, Moving weighted average (4); Months after surgery

Glaucoma Rx chart — Number of Meds baseline, Number of Meds, Moving weighted average (4); Months after surgery

Survival plot — Survival vs Survival time in months; 75%

	IOP	Δ IOP	# of Meds	Δ # Meds
Baseline	37.6 ± 6.6	—	3.4 ± 1.3	—
1D	14.3 ± 5.6	−23.2 ± 7.4	3.0 ± 1.6	−0.4 ± 1.4
1M	19.9 ± 7.8	−17.7 ± 10.3	3.2 ± 1.2	−0.2 ± 1.5
3M	20.0 ± 6.6	−16.8 ± 10.4	3.0 ± 1.2	−0.3 ± 1.5
6M	18.8 ± 6.0	−18.9 ± 8.7	2.5 ± 1.4	−1.0 ± 1.5
12 M	16.9 ± 2.4	−21.2 ± 7.9	1.8 ± 1.3	−1.9 ± 1.5

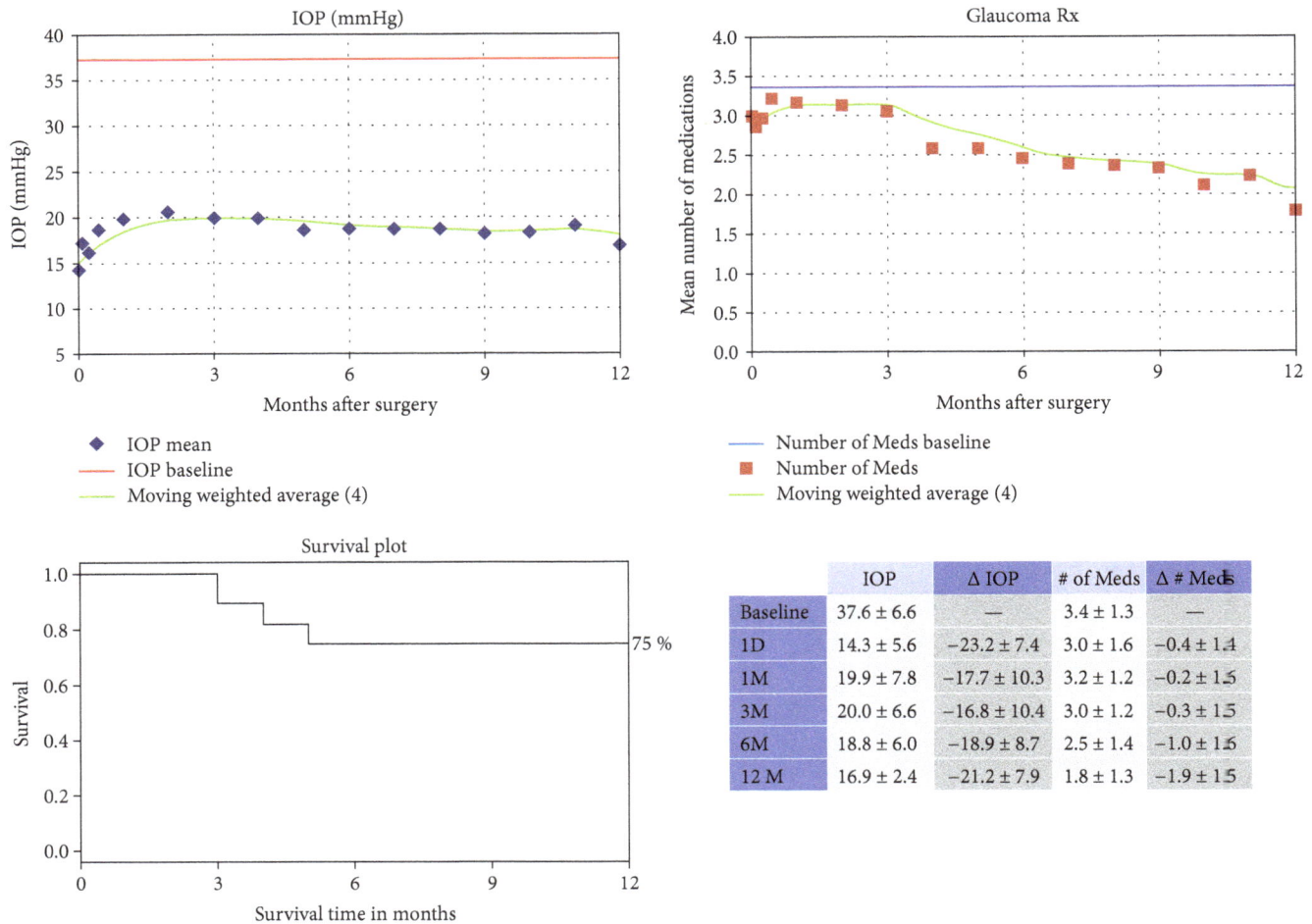

FIGURE 3: Intraocular pressure (IOP) and number of glaucoma medications data over time from the eyes with IOP> 30 mmHg and having undergone Trabectome-alone surgery. Kaplan-Meier survival curve of the success of the procedure defined as decrease in IOP of 20% or more or a decrease in glaucoma medications with no need for additional medications or glaucoma procedures.

A prospective nonrandomized study grouped open-angle glaucoma patients who underwent Trabectome procedures according to baseline IOP levels [13]. In the group with pre-operative IOP levels ≤17 mmHg, the IOP mean reduction was 7% mmHg with a 35% reduction in IOP-lowering medications. However, patients having IOP ≥ 30 mmHg showed IOP reduction as 48% with a 25% reduction in IOP-lowering medications.

Maeda et al. [14] also reported a decrease from mean pre-operative IOP of 26.6 ± 8.1 mmHg to 17.4 ± 3.4 mmHg after surgery. The number of IOP-lowering medications decreased from 4.0 ± 1.4 to 2.3 ± 1.2 at 6 months.

In our study, Trabectome surgery with or without cataract surgery achieved fairly good IOP levels from the values of 30 mmHg or higher to mid teens (16.8 ± 3.8). The number of IOP-lowering medications also decreased from 3.1 ± 1.3 to 1.8 ± 1.4 at 12 months.

The strengths of our study include having the Trabectome-alone group as controls to determine the IOP-lowering effect of procedures accurately and close monitoring of IOP, medications, and complications in a prospective fashion. Results are presented by differences in mean IOP and glaucoma medications as well as by a Kaplan-Meier survival curve. Our study covers high IOP cases with short-term follow-up; so, it might be valuable to compare the results with the long-term follow-up studies (Figure 4) [4, 6–8, 12, 14–16]. Severe complications like expulsive hemorrhage which may be caused by sudden drop of IOP after the surgery have not been reported yet; therefore, ab interno trabeculotomy using Trabectome might be safer compared to filtration procedures regarding the pressure changes. One of the major limitations of this study is the inclusion of the patients with a high initial IOP (presumably above the mean baseline of all patients undergoing Trabectome). One would anticipate that repeated IOP measurements in this group (even without Trabectome) would be closer to the mean (i.e., lower) on subsequent readings. The other limitations include the nonrandomized design of the study, with the inherent selection bias and drop-out issues. Although IOP and a number of medications were found to be lower during follow-up after the surgery, it cannot be claimed that the surgery itself lowered the pressure without a comparison group. Additionally, the patients who maintained a one-year follow-up may have a selection bias. In our study, we did not have a wash-out time interval for

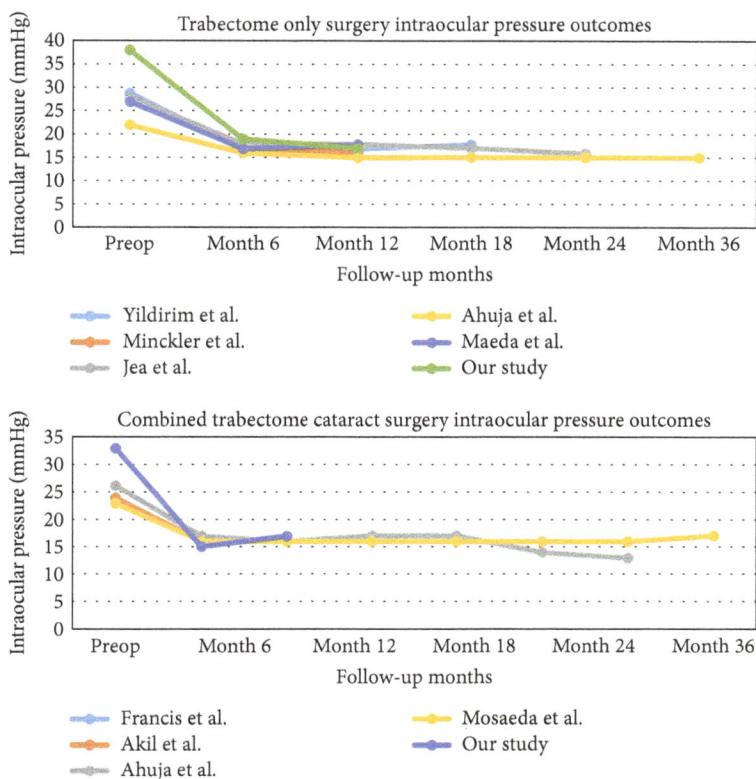

FIGURE 4: Intraocular pressure (IOP) changes over time after the Trabectome surgery with or without cataract extraction in different studies.

glaucoma medications before or after surgery; so, we cannot be certain as to the efficacy or necessity of the number of medications either pre- or posttreatment. We included a comparison group of glaucoma patients who had Trabectome-alone surgery. We encountered some differences between the groups in ethnicity, type of glaucoma, amount of visual field loss, prior surgeries, and degree of angle opening. However, these differences can be expected given the pathogenesis and epidemiology of cataract and glaucoma. The next step would be the establishment of randomized trials to determine the efficacy of Trabectome surgery compared with newer IOP-lowering surgeries for OAG, with one another, and with phacoemulsification alone (in the case of combined procedures).

In conclusion, the risk-to-benefit profile of trabeculotomy by internal approach in patients with high IOP levels has not been studied yet. The results of our study showed that the Trabectome, as a minimally invasive glaucoma surgery, might be considered as an alternative to standard filtration surgery in the surgical treatment of the open-angle glaucoma patients with higher IOP levels because of its internal approach, giving a good option for the combined cataract-glaucoma surgery, the low-risk profile, and the remaining of the future option for filtration surgery.

Disclosure

An earlier version of this work was presented as a poster at the 25th Annual Meeting of the American Glaucoma Society, 2015.

Conflicts of Interest

Dr. Brian A. Francis reports consulting agreements with Neomedix company (Trabectome). No other author has a financial or proprietary interest in any material or method mentioned.

References

[1] H. A. Quigley and A. T. Broman, "The number of people with glaucoma worldwide in 2010 and 2020," *The British Journal of Ophthalmology*, vol. 90, no. 3, pp. 262–267, 2006.

[2] J. F. Jordan, T. Wecker, C. van Oterendorp et al., "Trabectome surgery for primary and secondary open angle glaucomas," *Graefe's Archive for Clinical and Experimental Ophthalmology*, vol. 251, no. 12, pp. 2753–2760, 2013.

[3] B. A. Francis, "Trabectome combined with phacoemulsification versus phacoemulsification alone: a prospective, nonrandomized controlled surgical trial," *Clinical Surgery Journal Ophthalmology*, vol. 28, pp. 1–7, 2010.

[4] D. Minckler, S. Mosaed, L. Dustin, B. Francis, and the Trabectome Study Group, "Trabectome (trabeculectomy-internal approach): additional experience and extended follow-up," *Transactions of the American Ophthalmological Society*, vol. 106, pp. 149–159, 2008.

[5] E. Hodapp, R. K. Parrish II, and D. R. Anderson, *Clinical Decisions in Glaucoma*, Mosby–Year Book, St Louis, Mo, 1993.

[6] S. Y. Jea, S. Mosaed, S. D. Vold, and D. J. Rhee, "Effect of a failed Trabectome on subsequent trabeculectomy," *Journal of Glaucoma*, vol. 21, no. 2, pp. 71–75, 2012.

[7] Y. Ahuja, S. Ma Khin Pyi, M. Malihi, D. O. Hodge, and A. J. Sit, "Clinical results of ab interno trabeculotomy using the Trabectome for open-angle glaucoma: the Mayo Clinic series in Rochester, Minnesota," *American Journal of Ophthalmology*, vol. 156, no. 5, pp. 927–935, 2013.

[8] H. Akil, V. Chopra, A. Huang, N. Loewen, J. Noguchi, and B. Francis, "Clinical results of ab interno trabeculotomy using the Trabectome in patients with pigmentary glaucoma compared to primary open angle glaucoma," *Clinical & Experimental Ophthalmology*, vol. 44, no. 7, pp. 563–569, 2016.

[9] T. Mizoguchi, S. Nishigaki, T. Sato, H. Wakiyama, and N. Ogino, "Clinical results of Trabectome surgery for open-angle glaucoma," *Clinical Ophthalmology (Auckland, NZ)*, vol. 9, pp. 1889–1894, 2015.

[10] N. Mathalone, M. Hyams, S. Neiman, G. Buckman, Y. Hod, and O. Geyer, "Long-term intraocular pressure control after clear corneal phacoemulsification in glaucoma patients," *Journal of Cataract and Refractive Surgery*, vol. 31, no. 3, pp. 479–483, 2005.

[11] B. J. Shingleton, J. J. Pasternack, J. W. Hung, and M. W. O'Donoghue, "Three and five year changes in intraocular pressures after clear corneal phacoemulsification in open angle glaucoma patients, glaucoma suspects, and normal patients," *Journal of Glaucoma*, vol. 15, no. 6, pp. 494–498, 2006.

[12] B. A. Francis, D. Minckler, L. Dustin et al., "Combined cataract extraction and trabeculotomy by the internal approach for coexisting cataract and open-angle glaucoma: initial results," *Journal of Cataract and Refractive Surgery*, vol. 34, no. 7, pp. 1096–1103, 2008.

[13] S. D. Vold, "Ab interno trabeculotomy with the Trabectome system: what does the data tell us?" *International Ophthalmology Clinics*, vol. 51, no. 3, pp. 65–81, 2011.

[14] M. Maeda, M. Watanabe, and K. Ichikawa, "Evaluation of Trabectome in open-angle glaucoma," *Journal of Glaucoma*, vol. 22, no. 3, pp. 205–220, 2013.

[15] Y. Yildirim, T. Kar, E. Duzgun, S. K. Sagdic, A. Ayata, and M. H. Unal, "Evaluation of the long-term results of Trabectome surgery," *International Ophthalmology*, vol. 36, no. 5, pp. 719–726, 2016.

[16] S. Mosaed, "The first decade of global Trabectome outcomes," *European Ophthalmic Review*, vol. 8, pp. 113–119, 2014.

23

Retrospective Analyses of Potential Risk Factors for Posterior Capsule Opacification after Cataract Surgery

Shuang Wu,[1] Nianting Tong,[2] Lin Pan,[3] Xiaohui Jiang ®,[2] Yanan Li,[1] MeiLing Guo,[1] and Hehuan Li[1]

[1]Qingdao Municipal Hospital Affiliated to Qingdao University, No. 5 Donghaizhong Road, Shinan District, Qingdao, Shandong, China
[2]Department of Ophthalmology, Qingdao Municipal Hospital, No. 5 Donghaizhong Road, Shinan District, Qingdao, Shandong, China
[3]Dalian Medical University, No. 9 Lushunnan Road, Dalian, Liaoning, China

Correspondence should be addressed to Xiaohui Jiang; ocularjxh@163.com

Academic Editor: Ciro Costagliola

Purpose. To evaluate the potential risk factors of posterior capsule opacification (PCO) after cataract surgery. *Methods.* Data on PCO patients diagnosed from September 2015 to May 2017 were obtained from the Department of Ophthalmology at Qingdao Municipal Hospital, Qingdao, China. The factors associated with PCO were assessed using Pearson's χ^2 test for univariate analyses and logistic regression for multivariate analyses. *Results.* Eyes (652) from 550 patients were enrolled in this study. All patients were diagnosed with PCO/non-PCO and had <3 years of follow-up after surgery. The numbers of PCO and non-PCO were 108 eyes and 544 eyes, respectively. Statistically significant associations with PCO were found for age at the time of surgery ($\chi^2 = 78.504$; $p < 0.001$), diabetes ($\chi^2 = 4.829$; $p = 0.028$), immune diseases ($\chi^2 = 4.234$; $p = 0.004$), high myopia ($\chi^2 = 5.753$; $p = 0.016$), lens nucleus hardness ($\chi^2 = 11.046$; $p = 0.026$), surgery type ($\chi^2 = 11.354$; $p = 0.001$), a history of vitrectomy ($\chi^2 = 4.212$; $p = 0.004$), ocular inflammation ($\chi^2 = 6.01$; $p = 0.009$), and the intraocular lens (IOL) type ($\chi^2 = 8.696$; $p = 0.003$). Multivariable data analyses using logistic regression analyses of the variables showed that age at the time of surgery <60 years, diabetes, lens nucleus hardness of III–V, extracapsular cataract extraction (ECCE), postvitrectomy, and hydrophilic IOLs were significant independent risk factors associated with PCO. *Conclusions.* Age <60 years, diabetes, lens nucleus hardness of III–V, ECCE, postvitrectomy, and a hydrophilic IOL were significantly associated with the formation of PCO. Estimation of the incidence of and risk factors for PCO should help in patients counseling and in the design of treatment protocols to reduce or prevent its development.

1. Introduction

Cataract is the most common cause of blindness, and cataract surgery is the only cure method performed. Phacoemulsification and extracapsular cataract extraction (ECCE) are the most common types of surgery to treat cataracts. Posterior capsule opacification (PCO) is one of the most common complications after surgery. Decreased visual acuity induced by PCO is reported to occur in 20%–40% of patients 2–5 years after surgery [1]. PCO in the central visual axis is usually treated with neodymium : YAG (Nd : YAG) laser capsulotomy. The cumulative incidence of Nd : YAG

capsulotomy were 10.6%, 14.8%, 21.2%, and 28.6% in the patients after 1, 2, 3, and 4 years [2]. Because this treatment risks complications in other structures of the eye, the need for PCO prevention becomes increasingly important. During the past decades, various forms of prevention have been used, including general measures during surgery (e.g., surgical techniques, intraocular lens (IOL) materials, and designs), pharmacological prevention, and the prevention of PCO by interfering with the biological processes of epithelial-to-mesenchymal transition (EMT) in lens epithelial cells (LECs) [3]. This is a lack of quantified information on these processes, and the only effective method is mechanical prevention of PCO formation. A low incidence of PCO after IOL implantation is therefore a key objective of most cataract surgeries.

Many previous cohort or randomized controlled studies that have assessed PCO after cataract surgery had small sample sizes or had postoperative outcomes involving a few, mainly senior, surgeons. These studies did not adjust for different surgeons or different surgical experiences. It remains unclear whether such findings are applicable to other settings, such as that of large sample sizes in a public tertiary hospital where a large number of cataract procedures are performed using different ophthalmologic surgeons.

In this study, we assessed the incidence of PCO within 3 years after cataract surgery, to identify preoperative and surgical factors associated with PCO in the study population. Factors such as the general condition of the patient, ocular conditions, surgical techniques, and IOL types were considered. Our results should help with evaluations of the long-term prognosis of cataract surgery, and provide early diagnosis and treatment options for high-risk patients.

2. Materials and Methods

In this retrospective case-control study, the incidence and risk factors of PCO were evaluated in patients who underwent phacoemulsification or ECCE, with a follow-up time <3 years. The hospital's Institutional Review Board approved the study protocol. Informed consent was obtained from all patients or their guardians before the study, and the study was performed at Qingdao Municipal Hospital, Qingdao, China. The medical records of patients with PCO and who visited the outpatient department of the Department of Ophthalmology between September 2015 and May 2017 were retrospectively reviewed. A group of patients without PCO was identified using a cumulative sampling strategy. The patients complied with the criteria for the diagnosis of PCO and were selected at a 1 : 5 case : control ratio with the non-PCO group. Surgery was uncomplicated in all cases. Both groups of patients received antibiotic and glucocorticoid eye drops during the follow-up period within 4 weeks after the surgery according to the intraocular inflammation. There was no difference in postoperative care between the two groups of patients.

The PCO and lens nucleus hardness classification was evaluated by the same physician (XHJ). Visualisation of the posterior pole was assessed by examining the optic disc and macula using a Volk 90D lens. Visualisation of the optic disc was subjectively graded according to the following scale: 0—clear view of optic disc margin, blood vessels at the optic disc, and nerve fibre layer (NFL examined using the red-free filter); 1—clear view of optic disc margin, but disc blood vessels and/or nerve fibre layer are not clearly seen; 2—optic disc margin, as well as disc blood vessels, and nerve fibre layer are not clearly seen. Visualisation of the macula was subjectively graded according to the following scale: 0—clear view of foveal reflex, perifoveal blood vessels, and nerve fibre layer; 1—diminished foveal reflex, but clear view of perifoveal blood vessels and nerve fibre layer; 2—blurred foveal

reflex, perifoveal blood vessels, and/or nerve fibre layer. The totals for the visualisations of the optic disc and the macula were combined to produce a total posterior pole visualisation score (PolVS), ranging from 0 to 4 (Figures 1(a)–1(d)) in order of decreasing visualisation [4]. The degree of lens nucleus hardness was classified according to the Emery–Little classification (grade I–V). Patients were excluded if they underwent cataract surgery more than 3 years prior to the study, had a history of ocular trauma, had a history of glaucoma filtration surgery, had the primary aphakia after cataract extraction, had a history of repeated vitrectomy after cataract surgery, had the intraoperative posterior capsule rupture, had a history of extracapsular fixation of the IOL, were unable to cooperate with the inspector, or had incomplete clinical information. All patients presented with decreased visual acuity which was attributed to PCO during study period in our clinic. Nd : YAG laser capsulotomy was performed if it was clinically indicated by a decrease in visual acuity of two lines at least since previous examination or in the presence of a clinically opaque capsule. Nd : YAG laser capsulotomy was eventually performed in all 92 eyes.

The data collected included age at the time of surgery, sex, cataract duration, surgery type, IOL materials, ocular inflammation, lens nucleus hardness, family history of cataracts, and personal history of smoking, history of drinking, diabetes, hypertension, immune diseases, high myopia, and vitrectomy. Follow-up examinations included visual acuity measurement, intraocular pressure measurement using Goldman applanation tonometry, evaluation of IOL centration, and dilated fundus examination. The data analyses were performed using SPSS statistical software for Windows, version 19.0 (SPSS, Chicago, IL, USA). Pearson's χ^2 test was used to determine if there were statistically significant differences in PCO incidence for each factor. Then the factors that were statistically significant at a univariate level were entered into a stepwise multiple logistic regression model to identify independent risk factors affecting PCO. The 95% confidence interval (CI) and odds ratio (OR) were calculated. A value of $p < 0.05$ was considered statistically significant.

3. Results

This retrospective study reviewed the records of 103 eyes of 92 PCO patients in PCO group, including 52 females and 40 males, with a mean age of 65.47 ± 15.32 years. A total of 544 eyes of 458 patients, including 231 females and 227 males, with a mean age of 64.77 ± 10.12 years, were evaluated in the non-PCO group. There was no difference in the mean age between the PCO group and non-PCO group ($p = 0.041$). The period from surgery to the follow-up visit was on average 26.04 ± 8.14 months in PCO group and non-PCO group at 25.27 ± 7.67 months ($p = 0.65$). All comparative statistics are shown in Table 1. Patients with various PCO grades are listed in Table 2.

Table 3 shows the associations between PCO and clinical characteristics. No statistically significant differences were found between the two groups (PCO versus non-PCO) for sex, cataract duration, and history of smoking, history of

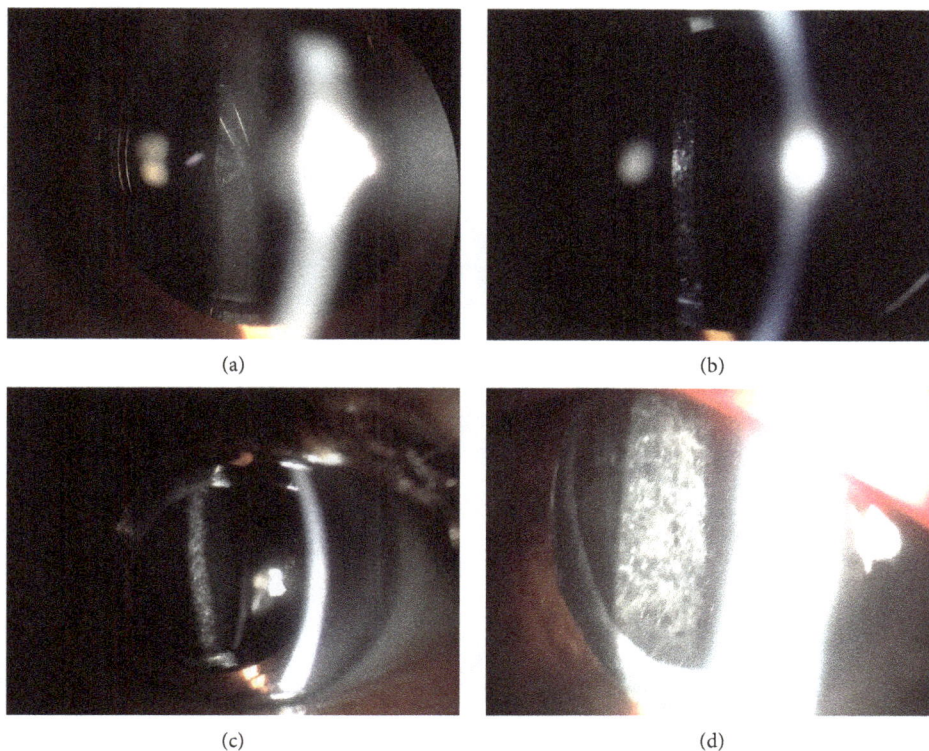

(a)

(b)

(c)

(d)

FIGURE 1: PCO grades by slit-lamp examination and a Volk 90D lens in this study: (a) Grade 0. (b) Grade 1. (c) Grade 2. (d) Grade 3.

TABLE 1: Patient demographics.

| Parameter | Group | | χ^2 | p value |
	Non-PCO	PCO		
Eye, n (patients)	544 (458)	108 (92)		
Age (y)	64.77 ± 10.12	65.47 ± 15.32	0.932	0.41
Laterality (OD/OS)	265/279	52/56	0.803	0.47
Period from surgery to the follow-up visit (m)	25.27 ± 7.67	26.04 ± 8.14	0.587	0.65

TABLE 2: Incidence and PCO grade among PCO and non-PCO patients.

	Incidence (%)	CDVA (logMAR) ± SD
Non-PCO		
Grade 0	544 (1)	0.06 ± 0.02
PCO		
Grade 1	46 (0.426)	0.27 ± 0.08
Grade 2	44 (0.407)	0.49 ± 0.13
Grade 3	18 (0.167)	0.74 ± 0.12

CDVA = corrected distance visual acuity; logMAR = logarithm of the minimum angle of resolution; SD = standard deviation.

drinking, hypertension, and cataracts. The χ^2 shown for clinical characteristics associated with PCO was based on univariate analyses. Variables with statistically significant differences were age at time of surgery, lens nucleus hardness, surgery type, ocular inflammation, IOL materials, and a history of diabetes, immune diseases, high myopia, and vitrectomy (Table 3). Variables with $p < 0.05$ were included in multiple logistic regression analyses (Table 4). Age at time

of surgery <60 years (OR, 0.149; 95% CI, 0.092–0.241; $p = 0.000$), diabetes (OR, 1.825; 95% CI, 1.042–3.197; $p = 0.035$), a lens nucleus hardness of III–V (OR, 0.508; 95% CI, 0.304–0.847; $p = 0.009$), ECCE (OR, 2.563; 95% CI, 1.242–5.290; $p = 0.011$), vitreous loss (OR, 1.905; 95% CI, 1.046–3.471; $p = 0.035$), and a hydrophilic IOL (OR, 1.672; 95% CI, 1.043–2.682; $p = 0.033$) were significant independent factors associated with PCO.

4. Discussion

PCO is caused by proliferation and migration of residual LECs, fibroblasts, macrophages, and iris-derived pigment cells on the posterior capsule. All of these processes are influenced by cytokines, growth factors, and extracellular matrix proteins. Clinically, there are two morphological types of PCO, including the fibrosis type and the pearl type. The fibrosis type is caused by the proliferation and migration of LECs, which undergo EMT, resulting in fibrous metaplasia and leading to significant visual loss because of folds and wrinkles in the posterior capsule. Pearl-type PCO is

TABLE 3: Univariate analyses of factors associated with PCO.

Variable	PCO ($n = 108$)	Non-PCO ($n = 544$)	χ^2	p value
Sex				
Male	46	276		
Female	62	68	2.39	0.122
Age at the time of surgery				
>60 years old	32	401		
<60 years old	76	143	78.504	<0.001
Cataract duration				
>3 years	79	390		
<3 years	29	154	0.064	0.8
History of smoking				
Yes	30	161		
No	78	383	0.144	0.705
History of drinking				
Yes	26	134		
No	82	410	0.015	0.902
History of hypertension				
Yes	52	287		
No	56	257	0.767	0.381
History of diabetes				
Yes	27	88		
No	81	456	4.829	0.028
History of immune diseases				
Yes	16	46		
No	92	498	4.234	0.04
High myopia				
Yes	13	31		
No	95	513	5.753	0.016
Family history of cataract				
Yes	33	175		
No	75	369	0.108	0.742
Lens nucleus hardness				
I grade	7	70		
II grade	22	145		
III grade	38	183		
IV grade	33	130		
V grade	8	16	11.046	0.026
Surgery type				
ECCE	18	37		
Phaco	90	507	11.354	0.001
History of vitrectomy				
Yes	23	74		
No	85	470	4.212	0.04
Ocular inflammation (aqueous cell)				
>15 cells	38	126		
<15 cells	70	418	6.01	0.009
IOL materials				
Hydrophilic	67	253		
Hydrophobic	41	291	8.696	0.003

TABLE 4: Significant risk factors for PCO based on variate logistic regression.

Variable	Regression coefficient	OR	95% CI		p value
Age at time of surgery					
>60 years old	Reference	0.149	0.092	0.24.	0.000
<60 years old	−1.904				
History of diabetes					
No	Reference	1.825	1.042	3.197	0.035
Yes	0.602				
History of immune diseases					
No	Reference	1.128	0.471	2.700	0.787
Yes	0.120				
History of high myopia					
No	Reference	2.344	0.884	6.217	0.087
Yes	0.852				
The lens nucleus hardness					
I-II grade	Reference	0.508	0.304	0.847	0.009
III-V grade	−0.678				
Surgery type					
Phaco	Reference	2.563	1.242	5.290	0.011
ECCE	0.941				
History of vitrectomy					
No	Reference	1.905	1.046	3.471	0.035
Yes	0.645				
Ocular inflammation (aqueous cell)					
<15 cells	Reference	1.286	0.757	2.182	0.352
>15 cells	0.251				
IOL materials					
Hydrophilic	Reference	1.672	1.043	2.682	0.033
Hydrophobic	0.514				

the posterior capsule. Remnants of the lens may become trapped, absorb water, and appear fluffy white. Folds or tears leading to mechanical distortion of the bag may cause irregularities in posterior capsule transparency. Posterior inflammation may lead to deposits of proteins and white blood cells on the capsule, while surgical trauma may lead to deposition of red blood cells and pigmented cells [5]. A number of potentially significant factors in the development of PCO have been identified, including IOL materials, design and placement, surgical techniques, cortical clean-up, and concomitant pathologies.

Young age is a known risk factor for PCO, as shown by several previous studies and confirmed by our study. There are more LECs on the anterior capsules of young patients. A higher percentage of LECs retain strong cellular proliferative activity in young patients compared to older patients. In addition, the levels of hormones and cytokines in the aqueous humor are more suitable for LECs growth. Previous studies have reported that the rate of LECs growth is age-dependent, and the rate in young patients <40 years of age is three times faster than that in patients >60 years of age [6]. Furthermore, the nuclear hardness of the lens gradually

caused by LECs located at the equatorial lens region (lens bow), causing regeneration of crystallin-expressing lenticular fibers and forming Elschnig pearls and Soemmering rings, which are responsible for most cases of PCO-related visual losses. At present, the molecular mechanisms influencing leftover LECs behavior after cataract surgery are not completely known. Many other mechanisms may also affect

increases with growth during aging, which may affect the choice of surgery.

Not even one surgical approach involving lens extraction is able to completely remove the residual LECs. It has recently been suggested that almost 100% elimination of residual LECs may be necessary to prevent LECs proliferation on the posterior capsule and the development of PCO [7]. A comparison of PCO formation using different surgical techniques in previous studies is therefore controversial. Previous studies have also found that phacoemulsification and cortical I/A lead to less residual LECs concentrations on the internal capsule surfaces than ECCE with manual nuclear expression [7]. In addition, Nishi and Nishi [8] reported that meticulous capsule vacuuming using ultrasound endocapsular cataract surgery significantly reduces the need for laser capsulotomy (in their study, from 10.8% to 3.7%). Furthermore, phacoemulsification reduces damage to the blood-aqueous barrier by requiring only a minor surgical incision compared to ECCE, particularly in patients with diabetes [9]. Phacoemulsification uses continuous curvilinear capsulorhexis to decrease the capsular space of proliferation and migration of residual LECs [10]. All of these factors are considered to increase the formation of PCO in ECCE compared to phacoemulsification. Our findings are similar to these previous clinical and basic studies. However, a different point was raised that cell survival and growth were dependent on the patient's general condition, rather than the surgical technique performed. Some other studies have also reported no significant differences between phacoemulsification and ECCE surgery in terms of the *in vitro* percentage of PCO formation using a human capsular bag model [11]. In our study, the patients were followed for different periods of time, which may have affected the results (due to the use of updated surgical materials and equipment). However, this protocol provided a means of studying clinically important factors.

There have been many previous studies on the relationship between diabetes and the development of PCO. Several studies have reported significantly greater PCO formation in diabetic patients compared to nondiabetic patients, while others have reported no difference or a lower incidence of PCO in diabetic patients. The difference between the formation mechanism of PCO in patients with diabetes and nondiabetic patients is presently unclear. Praveen et al. [12] performed an observational case-control study to compare the development of PCO between eyes with and without diabetes after phacoemulsification and implantation of a single-piece hydrophobic acrylic IOL, with a 4-year follow-up. They reported a higher incidence of PCO in diabetic patients for up to 12 postoperative months. At the 4-year follow-up, there were no significant differences between the two groups. They also reported that the duration of diabetes increased the risk for PCO and the severity of retinopathy but did not influence the development of PCO. Hayashi et al. [13] reported similar findings at 36 months of follow-up. However, Elgohary and Dowler [2] suggested that diabetic patients had a lower long-term incidence and decreased risk for PCO at 4 years. Zaczek and Zetterstrom [14] reported similar findings at 2 years. A possible explanation for the lower PCO in diabetic patients may be the decreased

density of LECs in the diabetic capsular bag [15] and/or the detrimental effects of accumulating intracellular sorbitol [16] and fructose, free radicals, and oxidative stress on their survival and proliferative capacities [17]. These effects may explain the decrease in the incidence of PCO in diabetic patients at longer follow-up periods. However, our study suggests that diabetic patients are at increased risk for developing PCO. Some studies have attributed this phenomenon to damage to the blood-aqueous barrier and increased inflammation in the aqueous chamber [18]. Several clinical and experimental studies have reported that the incidence of LECs proliferation increases in protein-rich environments [19], which may subsequently result in extensive PCO.

A limitation of the present study is that we did not record the stage of diabetic retinopathy or blood glucose levels, which may be correlated with the degree of PCO in diabetic patients. In previous studies, the observation time of the subjects was fixed for long-term follow-up after surgery, whereas the observation times of our patients varied within 3 years, which may partially explain these discrepancies. Although they appear to be related, it is likely that inflammation, LECs proliferation, and PCO formation are independent of each other.

In previous studies, the incidence of PCO was significantly higher after cataract surgery using vitrectomy than that after cataract surgery alone, particularly in diabetic patients [20]. We found that combined surgery with vitrectomy was also an independent risk factor for the progression of PCO, consistent with other reports. Most reports have concluded that combined surgery of eyes could result in severe postoperative inflammation, which presumably leads to more extensive PCO. Such studies have suggested that elevated levels of cytokines caused by postoperative inflammation accelerate LECs proliferation via autocrine and/or paracrine signaling. Furthermore, it has recently been reported that there is more extensive PCO formation using 20-gauge phacovitrectomy than when 23-gauge phacovitrectomy is used to lower postoperative inflammation [21]. In addition, posterior vitreous pressure, the hypoxic state, intraocular gas tamponade, and silicone oil tamponade are associated with LECs proliferation, migration, and transdifferentiation after combined surgery. Meanwhile, we cannot differentiate whether the formation of PCO influenced by the factors of other vitreo-retinal disease, for which combined surgery is necessary.

Previous studies have reported a high incidence of PCO and subsequent Nd:YAG laser posterior capsulotomy in highly myopic eyes. High myopia is pathologic and is associated with an increase in certain growth factors in the aqueous humor, which might influence the development of PCO. However, the degree of PCO and the incidence of Nd:YAG capsulotomy in myopia eyes may be relatively low [22]. Furthermore, Hayashi et al. [23] reported that a long axial length is not a risk factor for the formation of PCO. However, these results on the role of myopia in PCO might not be extrapolated from clinical studies that have defined myopia based on different standards, such as axial length, the power of the implanted IOL, and the preoperative refraction. In the present study, it was difficult to clearly correlate the development of PCO with the factors of age, refractive lens exchange, or solely myopia. Nonetheless, our results could help surgeons estimate the incidence of PCO in myopic eyes and make decisions on the timing of Nd : YAG to minimize the risk of PCO formation after cataract surgery.

In the present study, IOL materials were either hydrophobic or hydrophilic. Previous studies have reported that the incidence of PCO in patients implanted with hydrophilic lenses is higher than the in patients implanted with hydrophobic lenses [24]. However, some studies have reported that the incidence of PCO using hydrophilic lenses is less than in patients using hydrophobic lenses [25, 26]. In addition to the optic material of IOLs, there are many other IOL factors that might influence the formation of PCO, such as the overall length, optic diameter, optic edge, haptic design, haptic material, and incision size needed for implantation. In the study by Findl et al. [27], a sharp-edged optic inhibited lens epithelial cells growth and lowered the incidence of PCO and laser capsulotomy. Schriefl et al. [28] reported that microincision cataract surgery of IOLs has a higher PCO incidence than conventional IOLs. Previous studies of cadaveric eyes have reported that Acrysof® has a relatively low propensity to induce cell proliferation in the capsular bag. Therefore, our study has a significant limitation, because only IOL material factors were analyzed. However, our results still have some clinical significance, because the incidence of PCO was higher in hydrophilic than in hydrophobic IOLs. Because the hydrophilic acrylic lenses have a different water content, there is a greater probability of contacting the lens capsule, which is more suitable to the "no space no cells" theory [29].

Other factors are thought to contribute to the formation of PCO, including IOL decentration, capsulorhexis decentration, capsule tears, and insufficient zonules, but we did not analyze these factors. We only compared the outcomes of surgeries performed using different surgeons at different institutions, and the patients were followed up for different periods of time. Any differences that occurred in the incidences of PCO may have resulted from factors not included in this study. In addition, the independent variable was not comprehensive, which may have affected the results of the logistic regression model. In future studies, we need to collect more clinical records of cases to improve the independent variable and conduct multicenter logistic regression analyses on a larger sample using a prospective study design.

Conflicts of Interest

The authors declare that they have no competing interests.

Acknowledgments

Supported by Qingdao Outstanding Health Professional Development Fund.

References

[1] N. Awasthi, S. Guo, and B. J. Wagner, "Posterior capsular opacification: a problem reduced but not yet eradicated," *Archives of Ophthalmology*, vol. 127, no. 4, pp. 555–562, 2009.

[2] M. A. Elgohary and J. G. Dowler, "Incidence and risk factors of Nd:YAG capsulotomy after phacoemulsification in non-diabetic and diabetic patients," *Clinical and Experimental Ophthalmology*, vol. 34, no. 6, pp. 526–534, 2006.

[3] L. M. Nibourg, E. Gelens, R. Kuijer, J. M. Hooymans, T. G. van Kooten, and S. A. Koopmans, "Prevention of posterior capsular opacification," *Experimental Eye Research*, vol. 136, pp. 100–115, 2015.

[4] T. M. Aslam and N. Patton, "Methods of assessment of patients for Nd:YAG laser capsulotomy that correlate with final visual improvement," *BMC Ophthalmology*, vol. 4, no. 1, p. 13, 2004.

[5] T. M. Aslam, H. Devlin, and B. Dhillon, "Use of Nd:YAG laser capsulotomy," *Survey of Ophthalmology*, vol. 48, no. 6, pp. 594–612, 2003.

[6] I. M. Wormstone, C. S. Liu, J. M. Rakic, J. M. Marcantonio, G. F. Vrensen, and G. Duncan, "Human lens epithelial cell proliferation in a protein-free medium," *Investigative Ophthamology & Visual Science*, vol. 38, no. 2, pp. 396–404, 1997.

[7] M. G. Davidson, D. K. Morgan, and M. C. McGahar, "Effect of surgical technique on in vitro posterior capsule opacification," *Journal of Cataract & Refractive Surgery*, vol. 26, no. 10, pp. 1550–1554, 2000.

[8] O. Nishi and K. Nishi, "Intercapsular cataract surgery with lens epithelial cell removal. Part III: long-term follow-up of posterior capsular opacification," *Journal of Cataract & Refractive Surgery*, vol. 17, no. 2, pp. 218–220, 1991.

[9] J. G. Dowler, P. G. Hykin, and A. M. Hamilton, "Phacoemulsification versus extracapsular cataract extraction in patients with diabetes," *Ophthalmology*, vol. 107, no. 3, pp. 457–462, 2000.

[10] N. Mamalis, A. S. Crandall, E. Linebarger, W. K. Shefield, and M. J. Leidenix, "Effect of intraocular lens size on posterior capsule opacification after phacoemulsification," *Journal of Cataract & Refractive Surgery*, vol. 21, no. 1, pp. 99–102, 1995.

[11] C. Wertheimer, T. C. Kreutzer, M. Dirisamer et al., "Effect of femtosecond laser-assisted lens surgery on posterior capsule opacification in the human capsular bag in vitro," *Acta Ophthalmologica*, vol. 95, no. 2, pp. e85–e88, 2017.

[12] M. R. Praveen, A. R. Vasavada, G. D. Shah, A. R. Shah, B. M. Khamar, and K. H. Dave, "A prospective evaluation of posterior capsule opacification in eyes with diabetes mellitus: a case-control study," *Eye*, vol. 28, no. 6, pp. 720–727, 2014.

[13] K. Hayashi, H. Hayashi, F. Nakao, and F. Hayashi, "Posterior capsule opacification after cataract surgery in patients with diabetes mellitus," *American Journal of Ophthalmology*, vol. 134, no. 1, pp. 10–16, 2002.

[14] A. Zaczek and C. Zetterstrom, "Posterior capsule opacification after phacoemulsification in patients with diabetes mellitus," *Journal of Cataract & Refractive Surgery*, vol. 25, no. 2, pp. 233–237, 1999.

[15] H. G. Struck, C. Heider, and C. Lautenschlager, "Changes in the lens epithelium of diabetic and non-diabetic patients with various forms of opacities in senile cataract," *Klinische Monatsblatter fur Augenheilkunde*, vol. 216, no. 4, pp. 204–209, 2000.

[16] Y. Takamura, E. Kubo, S. Tsuzuki, and Y. Akagi, "Apoptotic cell death in the lens epithelium of rat sugar cataract," *Experimental Eye Research*, vol. 77, no. 1, pp. 51–57, 2003.

[17] E. Kubo, T. Urakami, N. Fatma, Y. Akagi, and D. P. Singh, "Polyol pathway-dependent osmotic and oxidative stresses in aldose reductase-mediated apoptosis in human lens epithelial cells: role of AOP2," *Biochemical and Biophysical Research Communications*, vol. 314, no. 4, pp. 1050–1056, 2004.

[18] P. Cortina, M. J. Gomez-Lechon, A. Navea, J. L. Menezo, M. C. Terencio, and M. Diaz-Llopis, "Diclofenac sodium and cyclosporin A inhibit human lens epithelial cell proliferation in culture," *Graefe's Archive for Clinical and Experimental Ophthalmology*, vol. 235, no. 3, pp. 180–185, 1997.

[19] M. G. Davidson, M. Wormstone, D. Morgan, R. Malakof, J. Allen, and M. C. McGahan, "Ex vivo canine lens capsular sac explants," *Graefe's Archive for Clinical and Experimental Ophthalmology*, vol. 238, no. 8, pp. 708–714, 2000.

[20] J. Toda, S. Kato, T. Oshika, and G. Sugita, "Posterior capsule opacification after combined cataract surgery and vitrectomy," *Journal of Cataract & Refractive Surgery*, vol. 33, no. 1, pp. 104–107, 2007.

[21] T. Iwase, B. C. Oveson, and Y. Nishi, "Posterior capsule opacification following 20- and 23-gauge phacovitrectomy (posterior capsule opacification following phacovitrectomy)," *Eye*, vol. 26, no. 11, pp. 1459–1464, 2012.

[22] A. R. Vasavada, A. Shah, S. M. Raj, M. R. Praveen, and G. D. Shah, "Prospective evaluation of posterior capsule opacification in myopic eyes 4 years after implantation of a single-piece acrylic IOL," *Journal of Cataract & Refractive Surgery*, vol. 35, no. 9, pp. 1532–1539, 2009.

[23] K. Hayashi, M. Yoshida, and H. Hayashi, "Posterior capsule opacification in myopic eyes," *Journal of Cataract & Refractive Surgery*, vol. 32, no. 4, pp. 634–638, 2006.

[24] R. S. Joshi, "Postoperative posterior capsular striae and the posterior capsular opacification in patients implanted with two types of intraocular lens material," *Indian Journal of Ophthalmology*, vol. 65, no. 6, pp. 466–471, 2017.

[25] L. Bai, J. Zhang, L. Chen, T. Ma, and H. C. Liang, "Comparison of posterior capsule opacification at 360-degree square edge hydrophilic and sharp edge hydrophobic acrylic intraocular lens in diabetic patients," *International Journal of Ophthalmology*, vol. 8, no. 4, pp. 725–729, 2015.

[26] S. M. Schriefl, R. Menapace, E. Stifter, D. Zaruba, and C. Leydolt, "Posterior capsule opacification and neodymium: YAG laser capsulotomy rates with 2 microincision intraocular lenses: four-year results," *Journal of Cataract & Refractive Surgery*, vol. 41, no. 5, pp. 956–963, 2015.

[27] O. Findl, W. Buehl, P. Bauer, and T. Sycha, "Interventions for preventing posterior capsule opacification," *Cochrane Database of Systematic Reviews*, no. 3, article CD003738, 2010.

[28] S. M. Schriefl, C. Leydolt, E. Stifter, and R. Menapace, "Posterior capsular opacification and Nd:YAG capsulotomy rates with the iMics Y-60H and Micro AY intra-ocular lenses: 3-year results of a randomized clinical trial," *Acta Ophthalmologica*, vol. 93, no. 4, pp. 342–347, 2015.

[29] S. Kang, M. J. Kim, S. H. Park, and C. K. Joo, "Comparison of clinical results between heparin surface modified hydrophilic acrylic and hydrophobic acrylic intraocular lens," *European Journal of Ophthalmology*, vol. 18, no. 3, pp. 377–383, 2008.

24

Analysis of Factors Associated with the Ocular Features of Congenital Cataract Children in the Shanghai Pediatric Cataract Study

Wenwen He,[1,2,3] Ting Sun,[4] Jin Yang,[1,2,3] Guoyou Qin,[4] Zhenyu Wu,[4] Xiangjia Zhu,[1,2,3] and Yi Lu[1,2,3]

[1]Department of Ophthalmology, Eye and Ear, Nose, and Throat Hospital of Fudan University, 83 Fenyang Road, Shanghai 200031, China
[2]Key Laboratory of Myopia, Ministry of Health, Shanghai 200031, China
[3]Shanghai Key Laboratory of Visual Impairment and Restoration, Shanghai 200031, China
[4]Department of Biostatistics, School of Public Health, Key Laboratory of Public Health Safety, Ministry of Education, Fudan University, Shanghai 200032, China

Correspondence should be addressed to Xiangjia Zhu; zhuxiangjia1982@126.com and Yi Lu; luyieent@126.com

Academic Editor: Tamer A. Macky

Purpose. To investigate the ocular features of children with congenital cataract in a tertiary referral eye center in East China. *Methods.* We retrospectively reviewed the clinical data of congenital cataract children who underwent cataract surgery between April 2009 and April 2014 at the Eye and ENT Hospital of Fudan University and identified factors associated with the axial length (AXL) and corneal curvature (K value). *Results.* We included 493 children, 210 with unilateral and 283 with bilateral cataract. The mean AXL was 22.03 ± 1.97 mm and the mean K value was 43.61 ± 1.86 D. Age showed a linear correlation with AXL in unilateral cataract eyes and a logarithmic correlation with AXL in bilateral cataract eyes (both $P < 0.001$). AXL was longer and the K value was smaller (both $P < 0.01$) in boys than in girls after adjusting for age and cataract laterality. AXL was longer in unilateral cataract eyes than in bilateral cataract eyes after adjusting for age and gender ($P = 0.004$). In children with unilateral cataract, AXL was significantly longer in the affected eye than in the contralateral eye ($P < 0.001$). *Conclusion.* Age, gender, and cataract laterality together contribute to the development of ocular features of congenital cataract children, especially for AXL.

1. Introduction

Congenital cataract is the leading cause of visual impairment worldwide according to the updated global report by the World Health Organization [1]. Cataract surgery with or without intraocular lens (IOL) implantation is still the most common treatment method for congenital cataract [2, 3]. The measurement of ocular features, especially axial length (AXL) and corneal curvature (K value), is essential for IOL power calculation [4]. However, the formulae used in IOL power calculation were derived from data in adults and may be inaccurate for children [5, 6]. Furthermore, although selection of the target refractive error is usually dependent on age [4, 7], other factors may influence the ocular development of children with congenital cataract that should also be considered. Thus, it is important to analyze these factors in order to choose the most suitable IOL for children with congenital cataract.

Although the AXL and K value in children with congenital cataract have been reported [8–10], few studies have determined these parameters in Chinese children or examined the correlation between AXL and K value. The

Eye and Ear, Nose and Throat (ENT) Hospital of Fudan University is the largest and best tertiary referral eye center in East China and is involved in the care of nearly all children with cataract in this region. Thus, the purpose of this cross-sectional study was to assess the AXL and K value of children with congenital cataract who underwent cataract surgery at ≤18 years of age at our hospital in 5 years. We also examined the factors associated with the AXL and K value, including age, gender, and laterality, and analyzed the relationship between the AXL and K value. Our results should provide a reference for IOL power selection in children undergoing cataract surgery in the future.

2. Methods

The Institutional Review Board of the Eye and ENT Hospital of Fudan University, Shanghai, China, approved this retrospective study affiliated to the Shanghai Pediatric Cataract Study. All procedures adhered to the tenets of the Declaration of Helsinki. The Shanghai Pediatric Cataract Study was registered at ClinicalTrials.gov (accession number NCT03063216).

2.1. Children. We retrospectively reviewed the medical records of children with congenital cataract who underwent cataract surgery with or without IOL implantation at the Eye & ENT Hospital of Fudan University between April 2009 and April 2014. Only children aged ≤18 years who were diagnosed with congenital cataract were enrolled. Children with systemic diseases, previous trauma, lens subluxation, or other conditions likely to affect the measurement of the AXL and K value were excluded. Other types of childhood cataracts due to trauma, exposure to radiations, metabolic and other acquired causes were excluded. We also excluded the eyes in which AXL was not measured. Data collected included the age at surgery, gender, cataract laterality (unilateral or bilateral), and the AXL and mean K values of both eyes.

2.2. Examinations. AXL was measured using an IOLMaster® 500 (Carl Zeiss AG, Oberkochen, Germany) before surgery in older children who cooperated with the procedure. If the AXL could not be measured in conscious infants, a contact A-scan (Tomey EM-3000, Nagoya, Japan) was performed after instillation of topical anesthetic and sedation with 10% chloral hydrate before surgery or under general anesthesia at surgery. The mean K value was only obtained in children who cooperated during measurements with the IOLMaster. Each eye was measured 5–10 times, and the mean value was recorded. The preoperative examinations were performed only by one special technician in biometry for children.

2.3. Main Outcome Measures. The main outcome measures were the AXL and K value of children with congenital cataract. In children with bilateral cataract, we randomly selected one eye for analysis to avoid correlation effects. The children were divided into four groups for further analyses according to their age at surgery: 0-1, 1-2, 2-6, 6–12, and 12–18 years old. The associations of age, gender, and cataract laterality

with the AXL and mean K value and the correlation between the AXL and K value were also determined.

2.4. Statistical Analysis. All statistical analyses were performed using SPSS version 11 (SPSS Inc., Chicago, IL, USA). Quantitative variables are presented as the mean ± standard deviation (SD), and categorical variables are described as the number and/or percent of children. Mean ± 3SD was set as the cut points of the quantitative variables, and data out of this range was excluded from analysis. Student's t-test was used to compare continuous variables, and the χ^2 test was used to compare categorical data between two groups. Univariate analysis of covariance (ANCOVA) was used to adjust for age, gender, and laterality. The correlation between AXL and mean K value was determined using Pearson's correlation analysis, while linear or logarithmic regression was also used to assess associations between these variables and other explanatory variables. P values of <0.05 were considered statistically significant.

3. Results

3.1. Characteristics of the Children. Overall, 493 children with congenital cataract satisfied our eligibility criteria and were included in this study. All of the children had complete AXL data for both eyes. There were 210 children with unilateral cataract and 283 with bilateral cataract. The mean age at surgery of all children combined was 4.72 ± 3.36 years and ranged from 0.25 to 17.40 years. The mean ages of children with unilateral and bilateral cataract were 4.93 ± 3.29 and 4.57 ± 3.40 years, respectively, and were not significantly different between these groups (Student's t-test, $P = 0.250$). The age distribution of children with congenital cataract is shown in Figure 1. There were more bilateral cases aged 0-1 year than unilateral cases (10.6% versus 4.3%, χ^2 test, $P = 0.010$). The largest subgroup was children aged 2–6 years (53.75%). Overall, 121 boys and 89 girls had unilateral cataract while 175 boys and 108 girls had bilateral cataract. The distribution of boys and girls was not significantly different between the two groups (χ^2 test, $P = 0.320$).

3.2. Correlations between Age, Gender, and Laterality with AXL and Mean K Value. After excluding cases with AXL out of cut points, there were 486 eyes used for further analysis. The excluded cases were all boys with bilateral cataract. The mean AXL of the 486 eyes with congenital cataract was 22.03 ± 1.97 mm and ranged from 16.61 to 30.32 mm. The logarithmic correlation between AXL and age in 486 children with congenital cataract is shown in Figure 2(a) ($R^2 = 0.255$, $P < 0.001$). We found a significant linear correlation between age and AXL in children with unilateral cataract (Figure 2(b), $R^2 = 0.223$, $P < 0.001$) and a significant logarithmic correlation between age and AXL in children with bilateral cataract (Figure 2(c), $R^2 = 0.287$, $P < 0.001$).

The mean K value was successfully measured in 201 children aged >2 years, of which 2 cases were out of cut points, and then, data from 87 unilateral cataract and 112 bilateral cataract were used. The mean K value of these children was 43.61 ± 1.86 D and ranged from 38.16 to 49.75 D. However,

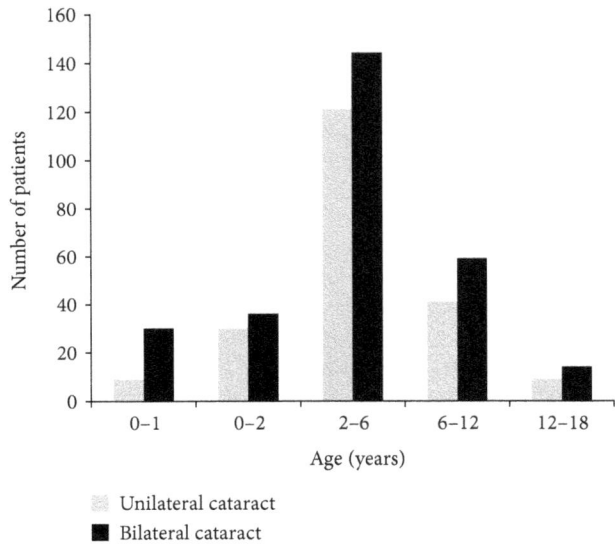

FIGURE 1: Distribution of children with congenital cataract according to the age at surgery and unilateral/bilateral cataract. There were more bilateral cases aged 0-1 year than unilateral cases (10.6% versus 4.3%, χ^2 test, $P = 0.010$).

age was not correlated with the mean K value in these children (linear regression, $R^2 < 0.001$, $P = 0.927$).

As shown in Table 1, AXL was significantly longer (ANCOVA, $P = 0.010$) and the mean K value (ANCOVA, $P < 0.001$) was significantly smaller in boys than in girls after adjusting for age and cataract laterality. The AXL and mean K value were also compared between boys and girls in age groups of children (Table 1). In these analyses, we found that AXL was significantly different between boys and girls in children aged 0-1 year (ANCOVA, $P = 0.037$), children aged 2-6 years (ANCOVA, $P = 0.036$), and children aged 6-12 years (ANCOVA, $P = 0.034$). The mean K value was significantly larger in girls than in boys aged 2-6 years old (ANCOVA, $P = 0.004$).

The AXL and mean K value are compared between children with unilateral cataract and children with bilateral cataract in Table 2. After adjusting for age and gender, AXL was significantly longer in children with unilateral cataract than in children with bilateral cataract (ANCOVA, $P = 0.004$). These differences were significant in children aged 1-2 and 6-12 years (ANCOVA, $P = 0.046$ and $P = 0.020$). The mean K value was not significantly different between children with unilateral cataract and children with bilateral cataract after adjusting for age and gender (ANCOVA, all $P > 0.05$).

The AXL and mean K value of affected eyes and contralateral eyes in children with unilateral congenital cataract are shown in Table 3. In all children, the AXL was significantly longer in the affected eye than in the contralateral eye (paired t-test, $P < 0.001$). This difference was also observed in all age groups (paired t-test, all $P < 0.05$), except in children aged 12-18 years (paired t-test, $P = 0.123$). By contrast, the K values were similar between the affected eye and the contralateral eye in all children and in each age group (paired t-test, all $P > 0.05$). In children with bilateral congenital

cataract, there were no differences in the AXL or K value between the randomly selected eye and the contralateral eye (Table 4, paired t-test, all $P > 0.05$).

3.3. Correlation between the AXL and K Value in Children with Congenital Cataract. After excluding cases with AXL and K value out of cut points, the K values were negatively correlated with AXL in all children, children with unilateral cataract, and children with bilateral cataract (Pearson's correlation analysis, $r = -0.314$, $P < 0.001$; $r = -0.237$, $P = 0.027$; and $r = -0.373$, $P < 0.001$, resp.).

4. Discussion

It is important to determine the ocular features in children with congenital cataract to understand the development of their affected eyes, to calculate the IOL power precisely, and to ensure that the target refractive error is correctly determined. Prior studies reported that age is significantly associated with ocular features [9, 11], as are gender and cataract laterality [9, 10]. However, most studies used univariate analyses and studied the effects of other factors in children who were only grouped by age [9, 12]. In our study, we used ANCOVA to adjust for each variable and identify which variables were independently associated with ocular features. This approach may be more reliable than the analyses used in prior reports [9, 12]. Furthermore, ocular features differed between races, but few studies have focused on Asian children [8-10]. Thus, our study could fill gaps in our knowledge, especially in terms of the ocular features of children with congenital cataract in East China. In this cross-sectional study, we analyzed the ocular characteristics of children with congenital cataract who underwent cataract surgery in our hospital at an age of ≤18 years. We found that age showed a linear correlation with AXL in children with unilateral cataract and a logarithmic correlation with AXL in children with bilateral cataract. Gender and cataract laterality were also associated with the AXL of children with congenital cataract. In children aged ≤12 years with unilateral cataract, the AXL of the affected eye was significantly longer than that of the contralateral eye. In addition, AXL showed a negative correlation with the mean K value in children with congenital cataract.

The mean age of the enrolled children was 4.72 ± 3.36 years, which was slightly older than the mean ages reported in previous studies [9, 12]. This may be due to the fact that children with cataract usually underwent IOL implantation after 1 year of age in our center. AXL was not available in younger children who underwent cataract surgery without IOL implantation; these children were excluded from this study and this is a limitation of our study. In addition, the operated age between unilateral and bilateral cases was not different in our study since some bilateral cases may have one-stage surgery without IOL implantation and AXL data under 1 year old. A study on baseline characteristics of children who underwent cataract surgery less than 13 years old in North America showed a mean operative age of 4.2 years, which was similar to ours, but this study has more unilateral

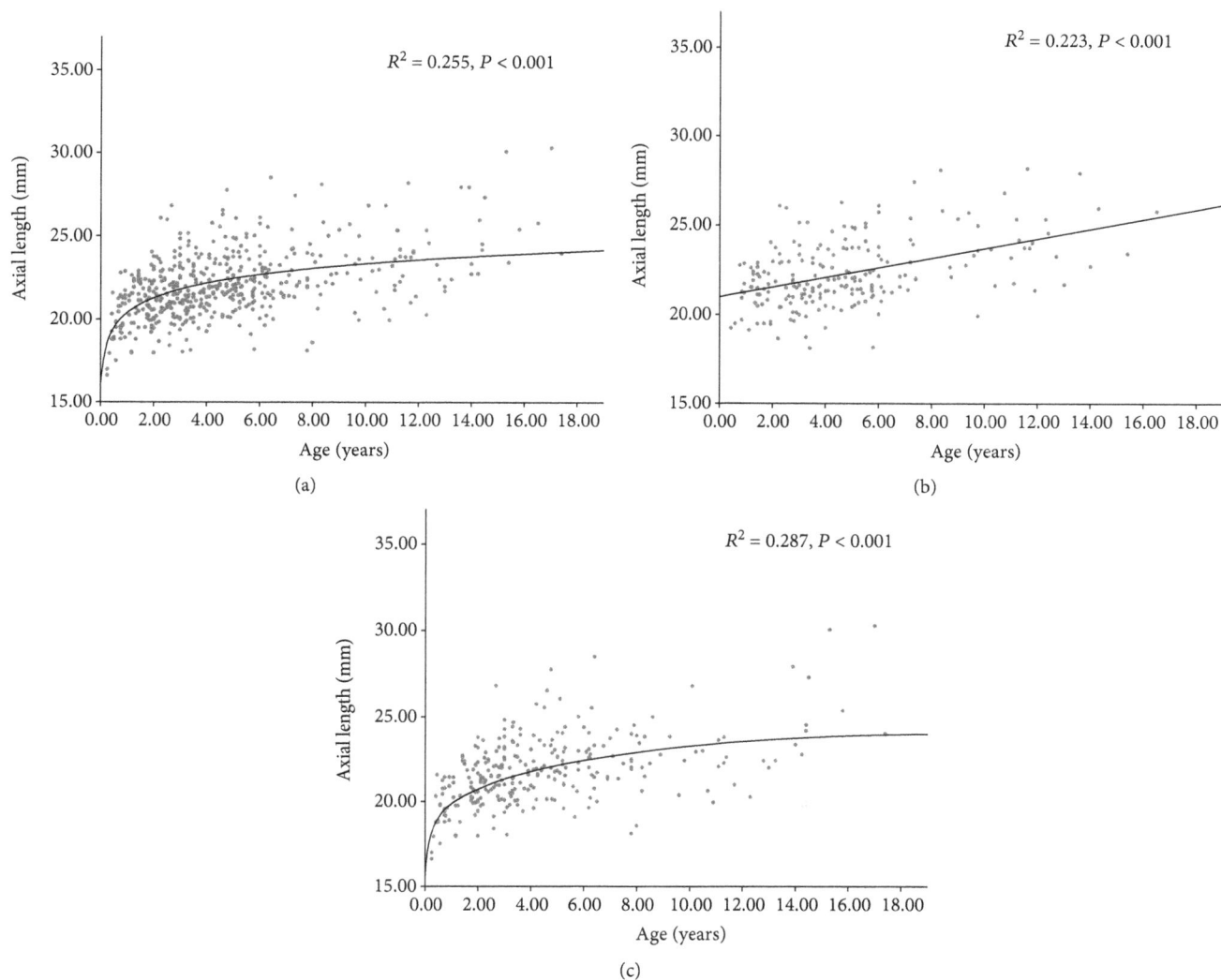

FIGURE 2: Correlations between age and the axial length of affected eyes in all children with congenital cataract ((a) logarithmic regression, $R^2 = 0.255$, $P < 0.001$), children with unilateral cataract ((b) linear regression, $R^2 = 0.223$, $P < 0.001$), and children with bilateral cataract eyes ((c) logarithmic regression, $R^2 = 0.287$, $P < 0.001$).

cases (59% versus 43%) and has more cases (34%) who underwent cataract surgery at 0-1 year [13].

We found a significant logarithmic correlation between age and AXL in all children and a marked increase in AXL in children aged ≤2 years, consistent with prior studies [9, 12, 14]. Trivedi and Wilson reported that the AXL at <1 year of age was significantly different from that of the other age groups and extended rapidly in the first year of age [9]. However, the earlier studies did not separate children with unilateral or bilateral cataract when analyzing the relationship between age and AXL [12, 14]. We found a significant linear correlation ($R^2 = 0.223$, $P < 0.001$) rather than a logarithmic correlation ($R^2 = 0.195$, $P < 001$) between age and AXL when the analysis was limited to children with unilateral cataract. This suggests that the eyeball may develop differently between children with unilateral and bilateral cataract. This finding may help explain why the visual acuity of the affected eye in children with unilateral cataract was

usually worse than that of the eyes in children with bilateral cataract in previous studies [15–17].

Previous studies revealed that AXL was longer in boys than in girls with congenital cataract [9, 12]. We confirmed this finding after adjusting for age and cataract laterality. This may be due to the positive correlation between AXL and head size reported elsewhere [18, 19]. According to the World Health Organization Child Growth Standards, at <5 years of age, boys have a larger head circumference than girls. This may explain the difference in AXL between boys and girls in children aged 0-1 year and 2–6 years.

After adjusting for age and gender, AXL was found to be longer in children with unilateral cataract than in children with bilateral cataract, especially in those aged 1 to 2 years. This is an important period of time for AXL development [20], and the AXL may increase quicker during this time in the affected eyes of children with unilateral cataract [12]. The growth of eyes affected by cataract may be influenced

TABLE 1: Comparison of axial length and mean K value between boys and girls after adjusting for age and the cataract laterality.

Age (years)	AXL (mm)			K value (D)		
	Boys	Girls	P	Boys	Girls	P
0-1	20.17 ± 1.59	19.56 ± 1.29	**0.037***	—	—	—
1-2	21.03 ± 1.23	21.19 ± 1.54	0.989	—	—	—
2–6	22.16 ± 1.73	21.73 ± 1.53	**0.036***	43.19 ± 1.69	44.11 ± 1.68	**0.004***
6–12	23.28 ± 1.97	22.33 ± 1.80	**0.034***	43.43 ± 1.90	44.31 ± 2.27	0.063
12–18	24.92 ± 4.22	24.58 ± 1.73	0.697	42.76 ± 1.41	44.23 ± 1.91	0.104
All children	22.23 ± 1.98	21.73 ± 1.93	**0.010***	43.22 ± 1.73	44.19 ± 1.90	**<0.001***

*Significantly different between boys and girls after adjusting for age and cataract laterality by analysis of covariance. Results are presented as the mean ± standard deviation. AXL = axial length.

TABLE 2: Comparison of axial length and K value between children with unilateral or bilateral congenital cataract after adjusting for age and gender.

Age (years)	AXL (mm)			K value (D)		
	Unilateral	Bilateral	P	Unilateral	Bilateral	P
0-1	21.03 ± 1.33	19.54 ± 1.37	0.093	—	—	—
1-2	21.43 ± 1.20	20.86 ± 1.45	**0.046***	—	—	—
2–6	22.11 ± 1.72	21.90 ± 1.62	0.494	43.66 ± 1.82	43.51 ± 1.69	0.763
6–12	23.48 ± 1.99	22.45 ± 1.82	**0.020***	43.60 ± 1.57	43.95 ± 2.45	0.385
12–18	24.53 ± 1.93	24.79 ± 3.07	0.722	43.18 ± 0.43	43.21 ± 2.08	0.896
All children	22.34 ± 1.89	21.79 ± 2.01	**0.004***	43.60 ± 1.65	43.62 ± 2.01	0.650

*Significantly different between children with unilateral and bilateral cataract after adjusting for age and gender using analysis of covariance. Results are presented as the mean ± standard deviation. AXL = axial length.

TABLE 3: Comparison of axial length and K value between the affected eye and the contralateral eye in children with unilateral congenital cataract.

Age (years)	AXL (mm)			K value (D)		
	Affected eye	Fellow eye	P	Affected eye	Fellow eye	P
0-1	21.03 ± 1.33	20.59 ± 1.21	0.243	—	—	—
1-2	21.43 ± 1.20	20.98 ± 0.74	**0.012***	—	—	—
2–6	22.11 ± 1.72	21.84 ± 0.89	**0.048***	43.69 ± 1.83	43.58 ± 1.52	0.547
6–12	23.48 ± 1.99	22.94 ± 1.40	**0.018***	43.60 ± 1.57	43.61 ± 1.52	0.940
12–18	24.53 ± 1.93	23.31 ± 1.97	0.123	43.18 ± 0.43	43.22 ± 0.48	0.843
All children	22.34 ± 1.89	21.94 ± 1.27	**<0.001***	43.61 ± 1.65	43.56 ± 1.46	0.621

*Significantly different between the affected eye and fellow eye using paired t-tests. Results are presented as the mean ± standard deviation. AXL = axial length.

TABLE 4: Comparison of axial length and K value between the randomly selected eye and the contralateral eye in bilateral congenital cataract children.

Age (years)	AXL (mm)			K value (D)		
	Selected eye	Fellow eye	P	Selected eye	Fellow eye	P
0-1	19.54 ± 1.37	19.70 ± 1.42	0.127	—	—	—
1-2	20.86 ± 1.45	20.93 ± 1.46	0.406	—	—	—
2–6	21.90 ± 1.62	21.94 ± 1.67	0.542	43.49 ± 1.70	43.40 ± 1.94	0.561
6–12	22.45 ± 1.82	22.67 ± 2.01	0.080	44.06 ± 2.50	44.19 ± 2.39	0.109
12–18	24.79 ± 3.07	24.83 ± 2.96	0.731	43.21 ± 2.08	42.95 ± 2.29	0.238
All children	21.79 ± 2.01	21.89 ± 2.06	0.053	43.64 ± 2.03	43.60 ± 2.15	0.648

Results are presented as the mean ± standard deviation. AXL = axial length.

by two mechanisms: form deprivation may lead to a longer AXL, whereas ocular anomalies may be associated with a shorter AXL. We surmise that unilateral cataract is a unilateral anomaly, which may be due to environmental factors rather than genetic factors, and develop into form-deprivation myopia. Besides, the AXL of the affected eye was also longer than that of the contralateral eye in our study, which was opposite to the results of some studies in Western countries [9]. Racial differences may explain these differences. Myopia and high myopia are more common in Asian populations than in Western populations [21, 22]. Thus, we think that form deprivation in unilateral cataract is more likely to lead to myopia or a longer AXL in Chinese children than in other races. What is more, a recent research from the Infant Aphakia Treatment Study showed this opposite result in unilateral cataract infants aged 1 to 7 months [23]. Compared with our study, which contained most unilateral cataract children aged over 2 years, it suggested that the occurrence of form deprivation myopia may need more than one year.

In our study, we did not find a correlation between age and the mean K value. One possible explanation may be that the mean K value could only be determined in children aged >2 years. It was previously reported that the K value was negatively correlated with age in children with congenital cataract aged <6 months old [10]. This means that the mean K value decreased significantly from birth to 6 months of age. However, this correlation disappeared in children aged >6 years [10].

Consistent with earlier studies, we found that the mean K value was smaller in boys than in girls with congenital cataract, [10] and may be due to the difference in head circumference between boys and girls. Previous studies reported that the K value in the affected eye of children with unilateral cataract was greater than that of children with bilateral cataract and the contralateral eye [10]. However, we did not observe a similar phenomenon. This may be due to the fact that the largest differences were observed in children aged 0–6 months [10], an age group excluded from our study.

We also examined the correlation between the AXL and mean K value in children with congenital cataract and found a negative correlation between these variables. This suggests that AXL is more strongly associated with the mean K value than age. Therefore, surgeons should consider the age, gender, and AXL when estimating the K value in children who did not cooperate with keratometry.

In conclusion, we determined the ocular features of children aged ≤18 years with congenital cataract who underwent cataract surgery in our hospital over a 5-year period. Age, gender, and cataract laterality together contribute to the development of ocular features, especially for AXL. We found different correlation types between age and AXL in children with unilateral cataract and bilateral cataract, which suggest that the eyeball may develop differently between children with these two types of congenital cataract. Unlike children in Western countries, Chinese children with unilateral congenital cataract usually have longer AXL in the affected eye than the fellow eye. Gender may have more influence on mean K value than age in children ≥2 years

old. In addition, the mean K value decreased with increasing AXL. Our study described the relationships between demographic characters and ocular features in Chinese congenital cataract children and may provide a reference for those who cannot cooperate with these measurements, especially in corneal curvature examination.

Conflicts of Interest

No author has conflicts of interest to report.

Authors' Contributions

Wenwen He, Xiangjia Zhu, and Yi Lu designed the study; Wenwen He conducted the study; Ting Sun and Jin Yang are responsible for the collection and management of the data; Wenwen He, Ting Sun, Zhenyu Wu, and Guoyou Qin analyzed and interpreted the data; and Wenwen He, Xiangjia Zhu, and Yi Lu prepared and reviewed the manuscript. All authors gave final approval of the manuscript. Wenwen He and Ting Sun contributed equally to this work.

Acknowledgments

Publication of this article was supported by the research grants from the National Natural Science Foundation of People's Republic of China (Grant nos. 81470613, 81100653, and 81270989), International Science and Technology Cooperation Foundation of Shanghai (Grant no. 14430721100), and National Health and Family Planning Commission of the People's Republic of China (Grant no. 201302015).

References

[1] S. Adhikari, M. K. Shrestha, K. Adhikari, N. Maharjan, and U. D. Shrestha, "Causes of visual impairment and blindness in children in three ecological regions of Nepal: Nepal pediatric ocular diseases study," *Clinical Ophthalmology*, vol. 9, pp. 1543–1547, 2015.

[2] M. C. Struck, "Long-term results of pediatric cataract surgery and primary intraocular lens implantation from 7 to 22 months of life," *The Journal of the American Medical Association Ophthalmology*, vol. 133, no. 10, pp. 1180–1183, 2015.

[3] M. E. Wilson Jr., L. R. Bartholomew, and R. H. Trivedi, "Pediatric cataract surgery and intraocular lens implantation: practice styles and preferences of the 2001 ASCRS and AAPOS memberships," *Journal of Cataract & Refractive Surgery*, vol. 29, no. 9, pp. 1811–1820, 2003.

[4] D. K. Vanderveen, R. H. Trivedi, A. Nizam, M. J. Lynn, S. R. Lambert, and Infant Aphakia Treatment Study Group, "Predictability of intraocular lens power calculation formulae in infantile eyes with unilateral congenital cataract: results from the infant aphakia treatment study," *American Journal of Ophthalmology*, vol. 156, no. 6, pp. 1252–1260 e2, 2013.

[5] V. Vasavada, S. K. Shah, V. A. Vasavada et al., "Comparison of IOL power calculation formulae for pediatric eyes," *Eye*, vol. 30, no. 9, pp. 1242–1250, 2016.

[6] S. Thanapaisal, P. Wongwai, W. Phanphruk, and S. Suwannaraj, "Accuracy of intraocular lens calculation by SRK/T formula in pediatric cataracts," *Journal of the Medical Association of Thailand*, vol. 98, Supplement 7, pp. S198–S203, 2015.

[7] M. E. Wilson Jr., R. H. Trivedi, E. G. Buckley et al., "ASCRS white paper hydrophobic acrylic intraocular lenses in children," *Journal of Cataract & Refractive Surgery*, vol. 33, no. 11, pp. 1966–1973, 2007.

[8] R. H. Trivedi and M. E. Wilson, "Axial length measurements by contact and immersion techniques in pediatric eyes with cataract," *Ophthalmology*, vol. 118, no. 3, pp. 498–502, 2011.

[9] R. H. Trivedi and M. E. Wilson, "Biometry data from Caucasian and African-American cataractous pediatric eyes," *Investigative Ophthalmology & Visual Science*, vol. 48, no. 10, pp. 4671–4678, 2007.

[10] R. H. Trivedi and M. E. Wilson, "Keratometry in pediatric eyes with cataract," *Archives of Ophthalmology*, vol. 126, no. 1, pp. 38–42, 2008.

[11] E. Ojaimi, I. G. Morgan, D. Robaei et al., "Effect of stature and other anthropometric parameters on eye size and refraction in a population-based study of Australian children," *Investigative Ophthalmology & Visual Science*, vol. 46, no. 12, pp. 4424–4429, 2005.

[12] H. Lin, D. Lin, J. Chen et al., "Distribution of axial length before cataract surgery in Chinese pediatric patients," *Scientific Reports*, vol. 6, article 23862, 2016.

[13] M. X. Repka, T. W. Dean, E. L. Lazar et al., "Cataract surgery in children from birth to less than 13 years of age: baseline characteristics of the cohort," *Ophthalmology*, vol. 123, no. 12, pp. 2462–2473, 2016.

[14] P. Capozzi, C. Morini, S. Piga, M. Cuttini, and P. Vadala, "Corneal curvature and axial length values in children with congenital/infantile cataract in the first 42 months of life," *Investigative Ophthalmology & Visual Science*, vol. 49, no. 11, pp. 4774–4778, 2008.

[15] Z. Rajavi, S. Mokhtari, H. Sabbaghi, and M. Yaseri, "Long-term visual outcome of congenital cataract at a tertiary referral center from 2004 to 2014," *Journal of Current Ophthalmology*, vol. 27, no. 3-4, pp. 103–109, 2015.

[16] A. L. Solebo, I. Russell-Eggitt, P. M. Cumberland, and J. S. Rahi, "Risks and outcomes associated with primary intraocular lens implantation in children under 2 years of age: the IoLunder2 cohort study," *The British Journal of Ophthalmology*, vol. 99, no. 11, pp. 1471–1476, 2015.

[17] X. Rong, Y. Ji, Y. Fang, Y. Jiang, and Y. Lu, "Long-term visual outcomes of secondary intraocular lens implantation in children with congenital cataracts," *PLoS One*, vol. 10, no. 7, article e0134864, 2015.

[18] S. M. Saw, L. Tong, K. S. Chia et al., "The relation between birth size and the results of refractive error and biometry measurements in children," *The British Journal of Ophthalmology*, vol. 88, no. 4, pp. 538–542, 2004.

[19] E. Ojaimi, D. Robaei, E. Rochtchina, K. A. Rose, I. G. Morgan, and P. Mitchell, "Impact of birth parameters on eye size in a population-based study of 6-year-old Australian children," *American Journal of Ophthalmology*, vol. 140, no. 3, pp. 535–537, 2005.

[20] R. N. Hussain, F. Shahid, and G. Woodruff, "Axial length in apparently normal pediatric eyes," *European Journal of Ophthalmology*, vol. 24, no. 1, pp. 120–123, 2014.

[21] M. T. Kang, S. M. Li, X. Peng et al., "Chinese eye exercises and myopia development in school age children: a nested case-control study," *Scientific Reports*, vol. 6, article 28531, 2016.

[22] C. W. Pan, T. Y. Wong, R. Lavanya et al., "Prevalence and risk factors for refractive errors in Indians: the Singapore Indian eye study (SINDI)," *Investigative Ophthalmology & Visual Science*, vol. 52, no. 6, pp. 3166–3173, 2011.

[23] M. E. Wilson, R. H. Trivedi, D. R. Weakley Jr., G. A. Cotsonis, S. R. Lambert, and Infant Aphakia Treatment Study Group, "Globe axial length growth at age 5 years in the infant aphakia treatment study," *Ophthalmology*, vol. 124, no. 5, pp. 730–733, 2017.

25

Effects of Residual Anterior Lens Epithelial Cell Removal on Axial Position of Intraocular Lens after Cataract Surgery

Seung Pil Bang [ID],[1] **Young-Sik Yoo,**[2] **Jong Hwa Jun** [ID],[1] **and Choun-Ki Joo** [ID][2,3]

[1]*Department of Ophthalmology, Dongsan Medical Center, Keimyung University School of Medicine, Daegu, Republic of Korea*
[2]*Catholic Institute for Visual Science, The Catholic University of Korea, Seoul, Republic of Korea*
[3]*Department of Ophthalmology and Visual Science, Seoul St. Mary's Hospital, College of Medicine,*
The Catholic University of Korea, Seoul, Republic of Korea

Correspondence should be addressed to Jong Hwa Jun; junjonghwa@gmail.com

Academic Editor: Usha P. Andley

Purpose. The aim of this study was to assess the effects of residual anterior lens epithelial cell (LEC) removal by anterior capsule polishing on the effective lens position (ELP) and axial position stability of the intraocular lens (IOL) after cataract surgery via postoperative measurement of the anterior chamber depth. *Methods.* We enrolled 30 patients (60 eyes) requiring bilateral cataract surgery for age-related cataracts. Meticulous anterior capsule polishing and removal of residual LECs under the capsule were performed using a bimanual irrigation/aspiration system for one randomly selected eye in each patient. The eye without polishing served as a control. ELP was measured at five different time points after surgery, and axial shifting of IOL was determined at each visit by comparison with the position at the previous visit. *Results.* The polishing and control groups showed significant differences with regard to the mean ELP at 1 (3.40 ± 0.29 versus 3.53 ± 0.32 mm, resp.; $p = 0.026$) and 2 months (3.42 ± 0.32 versus 3.61 ± 0.35 mm, resp.; $p = 0.001$) after surgery, the mean standard deviation for the five ELP values (0.087 ± 0.093 versus 0.159 ± 0.138 mm, $p = 0.001$), and the root mean square of the change in ELP at each follow-up visit (0.124 ± 0.034 versus 0.246 ± 0.038 mm, $p = 0.047$). The eyes in the control group exhibited a tendency for backward IOL movement with a concurrent hyperopic shift in refraction of approximately 0.2 diopter at 2 months after surgery. *Conclusion.* Our findings suggest that residual anterior LEC polishing enhances the axial position stability of IOLs, without any complications, after cataract surgery.

1. Introduction

In recent years, phacoemulsification with concurrent foldable intraocular lens (IOL) implantation has taken the place of refractive surgery, with the development and increase in the popularity of various refraction-correcting IOLs, including multifocal or toric IOLs. In addition to an accurate IOL power calculation formula and ocular biometry, the precise determination of the effective lens position (ELP) is essential to optimize the postoperative refractive outcomes [1, 2]. ELP, described as the distance between the anterior surface of the cornea and the IOL plane, indicates the axial position of IOL [3]. Forward movement of IOL from the estimated ELP results in

myopia, while backward displacement leads to a hyperopic shift in refraction [4, 5]. One study reported that inaccurate ELP prediction can account for 22% to 38% of the total refractive prediction error [6], while a postoperative shift in ELP could induce an unexpected refractive change apart from the prediction error. The reciprocal action between capsular fibrosis and bag fusion possibly accounts for the change in ELP after surgery [7].

Residual lens epithelial cells (LECs) after cataract surgery play a significant role in the development and progression of capsule fibrosis and contraction [8–10]. Several studies have reported that the removal of residual anterior LECs resulted in delayed or lesser capsular bag contraction and anterior capsule fibrosis [11–14].

We speculated that the removal of residual anterior LECs by anterior capsule polishing may minimize changes in ELP and the axial position of IOL induced by capsular bag contraction and anterior capsule fibrosis. Accordingly, we designed the present study to evaluate changes in ELP in order to identify the axial position stability of IOL and associated refractive alterations after cataract surgery with anterior capsule polishing.

2. Patients and Methods

2.1. Patients. We enrolled 30 patients (60 eyes) from January 2016 to April 2017. The research was performed at the Department of Ophthalmology in Dongsan Medical Center, which is affiliated with Keimyung University in Daegu, Republic of Korea. All studies and measurements were in accordance with the tenets of the Declaration of Helsinki, and the study protocol was reviewed and approved by the Ethics Committee of Dongsan Medical Center (Approval no. 2016-01-001). Informed consent for participation was obtained from all patients. The inclusion criteria were as follows: bilateral age-related cataract with a favorable clinical status and uneventful in-the-bag IOL implantation in both eyes. The exclusion criteria were as follows: a history of intraocular surgery or corneal laser surgery, a history of ocular trauma or uveitis, severe fundus pathology, an axial length (AL) of <22.0 mm or >24.0 mm, pseudoexfoliation syndrome (PEX), poor pupil dilation, zonular weakening or tension ring insertion, too large or too small continuous curvilinear capsulorhexis (CCC), eccentric CCC, radial tear in the anterior capsule, and inability to attend follow-up appointments on time.

2.2. Cataract Classification. Before surgery, the opacity in each eye was evaluated using the Lens Opacities Classification System III (LOCS III) [15] after pupil dilation with 0.5% tropicamide/0.5% phenylephrine fixed combination eye drops (Tropherine®, Hanmi Pharm, Seoul, Korea). A cataract surgery specialist graded every eye using slit-lamp examination for matching nuclear opalescence and color, cortical cataract, and posterior subcapsular cataract with opacities on standardized color photographs. Patients with a large discrepancy in the severity of cataract between the right and left eyes, those with brunescent or mature cataract, and those with anterior subcapsular opacity were excluded. Nuclear opalescence, cortical cataract, and posterior subcapsular cataract grades were used to confirm similarities between the polishing and control groups in terms of the cataract grade and evaluate the effect of cortical cataract on capsular contraction and fibrosis after surgery.

2.3. Surgical Procedure. All study patients underwent the necessary laboratory tests and clinical examinations. The IOL power was set to achieve postoperative refraction between +0.25 and −0.25 diopter (D) using optical low-coherence reflectometry (Lenstar LS900®, Haag-Streit AG, Bern, Switzerland). The preoperative best-corrected visual acuity (BCVA) was confirmed and converted to logMAR

units. The anterior chamber depth (ACD) was measured before surgery using A-scan (AXIS-II PR®, Quantel Medical Inc., Paris, France). Approximately 30 min before surgery, 0.5% tropicamide/0.5% phenylephrine fixed combination eye drops (Tropherine®, Hanmi Pharm) were instilled in the patients' eyes twice within 5 min for maximal pupil dilation. A single surgeon (JHJ) performed all surgeries with a 2.85 mm coaxial incision (Infiniti® vision system, Alcon Laboratories, Fort Worth, TX, USA). After topical anesthesia with 0.5% proparacaine eye drops (Paracaine®, Hanmi Pharm), a clear corneal incision was placed at the 9 o'clock (right eye) and 2 o'clock (left eye) positions. A centered CCC with a 5.5 mm diameter was prepared using capsulorhexis forceps. For the precise achievement of an equal CCC size, we used a 6 mm diameter capsulorhexis marker (K3-7850, Katena, Denville, NJ, USA) for a 5.5 mm diameter CCC; too large, too small, or eccentric CCCs were excluded. Subsequently, thorough hydrodissection was performed to freely rotate the nucleus, following which phacochop nucleofractis was used for emulsification and removal of the nucleus.

To eliminate any bias, the decision to perform anterior polishing or not was made only after the completion of cortex aspiration using an ordinary one-hand irrigation/aspiration system, without reference to the amount of visible residual LECs. Subsequently, the eyes were assigned to a polishing or control group using a table of random numbers generated by Microsoft Excel for Windows 2013, according to Monte Carlo calculations. For the control group eyes, no additional anterior capsular polishing was performed after routine cortex aspiration. For the polishing group eyes, residual LECs in the anterior capsule were aspirated using a bimanual irrigation/aspiration system (Figure 1). Accessibility to the entire capsule was achieved by the creation of two paracenteses at a distance of 180° from each other. Anterior capsule polishing was performed for the removal of all visible LECs. Following insertion of a hydrophobic one-piece IOL (Sensar® AAB00, Abbott Medical Optics Inc., Santa Ana, CA, USA) and aspiration of the ophthalmic viscosurgical device, the corneal wound was hydrated. Patients were treated with 0.5% moxifloxacin eye drops (Vigamox®, Alcon Laboratories) and 1% prednisolone acetate ophthalmic suspension (Pred Forte®, Allergan, Irvine, CA, USA) every 2 h for 3 days after surgery, following which the frequency was tapered to four times a day over 3 weeks or as clinically indicated.

2.4. ELP Measurements. ELP was defined as the distance from the anterior surface of the cornea to the anterior surface of IOL in the pupil center, along the optical axis. It was measured on an A-scan at 1 day, 3 days, 1 week, 1 month, and 2 months after surgery. Comparison of the mean ELP was considered inappropriate because forward and backward movements could be partly neutralized; therefore, we compared the mean standard deviation (SD) for the five ELP values, calculated at 2 months after surgery, between the two groups. Furthermore, on the basis of a report by Eom et al. [5], who reported that the root mean square (RMS) of

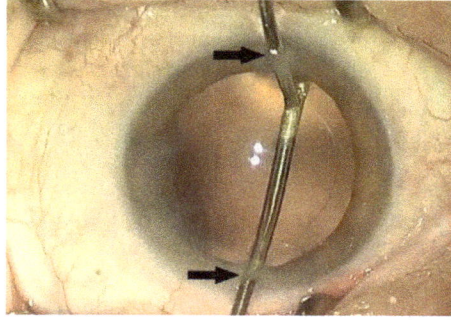

FIGURE 1: Residual anterior lens epithelial cell (LEC) removal using a bimanual irrigation/aspiration system during cataract surgery. Accessibility to the entire capsule is achieved by the creation of two paracenteses (arrows) at a distance of 180° from each other. Complete polishing of the anterior capsule is performed for the removal of all visible LECs under the capsule.

the change in ELP at each follow-up visit (ELP_{RMS}) could determine the axial position stability of IOLs more precisely than the mean ELP could; we calculated ELP_{RMS} for each group at 2 months after surgery using the following formula:

$$ELP_{RMS} = \sqrt{\frac{(ELP_{3D} - ELP_{1D})^2 + (ELP_{1W} - ELP_{3D})^2 + (ELP_{1M} - ELP_{1W})^2 + (ELP_{2M} - ELP_{1M})^2}{4}}. \quad (1)$$

Here, 1D, 3D, 1W, 1M, and 2M represent 1 day, 3 days, 1 week, 1 month, and 2 months after surgery, respectively.

2.5. Visual Acuity and Postoperative Refraction Error. The postoperative BCVA was recorded in logMAR units, and autorefraction (RK-F2, Canon Inc., Tokyo, Japan) was performed at each visit to evaluate the surgical outcomes. To demonstrate the discrepancy between the preoperatively calculated refraction (Lenstar LS900®) and the postoperative refraction at each time point, we calculated the postoperative refraction error (PRE) as the postoperative spherical equivalent (SE) minus the preoperative SE (SE = sphere + cylinder/2).

2.6. Specular Microscopy. The preoperative central corneal endothelial cell density (ECD), coefficient of variation (CV), and percentage of hexagonal cells were measured with a specular microscope (SP-9000, Konan Medical, Nishino-miya, Hyogo, Japan). To rule out the effect of anterior capsule polishing using a bimanual irrigation/aspiration system on corneal endothelial cell loss, the central corneal ECD, CV, and hexagonality were measured again at 1 and 2 months after surgery.

2.7. Statistical Analysis. The number of participants required to achieve a statistical power of 80% at a level of significance of 0.05 was 27. This sample size calculation was performed using the statistical freeware G∗Power (version 3.1.9.2) [16]. Data are reported as means and standard deviations. All statistical analyses were performed using SPSS for Windows (version 22.0, SPSS Inc.). Data normality was assessed using the Kolmogorov–Smirnov test. For intereye comparisons of

variables with a normal distribution, a paired *t*-test was used. A *p* value of <0.05 was considered statistically significant.

3. Results

Sixty eyes of 30 patients were included, and nine patients (33.3%) were men. All patients underwent uneventful surgeries with no intraoperative or postoperative complications and returned on time for measurements. The mean age of patients was 74.1 ± 8.9 years (range, 51 to 88 years). Table 1 shows the preoperative data, including BCVA; nuclear opalescence, cortical cataract, and posterior subcapsular cataract grades; ACD; AL; IOL power; and the predicted refraction, for both groups. There were no significant differences between groups in any of these parameters ($p > 0.05$).

Figure 2 shows the mean ELP at the different visits for each group. The mean ELP showed no significant difference between groups at 1 day, 3 days, and 1 week after surgery. However, significant differences were observed in the mean ELP at 1 and 2 months after surgery ($p = 0.026$ and 0.004, resp.). The mean SD for the five ELP values was significantly smaller for the polishing group (0.087 ± 0.093 mm) than that for the control group (0.159 ± 0.138 mm; $p = 0.001$). ELP_{RMS} was also significantly smaller for the polishing group (0.124 ± 0.034 mm) than that for the control group (0.246 ± 0.038 mm; $p = 0.047$; Table 2).

PRE was 0.29 ± 0.74, 0.23 ± 1.33, -0.03 ± 1.23, 0.02 ± 0.78, and 0.06 ± 0.60 D at 1 day, 3 days, 1 week, 1 month, and 2 months after surgery, respectively, in the polishing group. For the control group, these values were 0.27 ± 0.43, 0.25 ± 0.93, 0.13 ± 0.66, 0.23 ± 1.01, and 0.27 ± 0.93 D, respectively. There were no significant differences between the two groups (1 day: $p = 0.901$, 3 days: $p = 0.966$, 1 week: $p = 0.524$, 1 month: $p = 0.314$, 2 months: $p = 0.309$).

TABLE 1: Preoperative data for eyes with (polishing group) or without (control group) anterior capsule polishing during cataract surgery.

	Polishing group	Control group	p value*
Best-corrected visual acuity (logMAR)	0.61 ± 0.37	0.64 ± 0.37	0.695
Nuclear opalescence grade	3.03 ± 0.85	2.80 ± 0.85	0.335
Cortical cataract grade	2.27 ± 0.83	2.13 ± 0.82	0.489
Posterior subcapsular cataract grade	1.97 ± 0.85	2.10 ± 0.76	0.382
Anterior chamber depth (mm)	2.91 ± 0.25	2.97 ± 0.26	0.203
Axial length (mm)	22.92 ± 0.70	23.04 ± 0.75	0.392
Intraocular lens power (D)	22.25 ± 2.06	21.77 ± 2.21	0.306
Predicted refraction (D)	-0.15 ± 0.45	-0.20 ± 0.50	0.284

Values are presented as means ± standard deviations. *Statistical analysis was performed by using a paired t-test.

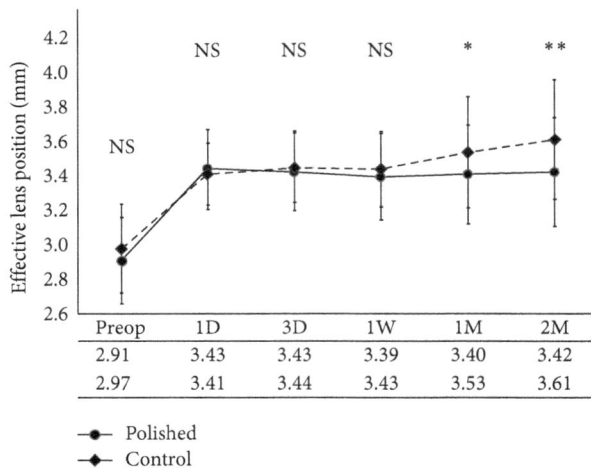

	Preop	1D	3D	1W	1M	2M
	2.91	3.43	3.43	3.39	3.40	3.42
	2.97	3.41	3.44	3.43	3.53	3.61

—•— Polished
—♦— Control

FIGURE 2: The mean effective lens position (ELP) at different visits in eyes with (polishing group) or without (control group) anterior capsule polishing during cataract surgery. There are no significant differences between groups in the mean ELP at 1 day, 3 days, and 1 week after surgery. The mean ELP at 1 and 2 months after surgery is significantly different ($p = 0.026$ and 0.004, resp.).

BCVA at 1 day, 3 days, 1 week, 1 month, and 2 months after surgery was 0.08 ± 0.10, 0.06 ± 0.09, 0.03 ± 0.06, 0.03 ± 0.06, and 0.02 ± 0.05, respectively, in the polishing group. These values were 0.07 ± 0.10, 0.05 ± 0.08, 0.03 ± 0.06, 0.02 ± 0.06, and 0.01 ± 0.04, respectively, in the control group. There were no significant differences between groups (1 day: $p = 0.489$, 3 days: $p = 0.662$, 1 week: $p = 0.573$, 1 month: $p = 0.745$, and 2 months: $p = 0.573$).

Table 3 shows the preoperative and postoperative ECD, CV, and hexagonality values for both groups. There were no significant differences in any variable between the two groups ($p > 0.05$).

4. Discussion

There are many studies concerning the influence of anterior capsule polishing during surgeries involving the implantation

of different IOLs on anterior capsule opacification (ACO), posterior capsule opacification (PCO), and the size of the capsulorhexis opening [11, 13, 14, 17]. However, few studies have assessed the effects of anterior capsule polishing on ELP or the axial position stability of IOL. Gao et al. [17] reported that anterior capsule polishing improved the axial position stability of the AcrySof IQ SN60WF IOL at 6 months after surgery, although no significant difference (no more than 0.06 mm) was detected in the mean ELP measured using anterior segment optical coherence tomography (AS-OCT) between the polishing and control groups. In our study, however, there were significant differences in the mean ELP at 1 month and 2 months after surgery between the polishing and control groups. We found that eyes that did not receive intraoperative anterior capsule polishing demonstrated a tendency for backward IOL movement by approximately 0.2 mm, with a concurrent hyperopic shift in refraction of approximately 0.2 D, at 2 months after surgery. Although this subtle change did not affect BCVA, the hyperopic shift after cataract surgery may be a problem, particularly for patients receiving refraction-correcting IOLs.

The mechanism underlying backward IOL movement in the absence of anterior capsule polishing remains uncertain. After cataract surgery, residual anterior LECs undergo fibrous metaplasia after contact with the anterior IOL surface [18]. These metaplastic LECs consist of α-smooth muscle actin elements that lead to anterior capsule contraction, constriction of the capsulorhexis and ACO [9]. This enhanced contractile force of the intrinsically elastic capsular membrane may result in a more potent centripetal capsular force and increased tensile force of the zonules attached to the capsule, eventually leading to backward shift of the IOL-capsule complex. In the present study, the number of eyes with anterior capsule fibrosis, which was measured using slit-lamp examination under pupil dilation at the last follow-up visit (2 months), was significantly lower in the polishing group (two eyes) than in the control group (nine eyes). Furthermore, anterior LECs migrate to the posterior capsule and result in fibrotic PCO as well as posterior capsule wrinkling [19]. In fact, there was no detectable posterior capsule fibrosis in any eye in the present study, probably because of the relatively short follow-up period. Constriction of the anterior and posterior capsules may synergistically result in a shift in the axial position of the IOL-capsule complex [8]. Therefore, the axial position of IOLs may remain more stable after the elimination of LECs under the anterior capsule during cataract surgery.

The axial position stability is also related to the mechanical characteristics of IOL, such as the design and material of the optic/haptic, optic-haptic angulation, and diameter [7]. In the present study, we used a single type of IOL, the Sensar AAB00 IOL, which has a hydrophobic acrylic optic with a diameter of 6.0 mm, an overall length of 13.0 mm, haptics of the same material, and no haptic angulation (0°). This hydrophobic, spherical, one-piece IOL demonstrated relatively little axial shift as well as a small refraction error and minimal BCVA changes during the follow-up period. This finding is consistent with those in previous studies showing that one-piece, hydrophobic,

TABLE 2: The postoperative effective lens position in eyes with (polishing group) or without (control group) anterior capsule polishing during cataract surgery.

Group	Mean ELP (mm)					Mean SD (mm)	Mean ELP$_{RMS}$ (mm)
	1 day	3 days	1 week	1 month	2 months		
Polishing	3.43 ± 0.23	3.43 ± 0.23	3.39 ± 0.25	3.40 ± 0.29	3.42 ± 0.32	0.087 ± 0.093	0.124 ± 0 .034
Control	3.41 ± 0.18	3.44 ± 0.20	3.43 ± 0.22	3.53 ± 0.32	3.61 ± 0.35	0.159 ± 0.138	0.246 ± 0.038
p value*	0.499	0.586	0.320	0.026	0.004	0.001	0.047

ELP, effective lens position; SD, standard deviation for ELP values obtained at the five time points; ELP$_{RMS}$, root mean square of the change in ELP at each time point. *Statistical analysis was performed by using a paired t-test.

TABLE 3: Pre-/postoperative (1 and 2 months after surgery) specular microscopy findings for eyes with (polishing group) or without (control group) anterior capsule polishing during cataract surgery.

Group	Mean ECD (cells/mm^2)			Mean CV			Mean hexagonality (%)		
	Preoperative	1 month	2 months	Preoperative	1 month	2 months	Preoperative	1 month	2 months
Polishing	2540.9 ± 426.7	2357.6 ± 497.9	2279.4 ± 575.3	28.83 ± 5.77	31.77 ± 5.82	32.10 ± 6.00	65.30 ± 6.29	64.03 ± 6.28	63.87 ± 6.79
Control	2430.9 ± 361.8	2323.8 ± 302.1	2259.2 ± 454.9	28.13 ± 5.69	29.63 ± 5.88	30.67 ± 6.96	66.07 ± 5.97	64.80 ± 6.60	64.40 ± 6.54
p value*	0.541	0.066	0.401	0.254	0.110	0.164	0.217	0.573	0.638

ECD, endothelial cell density; CV, coefficient of variation. *Statistical analysis was performed by using a paired t-test.

acrylic IOLs display little axial movement associated with stable postoperative refraction [5, 20]. The longer the overall length of IOL, the more it thrusts the equator of the capsule and the more stable is its axial position [21]. Furthermore, nonangulated IOLs show lesser postoperative axial movement than do angulated IOLs; a sharp optic edge design to prevent PCO has little influence on the axial position stability of IOL [11]. Not proven in the Sensar IOL, hydrophobic acrylic has bioadhesive characteristics that enhance the adhesion of IOL to the capsular bag and leads to less proliferation of LECs and anterior and posterior capsule fibrosis, with successive alleviation of capsule contraction and optic movement [22, 23]. Several studies have reported that anterior capsule contraction was significantly greater after hydrophilic IOL implantation than after hydrophobic IOL implantation [24–26]. We expect that more definite results may be found in further studies using hydrophilic acrylic IOLs instead of hydrophobic acrylic IOLs.

The main limitation of this study is the short follow-up period of 2 months after surgery, during which few instances of ACO, as well as no PCO, were detected. Moreover, our study population size is somewhat small despite the high statistical power of the paired t-test that we used. A larger population size, as well as follow-up periods that extend beyond 1 year (when most capsular events have already occurred), are necessary in future studies. Furthermore, we measured postoperative ELP using A-scan ultrasound images, not AS-OCT. Nemeth et al. [27] reported that the repeatability (intraobserver CV) of AS-OCT by two observers (0.8% and 1.9%) was superior to that of immersion A-scans (6.4% and 8.5%), whereas the reproducibility (interobserver CV) was comparable between the two modalities (0.23% and 0.88%, resp.).

However, AS-OCT was not available in our clinic; therefore, we repeated the measurements five times and used the average value to improve the repeatability. Finally, no significant discrepancy in the postoperative visual acuity and refraction error was detected between the polishing and control groups. The improvement in the axial position stability by anterior capsule polishing may not be noticed by patients, although it is imperative in refractive cataract surgery, which requires a remarkably high level of surgical accuracy. Larger study samples with the implantation of various refraction-correcting IOLs are necessary to clarify this aspect.

5. Conclusions

In the present study, we polished the anterior capsule to eliminate residual LECs using a bimanual irrigation/aspiration system to assess the effects of this procedure on the axial position stability of hydrophobic, spherical, one-piece IOLs. We found that anterior capsule polishing enhanced the axial position stability of IOL without any complications. Without anterior capsule polishing, IOL tended to move backwards by approximately 0.2 mm, with a concurrent hyperopic shift in refraction of approximately 0.2 D, at 2 months after surgery. With the advancement of various refraction-correcting IOLs, the axial position stability becomes an important aspect. Therefore, anterior capsule polishing using a bimanual irrigation/aspiration system during cataract surgery may be considered a useful procedure, particularly for eyes receiving refraction-correcting IOLs.

Disclosure

A summary of this paper was presented as a narrative at the 117th Spring Meeting of the Korean Ophthalmology Society, Gwangju, Korea (April 14-15, 2017).

Conflicts of Interest

The authors declare that there are no conflicts of interest regarding the publication of this paper.

Acknowledgments

This research was supported by the Keimyung University Research Grant of 2017. The authors acknowledge the sincere help and support of Myeong Jin Son for her great effort and all the facilities she provided for the study.

References

[1] K. J. Hoffer, J. Aramberri, W. Haigis et al., "Protocols for studies of intraocular lens formula accuracy," *American Journal of Ophthalmology*, vol. 160, no. 3, pp. 403–405, 2015.

[2] Y. Eom, S.-Y. Kang, J. Suk Song, Y. Yeon Kim, and H. M. Kim, "Effect of effective lens position on cylinder power of toric intraocular lenses," *Canadian Journal of Ophthalmology*, vol. 50, no. 1, pp. 26–32, 2015.

[3] I. Dooley, S. Charalampidou, J. Nolan, J. Loughman, L. Molloy, and S. Beatty, "Estimation of effective lens position using a method independent of preoperative keratometry readings," *Journal of Cataract & Refractive Surgery*, vol. 37, no. 3, pp. 506–512, 2011.

[4] J. Korynta, J. Bok, and J. Cendelin, "Changes in refraction induced by change in intraocular lens position," *Journal of Refractive Surgery*, vol. 10, no. 5, pp. 556–564, 1994.

[5] Y. Eom, S.-Y. Kang, J.-S. Song, and H. M. Kim, "Comparison of the actual amount of axial movement of 3 aspheric intraocular lenses using anterior segment optical coherence tomography," *Journal of Cataract & Refractive Surgery*, vol. 39, no. 10, pp. 1528–1533, 2013.

[6] T. Olsen, "Sources of error in intraocular lens power calculation," *Journal of Cataract & Refractive Surgery*, vol. 18, no. 2, pp. 125–129, 1992.

[7] O. Çekiç and C. Batman, "The relationship between capsulorhexis size and anterior chamber depth relation," *Ophthalmic Surgery, Lasers and Imaging Retina*, vol. 30, no. 3, pp. 185–190, 1999.

[8] P. J. McDonnell, M. A. Zarbin, and W. Richard Green, "Posterior capsule opacification in pseudophakic eyes," *Ophthalmology*, vol. 90, no. 12, pp. 1548–1553, 1983.

[9] D. Kurosaka, K. Kato, and T. Nagamoto, "Presence of alpha smooth muscle actin in lens epithelial cells of aphakic rabbit eyes," *British Journal of Ophthalmology*, vol. 80, no. 10, pp. 906–910, 1996.

[10] T. T. L. Wong, J. T. Daniels, J. G. Crowston, and P. T. Khaw, "MMP inhibition prevents human lens epithelial cell migration and contraction of the lens capsule," *British Journal of Ophthalmology*, vol. 88, no. 7, pp. 868–872, 2004.

[11] R. J. Hanson, A. Rubinstein, S. Sarangapani, L. Benjamin, and C. K. Patel, "Effect of lens epithelial cell aspiration on postoperative capsulorhexis contraction with the use of the AcrySof intraocular lens: randomized clinical trial," *Journal of*

Cataract & Refractive Surgery, vol. 32, no. 10, pp. 1621–1626, 2006.

[12] R. Menapace, "Posterior capsulorhexis combined with optic buttonholing: an alternative to standard in-the-bag implantation of sharp-edged intraocular lenses? A critical analysis of 1000 consecutive cases," *Graefe's Archive for Clinical and Experimental Ophthalmology*, vol. 246, no. 6, pp. 787–801, 2008.

[13] S. K. Shah, M. R. Praveen, A. Kaul, A. R. Vasavada, G. D. Shah, and B. R. Nihalani, "Impact of anterior capsule polishing on anterior capsule opacification after cataract surgery: a randomized clinical trial," *Eye*, vol. 23, no. 8, pp. 1702–1706, 2009.

[14] R. Baile, M. Sahasrabuddhe, S. Nadkarni, V. Karira, and J. Kelkar, "Effect of anterior capsular polishing on the rate of posterior capsule opacification: a retrospective analytical study," *Saudi Journal of Ophthalmology*, vol. 26, no. 1, pp. 101–104, 2012.

[15] L. T. Chylack, J. K. Wolfe, D. M. Singer et al., "The lens opacities classification system III," *Archives of Ophthalmology*, vol. 111, no. 6, p. 1506, 1993.

[16] F. Faul, E. Erdfelder, A.-G. Lang, and A. Buchner, "G∗Power 3: a flexible statistical power analysis program for the social, behavioral, and biomedical sciences," *Behavior Research Methods*, vol. 39, no. 2, pp. 175–191, 2007.

[17] Y. Gao, G.-F. Dang, X. Wang, L. Duan, and X.-Y. Wu, "Influences of anterior capsule polishing on effective lens position after cataract surgery: a randomized controlled trial," *International Journal of Clinical and Experimental Medicine*, vol. 8, no. 8, p. 13769, 2015.

[18] O. Nishi, "Intercapsular cataract surgery with lens epithelial cell removal Part II: Effect on prevention of fibrinous reaction," *Journal of Cataract & Refractive Surgery*, vol. 15, no. 3, pp. 301–303, 1989.

[19] O. Nishi and K. Nishi, "Intraocular lens encapsulation by shrinkage of the capsulorhexis opening," *Journal of Cataract & Refractive Surgery*, vol. 19, no. 4, pp. 544–545, 1993.

[20] R. Nejima, T. Miyai, Y. Kataoka et al., "Prospective intra-patient comparison of 6.0-millimeter optic single-piece and 3-piece hydrophobic acrylic foldable intraocular lenses," *Ophthalmology*, vol. 113, no. 4, pp. 585–590, 2006.

[21] M. Aose, H. Matsushima, K. Mukai, Y. Katsuki, N. Gotoh, and T. Senoo, "Influence of intraocular lens implantation on anterior capsule contraction and posterior capsule opacification," *Journal of Cataract & Refractive Surgery*, vol. 40, no. 12, pp. 2128–2133, 2014.

[22] T. Oshika, T. Nagata, and Y. Ishii, "Adhesion of lens capsule to intraocular lenses of polymethylmethacrylate, silicone, and acrylic foldable materials: an experimental study," *British Journal of Ophthalmology*, vol. 82, no. 5, pp. 549–553, 1998.

[23] X. Zhu, W. He, J. Yang, M. Hooi, J. Dai, and Y. Lu, "Adhesion of the posterior capsule to different intraocular lenses following cataract surgery," *Acta Ophthalmologica*, vol. 94, no. 1, pp. e16–e25, 2016.

[24] I. T. Tsinopoulos, K. T. Tsaousis, G. D. Kymionis et al., "Comparison of anterior capsule contraction between hydrophobic and hydrophilic intraocular lens models," *Graefe's Archive for Clinical and Experimental Ophthalmology*, vol. 248, no. 8, pp. 1155–1158, 2010.

[25] D. J. Apple, "Influence of intraocular lens material and design on postoperative intracapsular cellular reactivity," *Transactions of the American Ophthalmological Society*, vol. 98, p. 257, 2000.

[26] R. Zemaitiene, M. Speckauskas, B. Glebauskiene, and V. Jasinskas, "Comparison of postoperative results after implantation of hydrophilic acrylic or hydrophobic acrylic intraocular lens: data of one-year prospective clinical study," *Medicina*, vol. 44, no. 12, pp. 936–943, 2008.

[27] G. Nemeth, A. Vajas, A. Tsorbatzoglou, B. Kolozsvari, L. Modis, and A. Berta, "Assessment and reproducibility of anterior chamber depth measurement with anterior segment optical coherence tomography compared with immersion ultrasonography," *Journal of Cataract & Refractive Surgery*, vol. 33, no. 3, pp. 443–447, 2007.

Permissions

All chapters in this book were first published in JO, by Hindawi Publishing Corporation; hereby published with permission under the Creative Commons Attribution License or equivalent. Every chapter published in this book has been scrutinized by our experts. Their significance has been extensively debated. The topics covered herein carry significant findings which will fuel the growth of the discipline. They may even be implemented as practical applications or may be referred to as a beginning point for another development.

The contributors of this book come from diverse backgrounds, making this book a truly international effort. This book will bring forth new frontiers with its revolutionizing research information and detailed analysis of the nascent developments around the world.

We would like to thank all the contributing authors for lending their expertise to make the book truly unique. They have played a crucial role in the development of this book. Without their invaluable contributions this book wouldn't have been possible. They have made vital efforts to compile up to date information on the varied aspects of this subject to make this book a valuable addition to the collection of many professionals and students.

This book was conceptualized with the vision of imparting up-to-date information and advanced data in this field. To ensure the same, a matchless editorial board was set up. Every individual on the board went through rigorous rounds of assessment to prove their worth. After which they invested a large part of their time researching and compiling the most relevant data for our readers.

The editorial board has been involved in producing this book since its inception. They have spent rigorous hours researching and exploring the diverse topics which have resulted in the successful publishing of this book. They have passed on their knowledge of decades through this book. To expedite this challenging task, the publisher supported the team at every step. A small team of assistant editors was also appointed to further simplify the editing procedure and attain best results for the readers.

Apart from the editorial board, the designing team has also invested a significant amount of their time in understanding the subject and creating the most relevant covers. They scrutinized every image to scout for the most suitable representation of the subject and create an appropriate cover for the book.

The publishing team has been an ardent support to the editorial, designing and production team. Their endless efforts to recruit the best for this project, has resulted in the accomplishment of this book. They are a veteran in the field of academics and their pool of knowledge is as vast as their experience in printing. Their expertise and guidance has proved useful at every step. Their uncompromising quality standards have made this book an exceptional effort. Their encouragement from time to time has been an inspiration for everyone.

The publisher and the editorial board hope that this book will prove to be a valuable piece of knowledge for researchers, students, practitioners and scholars across the globe.

List of Contributors

Dilek Yaşa, Ufuk Ürdem, Alper Ağca, Yusuf Yildirim, Burçin Kepez Yildiz, Nilay Kandemir Beşek and Ahmet Demirok
Beyoğlu Eye Research and Training Hospital, Bereketzade Mah, No. 2 Beyoglu, Istanbul, Turkey

Ulviye Yiğit
Dr. Sadi Konuk Bakirkoy Research and Training Hospital, Zuhuratbaba Mah., Tevfik Saglam Cad., No. 21 Bakirkoy, Istanbul, Turkey

Alahmady Hamad Alsmman, Mohammed Ezzeldawla, Amr Mounir, Ashraf Mostafa Elhawary, Osama Ali Mohammed and Mahmoud Farouk
Department of Ophthalmology, Sohag Faculty of Medicine, Sohag University, Sohag, Egypt

Ahmed Mohamed Sherif
Department of Ophthalmology, Cairo Faculty of Medicine, Cairo University, Cairo, Egypt

Zi Ye, Zhaohui Li and Shouzhi He
Department of Ophthalmology, The PLA General Hospital, 28 Fuxing Road, Beijing 100853, China

Claudio Furino, Alfredo Niro, Maria Oliva Grassi and Giovanni Alessio
Department of Medical Science, Neuroscience and Sense Organs, Eye Clinic, University of Bari, Bari, Italy

Francesco Boscia, Ermete Giancipoli, Giuseppe D'amico Ricci and Francesco Blasetti
Department of Surgical, Microsurgical and Medical Sciences, Eye Clinic, University of Sassari, Sassari, Italy

Michele Reibaldi
Eye clinic, University of Catania, Catania, Italy

Sonia Gholami
Rotterdam Ophthalmic Institute, Rotterdam, Netherlands

Nicolaas J. Reus
Amphia Hospital, Breda, Netherlands

Thomas J. T. P. van den Berg
Netherlands Institute for Neuroscience and Royal Netherlands Academy of Arts and Sciences, Amsterdam, Netherlands

Domenico Schiano Lomoriello, Giacomo Savini and Valeria Bono
IRCCS Fondazione G.B. Bietti, Rome, Italy

Kristian Naeser
Regions Hospital Randers, Randers, Denmark

Rossella Maria Colabelli-Gisoldi and Augusto Pocobelli
Azienda Ospedaliera San Giovanni-Addolorata, Rome, Italy

Qingjian Li, Yiwen Qian, Yu Zhang, Gaoyuan Sun, Xian Zhou and Zhiliang Wang
Department of Ophthalmology, Huashan Hospital, Fudan University, Shanghai, China

Hisaharu Suzuki
Department of Ophthalmology, Nippon Medical School Musashikosugi Hospital, 1-396 Kosugi-cho, Nakahara-ku, Kawasaki City, Kanagawa 211-8533, Japan

Tsutomu Igarashi, Toshihiko Shiwa and Hiroshi Takahashi
Department of Ophthalmology, Nippon Medical School, 1-1-5 Sendagi, Bunkyo-ku, Tokyo 113-8603, Japan

Ali Kurt and Raşit Kılıç
Department of Ophthalmology, Faculty of Medicine, Ahi Evran University, Kırşehir, Turkey

Lihua Kang, Yuanyuan Tu, Lele Li, Bai Qin, Mei Yang and Huaijin Guan
Department of Ophthalmology, Affiliated Hospital of Nantong University, Nantong, Jiangsu 226001, China

Xinyue Shen
Department of Ophthalmology, Affiliated Hospital of Nantong University, Nantong, Jiangsu 226001, China
Department of Ophthalmology, Wuxi No. 3 People's Hospital, Wuxi, Jiangsu 214041, China

Manhui Zhu
Department of Ophthalmology, Affiliated Hospital of Nantong University, Nantong, Jiangsu 226001, China
Department of Ophthalmology, Lixiang Eye Hospital of Soochow University, Suzhou 215021, China

Rutan Zhang
Department of Chemistry, Fudan University, Shanghai 200433, China

Hang Song, Yingyu Li, Danna Shi and Xuemin Li
Department of Ophthalmology, Peking University ird Hospital, Beijing, China

Yan Zhang
Sino Japanese Union Hospital of Jilin University, Changchun, Jilin, China

Hui Xu, Li Zhu, Yu Wang and Yongzhen Bao
Department of Ophthalmology, Peking University People's Hospital, Eye diseases and Optometry Institute, Beijing Key Laboratory of Diagnosis and Therapy of Retina and Choroid Diseases, College of Optometry, Peking University Health Science Center, Beijing, China

Manuel Rodríguez-Vallejo, Javier Martínez and Ana Tauste
Department of Ophthalmology (Qvision), Vithas Virgen del Mar Hospital, 04120 Almería, Spain

Joaquín Fernández
Department of Ophthalmology (Qvision), Vithas Virgen del Mar Hospital, 04120 Almer´ıa, Spain
Department of Ophthalmology, Torrec´ardenas Hospital Complex, 04009 Almer´ıa, Spain

David P. Piñero
Department of Optics, Pharmacology and Anatomy, University of Alicante, Alicante, Spain
Department of Ophthalmology (OFTALMAR), Vithas Medimar International Hospital, Alicante, Spain

Eva-Maria Faschinger, Pia Veronika Vécsei-Marlovits and Birgit Weingessel
Department of Ophthalmology, KH Hietzing, Wolkersbergenstrasse 1, 1130 Vienna, Austria
Karl Landsteiner Institute of Process Optimization and Quality Management in Cataract-Surgery, Wolkersbergenstrasse 1, 1130 Vienna, Austria

Dieter Franz Rabensteiner
Department of Ophthalmology, Medical University of Graz, Auenbruggerplatz 4, 8036 Graz, Austria

Vincenza Bonfiglio, Antonio Longo, Teresio Avitabile, Andrea Russo, Matteo Fallico, Elina Ortisi and Michele Reibaldi
Eye Clinic, University of Catania, Catania, Italy

Mario D. Toro
Eye Clinic, University of Catania, Catania, Italy
Department of General Ophthalmology, Medical University of Lublin, Lublin, Poland

Robert Rejdak and Tomasz Choragiewicz
Department of General Ophthalmology, Medical University of Lublin, Lublin, Poland

Katarzyna Nowomiejska
Department of General Ophthalmology, Medical University of Lublin, Lublin, Poland

Institute for Ophthalmic Research, University Eye Hospital, Tuebingen, Germany

Agnieszka Kaminska
Faculty of Family Studies, Cardinal Stefan Wyszynski University, Warsaw, Poland

Stefano Zenoni
Life Clinic, Milano, Italy

Chenxi Fu, Naipin Chu, Xiaoning Yu and Ke Yao
Eye Center, Second Affiliated Hospital, School of Medicine, Zhejiang University, Hangzhou, China

Dominika Podkowinski, Ehsan Sharian Varnousfaderani, Christian Simader, Hrvoje Bogunovic, Ana-Maria Philip, Bianca S. Gerendas, Ursula Schmidt-Erfurth and Sebastian M. Waldstein
Christian Doppler Laboratory for Ophthalmic Image Analysis, Vienna Reading Center, Department of Ophthalmology, Medical University of Vienna, Spitalgasse 23, 1090 Vienna, Austria

Dandan Wang, Xiaoyu Yu, Zhangliang Li, Xixia Ding, Hengli Lian, Jianyang Mao, Yinying Zhao and Yun-E. Zhao
School of Optometry and Ophthalmology and Eye Hospital, Wenzhou Medical University, Wenzhou, Zhejiang, China
Key Laboratory of Vision Science, Ministry of Health P.R. China, Wenzhou, Zhejiang, China

Ana Martínez-Palmer, Daniel Martín-Moral and Janny Aronés-Santivañez
Department of Ophthalmology, Hospital Universitario del Mar and Hospital de la Esperanza, Pompeu and Fabra University, Barcelona, Spain

Agnieszka Dyrda
Department of Ophthalmology, Hospital Universitario del Mar and Hospital de la Esperanza, Pompeu and Fabra University, Barcelona, Spain
Institut Català de Retina, Barcelona, Spain

Amanda Rey and Antonio Morilla
Institut Catal`a de Retina, Barcelona, Spain

Miguel Castilla-Martí
Valles Ophthalmology Research, Hospital General de Catalunya, Barcelona, Spain

C. Lisa, R. M. Sanchez-Avila and J. F. Alfonso
Fernández-Vega Ophthalmological Institute, Oviedo, Spain

R. Zaldivar
Instituto Zaldivar, Mendoza, Argentina

A. Fernández-Vega Cueto
Centro de Oftalmología Barraquer, Barcelona, Spain

D. Madrid-Costa
Optics II Department, Faculty of Optics and Optometry, Universidad Complutense de Madrid, Madrid, Spain

Paolo Mora, Giacomo Calzetti, Matteo Forlini, Salvatore Tedesco, Viola Tagliavini, Arturo Carta and Stefano Gandolfi
Ophthalmology Unit, University Hospital of Parma, Parma, Italy

Stefania Favilla
Independent Researcher, Parma, Italy

Purva Date
Aditya Jyot Eye Hospital, Wadala, Mumbai, India

Rino Frisina
Department of Ophthalmology, University of Padova, Padova, Italy

Emilio Pedrotti
Eye Clinic, Department of Neurosciences, Biomedicine and Movement Sciences, University of Verona, AOUI-Policlinico G. B. Rossi, Verona, Italy

Handan Akil, Vikas Chopra, Alex S. Huang, Ramya Swamy and Brian A. Francis
Doheny Image Reading Center, Doheny Eye Institute, Los Angeles, CA, USA
Department of Ophthalmology, David Geffen School of Medicine, Los Angeles, CA, USA

Shuang Wu, Yanan Li, MeiLing Guo and Hehuan Li
Qingdao Municipal Hospital Affiliated to Qingdao University, No. 5 Donghaizhong Road, Shinan District, Qingdao, Shandong, China

Nianting Tong and Xiaohui Jiang
Department of Ophthalmology, Qingdao Municipal Hospital, No. 5 Donghaizhong Road, Shinan District, Qingdao, Shandong, China

Lin Pan
Dalian Medical University, No. 9 Lushunnan Road, Dalian, Liaoning, China

Wenwen He, Jin Yang, Xiangjia Zhu and Yi Lu
Department of Ophthalmology, Eye and Ear, Nose, and Throat Hospital of Fudan University, 83 Fenyang Road, Shanghai 200031, China
Key Laboratory of Myopia, Ministry of Health, Shanghai 200031, China
Shanghai Key Laboratory of Visual Impairment and Restoration, Shanghai 200031, China

Ting Sun, Guoyou Qin and Zhenyu Wu
Department of Biostatistics, School of Public Health, Key Laboratory of Public Health Safety, Ministry of Education, Fudan University, Shanghai 200032, China

Seung Pil Bang and Jong Hwa Jun
Department of Ophthalmology, Dongsan Medical Center, Keimyung University School of Medicine, Daegu, Republic of Korea

Young-Sik Yoo
Catholic Institute for Visual Science, The Catholic University of Korea, Seoul, Republic of Korea

Choun-Ki Joo
Catholic Institute for Visual Science, The Catholic University of Korea, Seoul, Republic of Korea
Department of Ophthalmology and Visual Science, Seoul St. Mary's Hospital, College of Medicine, The Catholic University of Korea, Seoul, Republic of Korea

Index